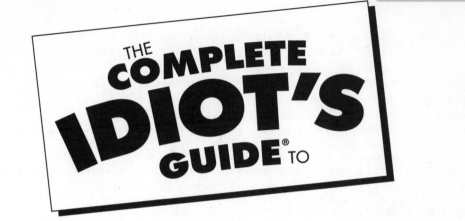

THE COMPLETE **IDIOT'S** GUIDE® TO

Vitamins and Minerals

Third Edition

by Dr. Alan H. Pressman, D.C., Ph.D., C.C.N., and Sheila Buff

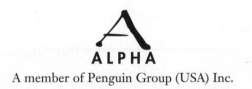

ALPHA

A member of Penguin Group (USA) Inc.

To my son Corey and my daughter Meghan because they are my life. —Alan H. Pressman
In loving memory of Grace Darling Griffin. —Sheila Buff

ALPHA BOOKS

Published by the Penguin Group

Penguin Group (USA) Inc., 375 Hudson Street, New York, New York 10014, U.S.A.

Penguin Group (Canada), 10 Alcorn Avenue, Toronto, Ontario, Canada M4V 3B2 (a division of Pearson Penguin Canada Inc.)

Penguin Books Ltd, 80 Strand, London WC2R 0RL, England

Penguin Ireland, 25 St Stephen's Green, Dublin 2, Ireland (a division of Penguin Books Ltd)

Penguin Group (Australia), 250 Camberwell Road, Camberwell, Victoria 3124, Australia (a division of Pearson Australia Group Pty Ltd)

Penguin Books India Pvt Ltd, 11 Community Centre, Panchsheel Park, New Delhi—110 017, India

Penguin Group (NZ), cnr Airborne and Rosedale Roads, Albany, Auckland 1310, New Zealand (a division of Pearson New Zealand Ltd)

Penguin Books (South Africa) (Pty) Ltd, 24 Sturdee Avenue, Rosebank, Johannesburg 2196, South Africa

Penguin Books Ltd, Registered Offices: 80 Strand, London WC2R 0RL, England

International Standard Book Number: 978-1-59257-609-8
Library of Congress Catalog Card Number: 2006934452

09 08 07   8 7 6 5 4 3 2 1

Interpretation of the printing code: The rightmost number of the first series of numbers is the year of the book's printing; the rightmost number of the second series of numbers is the number of the book's printing. For example, a printing code of 07-1 shows that the first printing occurred in 2007.

Printed in the United States of America

Note: This publication contains the opinions and ideas of its authors. It is intended to provide helpful and informative material on the subject matter covered. It is sold with the understanding that the authors and publisher are not engaged in rendering professional services in the book. If the reader requires personal assistance or advice, a competent professional should be consulted.

The authors and publisher specifically disclaim any responsibility for any liability, loss, or risk, personal or otherwise, which is incurred as a consequence, directly or indirectly, of the use and application of any of the contents of this book.

Most Alpha books are available at special quantity discounts for bulk purchases for sales promotions, premiums, fundraising, or educational use. Special books, or book excerpts, can also be created to fit specific needs.

For details, write: Special Markets, Alpha Books, 375 Hudson Street, New York, NY 10014.

Publisher: *Marie Butler-Knight*
Editorial Director: *Mike Sanders*
Managing Editor: *Billy Fields*
Executive Editor: *Randy Ladenheim-Gil*
Development Editor: *Jennifer Moore*
Production Editor: *Kayla Dugger*
Copy Editor: *Tricia Liebig*
Cartoonist: *Richard King*
Cover Designer: *Bill Thomas*
Book Designer: *Trina Wurst*
Indexer: *Angie Bess*
Layout: *Ayanna Lacey*
Proofreaders: *Mary Hunt, Donna Martin*

Contents at a Glance

Contents

Foreword

You don't have to be an idiot to understand how simple, easy, and beneficial this book is to your overall well-being. Dr. Alan Pressman has included all the information you need to help you decide which vitamins, minerals, and supplements you need for good health. This book serves that purpose.

Knowing that you're getting the right amount of nutrients is important whether you're 18 or 80. This book gives you the knowledge you need to look and feel better—it's just a matter of looking in the index and going to the right page. There you'll see a synthesized, easy-to-follow understanding to all your health questions.

Gary Null, Ph.D.

Gary Null, Ph.D., is host of the nationally syndicated *Gary Null Show*, which airs daily. In addition, Mr. Null is author of more than 50 books on health and nutrition, including *Get Healthy Now!*, *The Complete Encyclopedia of Natural Healing*, and *Kiss Your Fat Goodbye*.

Introduction: Live Better with Vitamins

Every year Americans spend more than $4 billion on vitamins, minerals, and other supplements. Why? They're seeking better health, perhaps a longer and more vigorous life, or maybe help for a painful health problem. Are they finding it? Yes! Can you? Yes! If you understand how important vitamins and minerals are and what they can—and can't—do, you too can achieve better health.

Why Are Vitamins So Important?

You need 13 different vitamins and at least 10 minerals. Vitamins and minerals are essential to your health—you have to have them to stay alive and to be healthy. Vitamins and minerals are also needed to make the thousands of enzymes, hormones, and other chemical messengers your body uses to grow, repair itself, make energy, remove wastes, defend against infection, and generally keep your body running smoothly. You also need them to keep your bones strong, your eyes sharp, and your brain alert. And most important of all, you need them to help protect you against cancer and heart disease.

The *only* way you can get all these vitamins and minerals into your body is to eat them. That's why we'll talk about your diet over and over again in this book—the foods you eat are the best way to get the nutrients you need. But even if you eat right all the time—which most people can't—you might still benefit from some extra vitamins and minerals.

Do You Really Need Vitamin Pills?

The short answer is yes—the long answers are found in each chapter of this book. Try as we might, most of us just can't eat a good, nutritious diet at every meal every day. We need the help vitamin and mineral supplements give. And sometimes we need a vitamin or mineral boost to help deal with health problems. Finally, some vitamins, such as Vitamin E, are most valuable in large doses—doses far greater (though very safe) than the amounts you could ever get only from your food.

Supplements are an easy, safe, and inexpensive way to make sure you're getting the vitamins and minerals your body needs for optimum health. Taking supplements can improve your health now and ensure it for the future.

About This Edition

Human health and nutrition is a complex and fascinating subject. There's so much great research going on about it that things change fast. We wrote the first edition of this book back in 1997 and updated it in 2000. In this third edition, we've had to change quite a bit. We've updated the information to include the latest official recommendations for the basic vitamins, minerals, and nutrients. We've also made many changes to reflect the latest scientific thinking. The chapter on Vitamin E, for instance, has been extensively revised. (Yes, this vitamin is still safe and valuable.) Likewise, based on new research, we discuss additional uses for some supplements (coenzyme Q_{10} for Parkinson's disease, for instance) and talk more about the use of soy products instead of hormone replacement therapy for women. We've tried to make this new edition as thorough, accurate, science-based, and up-to-date as we can.

How to Use This Book

We've divided this book into four parts:

In **Part 1, "The Vital Keys to Good Health,"** we explain the basics of vitamins and minerals: why you need them, how much you need, and the best ways to get them.

In **Part 2, "The A to K of Vitamins,"** we discuss each vitamin in detail, explaining how it works in your body, specific health problems it can help, and how to get the amounts you need.

In **Part 3, "Minerals: The Elements of Good Health,"** we do the same for minerals.

In **Part 4, "Exploring Other Supplements,"** we discuss many other nutritional supplements, such as essential fatty acids, flavonoids, and natural hormones. This part gives you the information you need to understand which supplements have real value, what conditions they can help, and how best to use them.

We end the book with a quick-reference chart for finding which supplements are helpful for particular health problems, a list of resources for finding more information, and a glossary.

To get the most from this book, we urge you to read through the first two chapters carefully. These give you the background you need to understand the overall importance of vitamins and minerals to your health.

Throughout this book, we give you plenty of charts, including many that list good food sources for the various vitamins, minerals, and other supplements. Look for Thumbs Up/Thumbs Down tables to get more details on the best ways to take your vitamins and minerals. We also give a lot of useful information and tips in sidebars.

Food for Thought

This box adds interesting bits of information, such as how some vitamins were discovered.

Warning!

Take these boxes seriously—they help you avoid problems such as overdoses or bad interactions with other drugs or supplements.

Quack, Quack

We also have a special sidebar reserved for debunking some of the sillier ideas about supplements. These boxes help you avoid supplements that don't work.

def•i•ni•tion

This sidebar expands the definitions of special terms and basic concepts.

Now You're Cooking

Here we give you tips on how to get the most from your foods and supplements.

Acknowledgments

We'd like to thank all the many people who have, over the years, shared their knowledge and enthusiasm with us. Thanks also to Gary Krebs for getting this project started in the first place. We thank our hardworking editors at Alpha Books—Nancy Mikhail and Linda Seifert—for their great work on the original edition of this book. For this revised and expanded edition, we thank our editor Randy Ladenheim-Gil (again); our development editor, Jennifer Moore; our production editor, Kayla Dugger; and our copy editor, Tricia Liebig.

Trademarks

All terms mentioned in this book that are known to be or are suspected of being trademarks or service marks have been appropriately capitalized. Alpha Books and Penguin Group (USA) Inc. cannot attest to the accuracy of this information. Use of a term in this book should not be regarded as affecting the validity of any trademark or service mark.

Part 1

The Vital Keys to Good Health

You've been hearing a lot about all the great things vitamins and minerals can do for your health, and you've decided to try them. Good decision. Now what?

What you need now is information—the knowledge that will let you unlock the door to good health. The knowledge you need isn't a secret and it's not hard to understand. In fact, after you've learned the basics of vitamins, minerals, and other supplements, you'll easily be able to decide what's right for you.

Your own good health, both for now and the future, is in your hands. Let's get started.

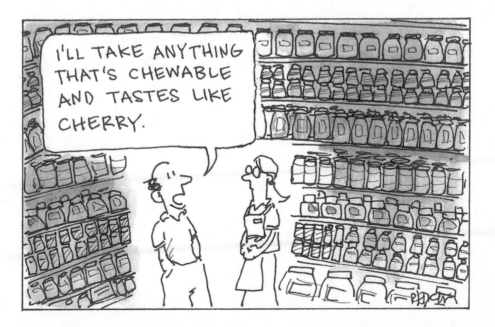

The Alphabet Soup of Nutrition

In This Chapter

◆ Needing vitamins and minerals

◆ Knowing how much you need

◆ Learning about vitamins, minerals, and your diet

◆ Protecting yourself from damaging free radicals with vitamins and minerals

Walk into any health-food store or drugstore and you're faced with shelf after shelf crammed with vitamins, minerals, and supplements of all sorts. What is all this stuff? How can you choose? What's best for *you?*

To decide wisely for your health, you need to understand what each vitamin does—and why you need them *all*. You need to understand what minerals do for you—and why you need them *all*. You need to understand how the vitamins and minerals in your food affect you—and how everything else in your food affects you as well. You need to understand which of those other supplements are valuable to your health—and which aren't.

Although all those bottles on the shelves may seem confusing and a little scary, they're really not. After you understand the basics of vitamins and minerals, you'll be able to pick the vitamin and mineral supplements that will help *your* health.

Vitamins: Why They're Vital

A *vitamin* is an organic (carbon-containing) chemical compound your body must have in very small amounts for normal growth, metabolism (creating energy in your cells), and health. You need vitamins to make *enzymes* and *hormones*—important substances your body uses to perform the many chemical reactions you need to live. You *must* get your vitamins from your food or from supplements—you can't make them in your body.

def•i•ni•tion

Enzymes are chemical compounds your body makes from various combinations of proteins, vitamins, and minerals. Enzymes speed up chemical reactions in your body. **Hormones** are chemical messengers your body makes to tell your organs what to do. Hormones regulate many activities, including your growth, blood pressure, heart rate, glucose levels, and sexual characteristics.

There are 13 vitamins in all, and you need every single one of them, no exceptions. Vitamins aren't food or a substitute for food. They have no calories and give you no energy directly—but your body needs vitamins, especially the B vitamins, to convert food to energy. We'll look at each vitamin in detail in the later chapters of this book, but for now we'll divide them into two groups: *fat-soluble* and *water-soluble*.

Fat-Soluble Vitamins

Fat-soluble vitamins are stored in your body, mostly in your fatty tissues and in your liver. Vitamins A, E, D, and K are fat-soluble—that is, they dissolve in fat but not water. Because you can store these vitamins, you don't have to get a supply of them every day. On the other hand, getting too much of these vitamins could make them build up in your body and cause problems.

Water-Soluble Vitamins

Water-soluble vitamins can't really be stored in your body for very long. That's because these vitamins dissolve in water, so any extra is carried out of your body. Vitamin C and all the B vitamins are water-soluble. Because you can't store these vitamins, you need to get a fresh supply every day. You can't really overdose on water-soluble vitamins. Unless you take truly massive doses, the extra just washes out harmlessly.

How Much Do You Need?

How much you need of each vitamin is a question that has a lot of different answers, depending on who you are and whom you ask. For now, we're going to tell you what the doctors and scientists at the Food and Nutrition Board of the Institute of Medicine think is enough to meet your basic needs for each vitamin, assuming you're an average, healthy, adult man or woman. The Institute of Medicine is the group that brings you what are called the Recommended Dietary Allowances, better known as RDAs. The RDAs are part of what is now officially called the Dietary Reference Intakes, or DRIs. Every 5 to 10 years, the Institute of Medicine looks at the standards and revises them up or down as needed, based on the latest scientific research. Since 2000, the RDAs for several vitamins and minerals have been updated. (We'll talk a lot more about RDAs, DRIs, and other ways of looking at your vitamin and mineral needs in Chapter 2.) Check out the chart to see the latest RDAs for vitamins. These are the *minimum* amounts you should be getting every day, preferably from your food (and from vitamin pills, if needed).

Adult RDAs for Vitamins

Vitamin	RDA for Men	RDA for Women
Fat-Soluble		
Vitamin A	900 mcg RAE* 3,000	700 RAE 2,330
Vitamin E	15 mg or 22 IU**	15 mg or 22 IU
Vitamin K	80 mcg	65 mcg
Water-Soluble		
Vitamin C	90 mg	75 mg
B Vitamins:		
Thiamin	1.2 mg	1.1 mg
Riboflavin	1.3 mg	1.1 mg
Niacin	16 mg	14 mg
Pyridoxine	1.3 mg	1.3 mg
Folic acid	400 mcg	400 mcg
Cobalamin	2.4 mcg	2.4 mcg

*RAE = Retinol Activity Equivalent **IU = International Unit*

If you were counting, you'd notice that the chart listed only 10 vitamins, even though we said you need 13. Three B vitamins—biotin, pantothenic acid, and choline—aren't listed. That's because even though you need them, they don't have RDAs. Why not? Because you get these vitamins so easily from your food, even if you have incredibly bad eating habits, it's rare to really be deficient in them. And if no one's ever deficient, there's no point in bothering to set an RDA.

In 1999, however, the Institute of Medicine decided on an Adequate Intake (AI) amount for choline, an amount that varies depending on your age. It's one of the B vitamins, with 550 mg a day for an adult male and 425 mg a day for an adult female. The B vitamins are so important that we give each one its very own chapter—we'll go more into the details there.

Food for Thought

For centuries we've known that there's a relationship between our diet and certain kinds of diseases. It was only in the early 1900s that research really got going on exactly what it was in food that prevented certain diseases. By 1912, researchers had decided that the vital substances, whatever they were, had to be amines—chemicals that contain nitrogen, hydrogen, and carbon. The Polish biochemist Casimir Funk coined the word "vitamine," from vital and amine. As it turns out, not all vitamins are amines, so to avoid confusion the word was changed to "vitamin" in 1920.

We also didn't give a listing for Vitamin D. In 1997, the Institute of Medicine stopped having an RDA for this vitamin and instead listed an Adequate Intake for it. We'll explain all about this in Chapter 14. For now, we'll just tell you that the range for adults is between 5 and 15 mcg, or 200 and 600 IU.

Food for Thought

The Food and Nutrition Board of the Institute of Medicine first established Recommended Dietary Allowances (RDAs) for vitamins and minerals in 1941. The RDAs, and the newer Adequate Intakes (AIs), are revised and changed as needed about once every 5 to 10 years. The parent organization of the Institute of Medicine is the National Academy of Science, a private, nonprofit, self-perpetuating society of distinguished scholars. Founded by Congressional charter in 1863, the NAS has a mandate to advise the federal government on scientific and technical matters.

The Measure of Good Health

The other thing you may have noticed about the vitamin chart is the way we gave the RDAs in funny measurement units: mg and mcg. Usually the amounts of vitamins (and minerals and other supplements) are given using the metric system. (We'll explain about RAEs and IUs in Chapter 3, and about IUs in Chapter 15.)

Most of us stubbornly refuse to use metric measurements unless we really have to. But when it comes to vitamins, minerals, and supplements, you have to. Here's how to understand the measurements:

One gram (g) contains 1,000 milligrams (mg). A gram is roughly equivalent to ¼ teaspoon, or 0.035 of an ounce. There are about 4,000 mg in a teaspoon—roughly equal to the amount of sugar found in one of those little packets.

One milligram contains 1,000 micrograms (mcg). That means a microgram is 1/1,000 milligram, or 1/1,000,000 (yes, one millionth) gram. That's less than the amount that would fit on the head of a pin.

> ### Quack, Quack
>
> The only thing a vitamin can cure is a deficiency disease caused by a shortage of that vitamin. In other words, Vitamin C cures scurvy. It doesn't cure the common cold, although it can help shorten how long you're sick. Megadoses of vitamins can help prevent or treat health problems such as heart disease and diabetes, but they don't cure them.

Beyond the Basics

Throughout this book, we'll use the RDA or AI as the rock-bottom, bare-minimum amount you need to get every day for a particular vitamin or mineral. That's because the RDAs and AIs are only the amounts needed to prevent disease in ordinary, healthy people. They are, in our opinion and the opinion of many other nutritionists, doctors, and researchers, the *least* you should get. In many cases we believe the RDAs and AIs are far from the amount you need to reach optimal good health or to prevent many serious health problems, such as heart disease. As you'll discover in the chapters to come, there are many, many good reasons for taking more—sometimes much more—than the RDA or AI. There are also sometimes many good reasons to stick to the RDA or AI and *not* take any extra—and we'll cover those issues as well.

Minerals: Essential Elements of Health

A *mineral* is an inorganic chemical element, such as calcium or potassium, which your body must have in very small amounts for normal growth, metabolism, and health, and to make many enzymes and hormones. As with vitamins, you must get your minerals from your food.

We use the word "mineral" in a broad sense to mean all the many inorganic substances you need every day, but we should really be a little more exact. Nutritionally speaking, a mineral is an inorganic substance that you need every day in amounts of more than 100 mg. If you need less than 100 mg a day, we call the mineral a *trace mineral* or *trace element*. Even though the amounts you need for a trace mineral are very small—sometimes no more than 50 mcg—they're just as important to your health as the major minerals.

Minerals: How Much Do You Need?

The minerals you need every day include calcium, chloride, magnesium, phosphorus, potassium, sodium, and sulfur. We deal with all these in separate chapters (potassium, sodium, and chloride are combined in Chapter 20). Take a look at the chart to see the RDAs for the major minerals.

Adult RDAs for Minerals

Mineral	RDA for Adults
Calcium	1,000 to 1,200 mg
Chloride	2,300 mg
Fluoride	.03 to 4.0 mg
Magnesium	320 to 460 mg
Phosphorus	700 mg
Potassium	4,700 mg
Sodium	1,500 mg

One mineral is missing from the chart: sulfur. You need more than 100 mg of sulfur a day, but this mineral is so common in foods that nobody is ever deficient. As with biotin and pantothenic acid in the B vitamins, there's no real need to set an RDA for sulfur, so nobody has.

Trace Minerals: How Much Do You Need?

How many trace elements you need to get and in what amounts is open to a lot of discussion (see Chapter 21). We know for sure that you need very small amounts of arsenic, boron, chromium, copper, iodine, iron, manganese, molybdenum, nickel, selenium, silicon, vanadium, and zinc. What about the tiny, tiny amounts of other minerals, such as aluminum and lithium, which are found in your body? We don't really know why you have them or how much you need.

A lot of the trace minerals don't have RDAs—we just don't know enough about them to set any. Your need for boron, for example, was discovered only in the mid-1980s, and researchers are still trying to figure what the DRI should be. Instead, some of these minerals have AIs. These are best guesses as to how much you probably need. The chart lists the RDAs or AIs for the trace minerals that have them—we've left off the ones that don't.

Adult RDAs or AIs for Trace Minerals

Trace Mineral	RDA	AI
Chromium		25 to 35 mcg
Copper	900 mcg	
Iodine	150 mcg	
Iron	10 to 15 mg	
Manganese		1.8 to 2.3 mg
Molybdenum	45 mcg	
Selenium	55 mcg	
Zinc	8 to 11 mg	

What's missing from the chart? Boron, cobalt, nickel, silicon, and vanadium. You easily get these trace minerals from your food. Very few people will ever be deficient in them.

Do You Need Vitamin and Mineral Supplements?

The average person can get the RDAs or AIs for vitamins and minerals simply by eating a reasonable diet containing plenty of whole grains and fresh fruits and vegetables. Yeah, right. First of all, who's that mythical average person? Not anyone we know.

The RDAs/AIs assume you're an adult younger than age 60 who's in good health, has perfect digestion, isn't overweight, leads a totally stress-free life, doesn't ever have any sort of medical problem, and never needs to take any sort of medicine. The RDAs/AIs also assume that you really manage to eat a good diet every day.

Now You're Cooking

A lot of the vitamins in fruits and vegetables are lost between the farm and your plate. The longer the foods are stored before you eat them, the more nutrients are lost. Heat, light, and exposure to air all reduce the amount of vitamins, especially Vitamin C, thiamin, and folic acid.

Because frozen vegetables are processed right after they're picked, they may actually have more vitamins than fresh vegetables that were picked several days or more before you buy them at the grocery store.

Let's get real here: even on a good day, you can't always manage a completely healthful diet. Who has the time or energy to do all that shopping and food preparation? On any given day, half of us eat at least one meal away from home anyway. You just can't always eat healthfully, even when you try.

The fact is, most of us don't try all that hard, and most of us don't meet all the RDAs/AIs from our diet. Just look at the results of the Department of Agriculture's Healthy Eating Index from 1999 to 2000:

◆ A whopping 90 percent of Americans had a diet that was poor or needed improvement!

◆ Only 17 percent of all Americans ate at least two servings of fruit daily.

◆ Only 28 percent of all Americans ate at least three servings of vegetables daily.

And according to the results from the Department of Agriculture's National Health and Nutrition Examination Survey (NHANES) 2001 to 2002, we're not doing very well on getting the minimums from food alone:

◆ Most of us—93 percent—had an inadequate intake of Vitamin E.

◆ More than half of all Americans—56 percent—had an inadequate intake of magnesium.

◆ For Vitamin K and calcium, more than one in four Americans met the Adequate Intake.

- Most adult women don't meet the RDAs for iron, zinc, Vitamin B$_6$ (pyridoxine), calcium, magnesium, and Vitamin E.

- Most adult men don't meet the RDAs for zinc and magnesium.

And that's not all. According to a 2000 article in the leading journal *Pediatrics*, many children in the United States between ages 1 and 2 don't consume enough iron, zinc, and Vitamin E. This puts them at an increased risk of slowed growth and mental development, along with an increased risk of illness. And according to a 1998 study in *Pediatrics*, they get most of their vitamins and minerals from fortified breakfast cereals, not from fruits, vegetables, and other foods. If it's that hard to meet the RDAs/AIs through diet, what about reaching the higher amounts of vitamins and minerals many health professionals now recommend? You could just try harder to eat better or differently. For example, women between the ages of 25 and 50 should get at least 1,000 mg of calcium every day to keep their bones strong. That's the calcium in three glasses of milk a day. You could easily drink that much milk, but would you? Do you even like milk? What if you hate the stuff or have trouble digesting it?

One of the biggest problems with the RDAs/AIs is that they assume you're in good health and eat about 2,000 calories a day. What if you don't eat that much? Many women don't—and even if they do, women who follow the official nutritional advice to eat a low-fat diet often end up being shortchanged on nutrients. A 1998 study by the USDA showed that more than half the women who reduce their fat intake to less than 30 percent of their daily calories don't get the recommended daily intake of Vitamin A, Vitamin E, folic acid, calcium, iron, and zinc! And in our weight-conscious society, at any given time, one in six Americans is dieting—usually in a way that doesn't provide good nutrition. There's no way these people are getting the vitamins and minerals they need from their food.

We'd be the first to tell you that vitamin and mineral supplements aren't a substitute for healthy eating. They're also not a magic shield against the effects of bad health habits, such as smoking or not getting much exercise, and they don't make you lose weight. But we know that you can't always eat as you should—and that sometimes you need more vitamins or minerals than you can reasonably get just from food.

That's why vitamin and mineral supplements are so important. Taking a daily multivitamin and mineral supplement is sensible insurance—it makes sure you get everything you need. You may also need extra of one or more vitamins or minerals—more than you could get from your diet. Here, too, supplements make sure you're getting enough.

Generally speaking, vitamin and mineral supplements are safe, even in large doses. To put that statement into perspective, in 1998 the *Journal of the American Medical Association* reported that adverse reactions to prescription drugs killed more than 106,000 hospital patients in 1997 and caused serious side effects in 2 million more. In all the 1990s, only about 50 deaths could be attributed to dietary supplements of all kinds.

More isn't always better, though, and some supplements can be harmful in big doses. Use your common sense. Read what we have to say about the vitamins and minerals, talk it over with your doctor, and then decide which supplements are best for you.

On the Edge: Marginal Deficiencies

If you don't get a particular vitamin for a long time, you develop a *deficiency*. If the deficiency goes on long enough, you get a deficiency disease. The classic example of a deficiency disease is scurvy, caused by a lack of Vitamin C (we'll explain more about this in Chapter 13). Long before you start having any of the signs of a deficiency disease—and long before the deficiency shows up in the usual medical tests—you could be *marginally deficient* in a vitamin or mineral.

def•i•ni•tion

If you go for a long period without getting enough of a vitamin or mineral, you become deficient. A **marginal** or **subclinical deficiency** is an early stage. Your body's supply of a vitamin or mineral is gradually drained and your body's normal workings are gradually impaired. If a marginal deficiency goes on long enough, you will get a deficiency disease.

Here's a very good example: many older adults are marginally deficient in cobalamin (Vitamin B_{12}). The main symptom of classic cobalamin deficiency is anemia, which a doctor can easily diagnose with a simple blood test. Long before anemia sets in, though, marginal cobalamin deficiency leads to depression, confused thinking, and other mental symptoms that look a lot like senility. So is your Uncle George ga-ga from old age, or is he just low on B vitamins from the overprocessed, overcooked food he gets at the nursing home? Chances are good that poor diet is playing a bigger role in his mental condition than you or his doctor might realize. Chances are also good that a supplement containing all the B vitamins could do a lot to restore Uncle George to his old self.

What about you? You might be marginally deficient if …

◆ You rarely eat fresh fruits and vegetables. They are the best natural sources of vitamins and minerals.

◆ You've been going through a long period of high stress or overwork. You're probably not eating right, plus you're using up a lot of vitamins and minerals to make extra stress hormones. Think of yourself as a battery running down.

◆ You're sick with something—bronchitis, say—or you're recovering from surgery. At a time when you probably don't feel much like eating, you need lots of extra vitamins and minerals to help you heal faster.

◆ You have a chronic disease such as asthma or diabetes. Low levels of a vitamin or mineral might be causing the problem or making it worse. Many people with asthma are low on magnesium, for example; many people with diabetes are very low on Vitamin C. Chronic diseases change how well your body absorbs and uses vitamins and minerals, so your needs change as well.

◆ You're pregnant or nursing. You need extra vitamins and minerals because you're passing some of yours on to your baby.

◆ You're seriously depressed. When you're depressed, you don't eat well. That can make the depression worse, because marginal deficiencies of many vitamins and minerals *cause* depression.

◆ You smoke. Smoking sharply increases your need for vitamins, especially Vitamin C.

◆ You drink a lot of alcohol. Heavy drinkers are often marginally deficient in almost all the vitamins and minerals, especially B vitamins.

How do you know you have a marginal deficiency? Deficiencies can be hard to pin down. You might just be feeling a little under par, or more tired than usual. That's easy to blame on all sorts of things, so you might not think a vitamin or mineral deficiency is the problem. Even if you go to your doctor with other deficiency symptoms, such as irritability, anxiety, or insomnia, you're more likely to come home with a prescription for Valium than for a vitamin supplement. If you feel your health isn't what it could be—if you get frequent minor illnesses, for example, or bad colds you just can't seem to shake—ask yourself whether you're getting enough of the vitamins and minerals you need.

The Antioxidant Revolution

You need vitamins and minerals to make all those thousands of enzymes, hormones, and other chemicals your body needs to work right. But vitamins and minerals have another crucial role in your body: they act as powerful *antioxidants* that capture *free radicals* in your body. It's only in the past few decades that we've begun to understand how damaging free radicals can be and how important it is to have plenty of antioxidants in your body to neutralize them.

def•i•ni•tion

Antioxidants are enzymes that protect your body by capturing free radicals and, in a complex series of steps, escorting them out of your body before they do any additional damage.

Free radicals are unstable oxygen atoms created by your body's natural processes and by the effects of toxins such as cigarette smoke. Free radicals, especially the types called "singlet oxygen" and "hydroxyl," are very reactive and cause a lot of damage to your cells, but they're not all bad. You use free radicals as part of your immune system to defend against invading bacteria.

Radicals on the Loose

When you drive your car, you burn gasoline by combining it with oxygen in the pistons of the engine. Your car zips along on the released energy, but it also gives off exhaust fumes as a byproduct. Something very similar happens in the cells of your body. When oxygen combines with glucose in your cells, for example, you make energy—and you also make free radicals, your body's version of exhaust fumes. Free radicals are oxygen atoms that are missing one electron from the pair the atom should have. When an atom is missing an electron from a pair, it becomes unstable and very reactive. That's because a free radical desperately wants to find another electron to fill in the gap, so it grabs an electron from the next atom it gets near. But when a free radical seizes an electron from another atom, the second atom then becomes a free radical, because now it's the one missing an electron. One free radical starts a cascade of new free radicals in your body. The free radicals blunder around, grabbing electrons from your cells—and doing a lot of damage to them at the same time. If free radicals damage the DNA in your cells often enough, they can cause the genetic changes that trigger cancer. If free radicals oxidize cholesterol in your blood, they can cause the artery-clogging plaque that leads to heart disease.

Fighting Back with Antioxidants

Antioxidants are your body's natural defense against free radicals. Antioxidants are enzymes that patrol your cells looking for free radicals. When they find one, they grab hold of it and neutralize it without being damaged themselves. The antioxidant enzymes stop the invasion and remove the free radical from circulation.

You have to have plenty of vitamins and minerals—especially Vitamin A, beta carotene, Vitamin C, Vitamin E, and selenium—in your body to make the antioxidant enzymes that do the neutralizing. If you're short on the right vitamins and minerals, you can't make enough of the antioxidant enzymes. That lets the free radicals get the upper hand and do extra damage to your cells before they get quenched.

Oxidation isn't the only thing that can cause free radicals in your cells. The ultraviolet light in sunshine can do it—that's why people who spend too much time in the sun are more likely to get skin cancer and cataracts. Toxins of all sorts—tobacco smoke, the natural chemicals found in our food, the poisonous wastes of your own metabolism, and man-made toxins such as air pollution and pesticides—trigger free radicals as well.

On average, every cell in your body comes under attack from a free radical once every 10 seconds. Your best protection is to keep your antioxidant levels high. How? That's what we're going to explain in just about every chapter for the rest of this book.

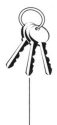

Food for Thought

According to a 1998 study, people who get above-average amounts of the important antioxidants Vitamin C, Vitamin E, beta carotene, and selenium from their food have better lung function than those who consume below-average amounts. The difference between the highest and lowest groups is about the same as the difference between nonsmokers and those who have smoked a pack a day for 10 years!

The Least You Need to Know

- Vitamins (organic substances) and minerals (inorganic substances) are necessary for life and good health.

- Vitamins A, D, E, and K are fat-soluble: they're stored in your body's fatty tissues.

- The B vitamins and Vitamin C are water-soluble: your body can't store them, so you need some every day.

- Vitamins and minerals are needed to make the thousands of different enzymes your body needs to live.

◆ Free radicals are unstable oxygen atoms made in your body as part of normal metabolism. They are very reactive and can damage your cells.

◆ Antioxidant enzymes capture and neutralize free radicals.

Choosing What's Right for You

In This Chapter

- ◆ Interpreting the Dietary Reference Intake (DRI) and Recommended Dietary Allowance (RDA)

- ◆ Determining vitamins and minerals needs for kids, adults, older adults, and vegetarians

- ◆ Understanding how vitamins and minerals can help common health problems

- ◆ Saving money on vitamin and mineral supplements

- ◆ Getting the most from your supplements

Your next-door neighbor tells you that a friend of her mother's feels a thousand times better since she started taking this new vitamin pill. Should you take the same pill? Of course not! You need real information, not third-hand stories, to make a good choice about which supplements are right for *you*.

It's not hard to make good choices. All you need is some reliable information based on real research, not anecdotes you hear by the supplements counter at your local health-food store. That's what we're here for. In this chapter, we give you the basics you need to select the vitamins and minerals that are best for you, choose products you can rely on, and get the most out of them.

Who Decides This Stuff, Anyway?

Two major players set the national standards for your daily vitamins and minerals: the nonprofit, independent Institute of Medicine and the federal Food and Drug Administration (FDA). The FDA is an agency within the Public Health Service, which in turn is part of the Department of Health and Human Services. One big part of the FDA's job is to make sure foods are safe and are labeled truthfully with useful information. The two organizations use similar abbreviations to explain their recommendations, which have created a lot of confusion among consumers. Here's what all those initials mean:

◆ **RDA.** As we explained in Chapter 1, the Food and Nutrition Board of the Institute of Medicine, an arm of the nonprofit National Academy of Sciences, sets the Recommended Dietary Allowances—the national guidelines for the minimum amounts you need every day. They're the basis for all the scientific research on nutrition—and for the information we give in this book.

◆ **DRI.** Starting in 1997, the Institute of Medicine created a set of comprehensive guidelines called the Daily Reference Intake, or DRI. For each vitamin and mineral, the DRI indicates the estimated average requirement (EAR), the RDA or the adequate intake (AI), and the tolerable upper intake level. DRIs provide more information than RDAs alone.

◆ **USRDA.** These are the "other" RDAs, set by the FDA. US stands for United States, of course, but this time RDA stands for Recommended Daily Allowance. The USRDAs are really just somewhat simplified versions of the Institute of Medicine's RDAs. This standard is being phased out in favor of a new one called RDI.

◆ **RDI.** Get used to this one, because it will eventually replace USRDA on all food and supplement labels. RDI stands for Reference Daily Intake. The amounts are still pretty much the same as the old USRDAs, which are pretty much the same as the RDAs, which are now called the DRIs. With us so far?

◆ **DRV.** Now it starts to get complicated. DRV stands for Daily Recommended Values. The FDA created this new standard to cover energy-producing nutrients, which aren't covered in the RDIs. The DRVs are the amounts of fats, carbohydrates, fiber, protein, cholesterol, sodium, and potassium you should get every day. As you can see from the following chart, the DRVs are percentages based on a diet that contains 2,000 calories.

◆ **DV.** In its wisdom, the FDA has combined the RDIs and DRVs into one, easy-to-understand standard called the Daily Value (DV). This is the basis for the detailed labels you now see on food packages. The labels include the DRVs and selected RDIs for some vitamins and minerals, usually Vitamin A, Vitamin C, calcium, and iron, but sometimes others (depending on whether the food is a good source of those nutrients). The label gives both the total amount of each nutrient per serving and what percentage of your recommended daily intake that amount is.

Daily Recommended Values for Adults

Nutrient	Portion of Daily Diet
Total fats	30 percent, 65 g, or 600 calories
Saturated fat	10 percent, 20 g, or 200 calories
Cholesterol	300 mg
Carbohydrates	60 percent, 300 g, or 1,200 calories
Protein	10 percent, 50 g, or 200 calories
Fiber	25 g
Sodium	2,400 mg
Potassium	3,500 mg

Note: Based on a daily diet of 2,000 calories. If you eat fewer or more calories, the percentages remain the same. Saturated fat should be no more than 10 percent of total fat. Children under age 4, and pregnant and nursing women, need more protein.

The Institute of Medicine (IOM) doesn't agree with the amounts in the DRV chart. For instance, the IOM sets the DRI for carbohydrates at just 130 g a day for an adult. The IOM is noncommittal about dietary fat, saying only that dietary cholesterol and saturated fat should be "as low as possible while consuming a nutritionally adequate diet."

Other agencies and organizations also get into the standards act. The nonprofit American Heart Association, for example, says your daily cholesterol intake should be no more than 300 mg a day—the same as the DRV. The federal National Institutes of Health recommends 1,000 mg of calcium for women aged 25 to 50 and 1,500 mg for women older than age 65. The amount for older women is higher than the current RDI. These recommendations don't have the force of law the way the ones from the FDA do, but they carry a lot of weight in the medical community.

No matter how you look at it—RDA, RDI, DV—there's still one big problem. In the opinion of many health professionals, the amounts for vitamins and minerals are too low. More and more research tells us that larger doses of some vitamins and minerals not only keep us healthier now, they can also help diseases from getting started and can help control them when they do.

What Are Your Needs?

Everybody's different, which is one reason minimum averages such as RDAs/AIs aren't always helpful. In many cases, you might want to take supplements to get more than the RDAs/AIs. But how can you decide what's best for you?

> **Food for Thought** _____
>
> According to Harvard Medical School's ongoing Physician's Health Study, people who take a daily multivitamin have a 25 percent lower risk of developing a cataract.
>
> In 2000, a major report from the federal Centers for Disease Control showed that adults who take a daily multivitamin along with additional Vitamin A, Vitamin C, or Vitamin E had a 15 percent lower risk of dying from a heart attack or stroke compared to adults who didn't take any vitamins at all.

We can't tell you exactly how much to take of anything. What we can do is explain, in the chapters on the individual vitamins and minerals, why you might want more of each and how much more is safe. The amounts you decide to take will depend on your personal health, family medical history, age, sex, and other factors. We also explain why it's safe to take supplements of some vitamins and minerals and why sometimes you should stick to the DRI or RDA.

You won't see instant changes in your health as soon as you start taking more vitamins and minerals. The improvements come slowly, over a period of a few weeks or even months. You may notice that you just feel better overall—more energetic and more optimistic. Nagging problems, such as a lingering cold or minor skin rash, may finally clear up. If you have a chronic disease such as diabetes, you may find that your symptoms are easier to deal with and some side effects and complications improve.

Warning! _____
Never stop taking a prescription medicine on your own. Always consult your doctor!

What may be most important about supplements, though, are the things that *won't* happen. By taking extra vitamins and minerals as part of a healthy diet, you may be preventing or delaying future problems, such as osteoporosis, cancer, heart disease, stroke, and senility.

Tests for Vitamin and Mineral Deficiencies

Today many doctors routinely check your blood for some vitamin and mineral deficiencies, especially iron and Vitamin B_{12} (cobalamin). There are blood and urine tests for most vitamins and minerals, but some are complicated or inconvenient, to say nothing of the costs. Generally, there's no real reason to do them, unless you have a medical problem that affects your ability to absorb nutrients.

Nutritionally Oriented Health Care

Nutritionally oriented doctors often describe their approach as *functional medicine* or sometimes *orthomolecular medicine*. They believe that fixing the underlying biochemical imbalance that is causing an illness is just as important as treating the symptoms. Vitamins, minerals, and other nutrients, along with lifestyle changes, are important parts of functional medicine.

Prestigious institutions such as the Harvard Medical School and the National Institutes of Health are now seriously studying the value of alternative treatments. Many doctors today have come to realize how important diet and vitamins and minerals are to their patients' health. Sadly, many more haven't. If your doctor is among the unenlightened, you may want to consult a nutritionally oriented doctor, nutritionist, or other health-care professional. We list several national professional organizations in Appendix B. These groups can help you find a qualified professional in your area.

def•i•ni•tion

The great Linus Pauling, two-time winner of the Nobel Prize, coined the term **orthomolecular medicine.** The prefix *ortho-* means "right" or "correct." Many doctors today prefer the term **functional medicine,** meaning they use supplements along with other treatments to restore a patient's body to its proper functioning.

Whenever you visit a health-care professional, be sure to bring a list of everything you take—including *all* prescription and nonprescription drugs and *all* vitamins, minerals, herbs, and other supplements. Otherwise, you might end up with an accidental bad reaction to a drug.

Quack, Quack

One in three Americans will seek an "alternative" therapy for a serious illness. These people are easy targets for unscrupulous companies and unlicensed "natural medicine" practitioners peddling phony treatments and formulas that "cure" ailments such as arthritis or Alzheimer's disease. If the advertising pitch includes words such as *special, instant relief, secret, miracle, rediscovered,* or *ancient,* beware! The only thing miraculous about these products is how quickly your money vanishes.

Vitamins and Minerals for Everyone

Almost everyone can benefit from vitamins and minerals beyond the RDAs/AIs. To help you decide how much more, we've compiled a very conservative chart showing the safe ranges for healthy adults. Remember, more isn't always better. When in doubt, less is always best. Don't exceed the maximum safe dosage!

Safe Dosage Ranges for Vitamins and Minerals for Healthy Adults

Vitamins	Safe Daily Dosage Range
Vitamin A	5,000 to 25,000 IU
B Vitamins:	
Thiamin	2 to 100 mg
Riboflavin	50 to 100 mg
Niacin	20 to 100 mg
Pyridoxine	3 to 50 mg
Folic acid	800 mcg to 2 mg
Cobalamin	500 to 1,000 mcg
Pantothenic acid	4 to 7 mg
Biotin	30 to 100 mcg
Vitamin C	500 to 2,000 mg
Vitamin D	400 to 600 IU
Vitamin E	200 to 400 IU

Minerals	Safe Daily Dosage Range
Calcium	1,000 to 1,500 mg
Copper	1.5 to 3.0 mg
Chromium	50 to 200 mcg
Iron	15 to 30 mg
Magnesium	300 to 500 mg
Manganese	2.5 to 5.0 mg
Molybdenum	75 to 250 mcg
Potassium	2,000 to 3,500 mg
Selenium	70 to 200 mcg
Zinc	15 to 50 mg

Special Needs of Older Adults

As you get older, your nutritional needs change. By the time you're 65, for instance, you just don't absorb Vitamin D and some B vitamins as well as you used to. If you're an older woman, you need more calcium and less iron. And by the time you're 65, you may well be taking at least one prescription drug to treat some sort of chronic condition. In fact, nearly half of all people older than age 75 take three or more prescription drugs every day. As you'll learn in later chapters of this book, some common prescription drugs can seriously affect your vitamin and mineral levels—and some vitamins and minerals could keep the drugs from working correctly.

Many older people just don't eat right or eat enough. Many older women eat only 1,250 to 1,500 calories a day, while many older men eat only about 1,600 to 1,900 calories daily. Even worse, studies show that 30 percent of elderly people regularly skip at least one meal a day. If you're not taking in enough good, nutritious calories, you're not taking in enough vitamins and minerals from your food.

Food for Thought

A 1997 international study showed that women who took multivitamin supplements throughout their pregnancy had children who were 40 percent less likely to get brain tumors. Vitamins A, C, and E and folic acid seemed to be the most important for providing the protection. If you're planning a family or are already pregnant, talk to your doctor about which vitamins and minerals to take. And be sure to read about folic acid in Chapter 9.

If you're older than 65, discuss your vitamin and mineral needs with your doctor. Look carefully at your diet and be sure you're getting all the B vitamins, but especially thiamin (Vitamin B_1), riboflavin (Vitamin B_{12}), pyridoxine (Vitamin B_6), and cobalamin (Vitamin B_{12}). Because your ability to absorb the B vitamins drops with age, consider taking a complete B-vitamin supplement. You also need to be sure you're getting enough Vitamin E, Vitamin C, iron, calcium, magnesium, and zinc. Supplements could help here as well.

The RDAs/AIs for many vitamins and minerals are somewhat different for adults older than age 70—check the RDA/AI charts in the chapters of this book for the specific amounts. We suggest talking to your doctor about daily doses of 250 IU of Vitamin D, 1,000 mcg of cobalamin, and 500 mg of calcium, along with the other supplements previously mentioned.

Vitamins for Kids and Teens

Kids and teenagers grow fast. To fuel that growth, they need good nutrition, including plenty of vitamins and minerals. Unfortunately, kids today don't always get what they need. One out of every 10 toddlers is low on iron, for example, and teenage girls need extra. Many teens, male and female, are low on zinc.

How can you be sure your kids are getting their vitamins? The standard answer is to make sure they eat a variety of foods, including lots of fresh fruits and vegetables. That's easy for the nutritionists to say. Anyone who's ever been a parent knows that it's a *lot* harder to do. It's tough enough to get a 6-year-old to eat vegetables—just try getting a 16-year-old to eat them!

Vitamin and mineral supplements can be very helpful here. Give children younger than 2 vitamin and mineral supplements only if your doctor recommends them. Many doctors do suggest an iron supplement or a formula containing iron for babies younger than 24 months, especially if you're breastfeeding. For young children older than age 2, liquid multi-supplements are convenient—all you have to do is add a squirt to their morning milk or juice. Older kids like chewable tablets, and you might even be able to get your teenagers to swallow a daily supplement. There are a lot of different brands from which to choose. We suggest looking for one that has the RDA/AI for your child's age group and is made without artificial colorings and preservatives. As a rule, there's no real reason to give a child or teen supplements of individual vitamins and minerals—stick to a good multi instead.

Warning!

Keep all supplements and drugs of any sort safely away from small children. The amount of iron in just three or four adult iron supplements, for example, could cause serious poisoning in a young child.

Vitamins for Vegetarians

Because they don't eat meat—and sometimes don't eat any animal foods at all—*vegetarians* and *vegans* need to be sure they're getting enough vitamins and minerals from their food. This is fairly easy to do with a little planning and a good understanding of nutrition. Even so, vegetarians and vegans may end up on the low side for some nutrients, especially the B vitamins, calcium, and iron. To be on the safe side, we recommend a good daily multi-supplement, especially for kids who don't eat animal foods.

def•i•ni•tion

Vegetarians are people who don't eat meat. Most vegetarians eat eggs and dairy foods, and some eat fish. **Vegans** are people who don't eat any animal foods at all.

Supplements and Common Health Problems

We're going to talk a lot in this book about how vitamins, minerals, and other supplements can help high cholesterol, high blood pressure, and diabetes. Rather than explain these very common health problems over and over, we're going to deal with them here.

High Cholesterol

We worry so much about our cholesterol these days that we sometimes forget that you need cholesterol to live. Cholesterol is a waxy fat your body needs to make your cell membranes and many hormones, among other important roles. You make most of your cholesterol in your liver, but you also get some from eating animal foods. Just like oil and water, cholesterol and blood don't mix. To get the cholesterol to where it has to go, your liver coats it with a layer of protein. The protein keeps the cholesterol together so that it doesn't just float around in your blood. The technical name for the cholesterol-protein package is *lipoprotein*.

There are several different kinds of lipoproteins, but the two most important are *low-density lipoprotein (LDL)* and *high-density lipoprotein (HDL)*. Most of the cholesterol in your blood is carried as LDL cholesterol; only about a third to a quarter is carried as

def•i•ni•tion

Low-density lipoprotein (LDL) is a form of cholesterol and is often called "bad" cholesterol because excess amounts in your blood can lead to health problems, including heart disease. **High-density lipoprotein (HDL)** is another form of cholesterol and is often called "good" cholesterol because it can help remove LDL cholesterol from your blood.

def•i•ni•tion

Atherosclerosis happens when fatty deposits called plaques build up inside one of your arteries, often an artery that nourishes your heart or leads to your brain. Many researchers today believe that plaque forms when LDL cholesterol is oxidized by free radicals. Keeping your antioxidant levels high may help prevent atherosclerosis.

HDL cholesterol. But too much LDL cholesterol in the blood can lead to *atherosclerosis*—"clogging" of the arteries—which can lead to heart disease, stroke, and other problems. That's why LDL cholesterol is often called "bad" cholesterol. HDL cholesterol actually helps remove cholesterol from the blood—that's why it's often called "good" cholesterol. Ideally, you want to have a relatively low LDL level and a relatively high HDL level.

What's a good level and how do you know? To measure your blood cholesterol levels, your doctor sends a sample of your blood to a laboratory, where the amounts of LDL and HDL in it are measured. (To make sure the results are accurate, don't eat for 12 hours before the test.) The results come back as milligrams per deciliter, abbreviated as mg/dL (a deciliter is one tenth of a liter). Usually there are two numbers: your total cholesterol (LDL plus HDL) and your LDL stated separately. In general, if your total cholesterol is below 200 mg/dL, you don't have to worry. If it's more than 200 mg/dL but below 240 mg/dL, you have borderline high cholesterol. If it's more than 240 mg/dL, you have high cholesterol. If your LDL is 130 mg/dL or lower, that's desirable; LDL between 130 and 159 mg/dL is borderline; and LDL above 160 mg/dL is high. Your HDL number should be more than 35 mg/dL; anything lower is undesirable.

If your total or LDL cholesterol is borderline high or high, lowering it by even 10 percent could prevent a heart attack or stroke. Eating less fat, getting more exercise, and quitting smoking are the most important steps, along with taking cholesterol-lowering drugs if your doctor recommends them. In addition, throughout this book we talk about how vitamins, minerals, and other supplements, along with diet and lifestyle changes, can help.

High Blood Pressure

Every time your heart beats (about 60 to 70 times a minute when you're resting), it pumps blood out through large blood vessels called arteries. Blood pressure is the force of that blood as it pushes against the walls of the arteries. Your blood pressure is at its highest when your heart beats and pushes the blood out—doctors call this the *systolic* pressure. When the heart is at rest between beats, your blood pressure falls. This is called *diastolic* pressure. Blood pressure is always given as two numbers: first the systolic and then the diastolic pressure.

In 2003, the National High Blood Pressure Education Program, part of the National Heart, Lung, and Blood Institute, changed the official guidelines for diagnosing high blood pressure, also known as *hypertension*. Here's how your blood pressure measures up now:

♦ Normal: below 120 systolic and below 80 diastolic

♦ Prehypertension: 120–139 systolic and 80–89 diastolic

♦ Hypertension Stage 1: 140–159 systolic and 90–99 diastolic

♦ Hypertension Stage 2: 160 and higher systolic and 100 and higher diastolic

def•i•ni•tion

Hypertension, or high blood pressure, is a disease with many causes, no symptoms at first, and no cure. Your doctor looks at two numbers when checking your blood pressure. The **systolic** pressure is the pressure against your arteries when your heart pumps out blood. The **diastolic** pressure is the pressure when your heart is at rest between beats. If your pressure is 140/90 or more, you have hypertension.

High blood pressure gets more serious as the numbers get higher. Your risk of heart attack, stroke, and kidney disease go up along with your blood pressure.

If your blood pressure is high, there are many lifestyle steps you can take to lower it, such as losing weight, getting more exercise, avoiding salt, giving up cigarettes, and drinking less alcohol. If your blood pressure stays high even when you do all that, your doctor may prescribe drugs to bring it down. As you'll learn in the rest of this book, vitamins, minerals, and other supplements, along with diet and lifestyle changes, can help.

Diabetes

The recommendations in this book are for the millions of Americans who have Type 2 diabetes (also known as noninsulin-dependent diabetes or adult-onset diabetes). People with this disease have trouble getting glucose—the body's main fuel—from their blood into their cells, where it can be turned into energy. Diabetes can lead to serious complications. It's the single biggest cause of kidney disease, for example; it's also a leading cause of blindness. People with diabetes have double the risk of the general population for heart attack and stroke. Vitamins, minerals, and supplements can reduce many of the problems caused by diabetes.

According to the American Diabetes Association, about 18 million Americans have Type 2 diabetes—but anywhere from 5 to 8 million of them don't know it yet. Many will find out when they're in a hospital emergency room for a heart attack. If you're overweight, have a sedentary lifestyle, or have a family history of diabetes, you are at serious risk of diabetes. Your doctor can easily diagnose diabetes with a simple blood test to check for glucose (sugar) in your blood. If your fasting blood sugar level is 126 mg/dL or higher, you may have diabetes.

Getting the Most from Supplements

We hope by now we've made a pretty good case for taking extra vitamins and minerals every day. The best way to do that is with a good multivitamin/mineral supplement. According to the Dietary Supplement Health and Education Act (DSHEA) of 1994, a dietary supplement is a product that contains one or more dietary ingredients, such as vitamins, minerals, herbs, amino acids, or other ingredients used to supplement the diet.

When purchasing a multivitamin/mineral supplement, check the label for this information:

◆ A formula that contains all the vitamins except Vitamin K. Be sure the supplement contains all the B vitamins, including cobalamin (Vitamin B_{12}).

◆ A formula that contains mixed carotenoids along with Vitamin A. (See Chapters 3 and 25 to learn why.)

◆ A formula that contains *chelated* forms of calcium, magnesium, potassium, selenium, and zinc, along with boron, chromium, manganese, and molybdenum. Because a tablet that has the RDAs for calcium and the other minerals would be too large to swallow, it's okay if the formula doesn't have the full amounts. Just be sure you're getting some calcium from your diet as well and take a separate calcium supplement in addition if necessary.

◆ A formula that contains iron, if you want to take extra of this mineral, or is iron-free if you don't. (See Chapter 21 to decide.)

def•i•ni•tion

Chelated minerals have been treated to alter their electrical charge, usually by binding them chemically to a harmless salt such as gluconate, citrate, picolinate, aspartate, or another -ate substance. That's why the label often reads "zinc picolinate" or "magnesium citrate" rather than just plain zinc or magnesium. You absorb minerals better if they've been chelated.

◆ A formula that contains the minerals in forms you can easily absorb. We go into that in more detail in each mineral chapter, but here's an easy rule of thumb: the calcium should be in the form of calcium citrate or an amino acid chelate. If it's not, choose a different brand.

Taking Your Vitamins

Many people like the convenience of taking a one-a-day supplement—a pill you can pop first thing in the morning and not have to think about again. One-a-days have some drawbacks, though. First, many one-a-days just don't have enough in them. To keep them small enough to swallow easily, they don't have the RDAs for calcium, magnesium, or potassium. Most don't have the RDA for selenium, either. Another problem is that the water-soluble B vitamins and Vitamin C will be washed from your body fairly quickly if you take them all at once.

It's much more effective to take your vitamins and minerals in divided doses through-out the day. That way, you can easily get the full RDAs/AIs for calcium and other minerals without having to swallow big pills, and your levels of the water-soluble vita-mins remain high throughout the day. You'll get the most from your supplements if you make a habit of taking them with meals.

Choosing a Good Product

There's unfortunately very little regulation of dietary supplements—no U.S. govern-ment agency requires them to be tested for safety or purity. To be sure of purchasing consistently high-quality products made by reputable manufacturers, look for the Good Manufacturing Practices (GMP) certification on the label. Reliable, indepen-dent GMP seals are currently provided by the following trade associations:

◆ Natural Products Association (NPA), formerly known as the National Nutritional Foods Association; www.naturalproductsassoc.org

◆ NSF International; www.nsf.org

◆ U.S. Pharmacopoeia (USP); www.usp.org

◆ ConsumerLab.com

The Least You Need to Know

◆ The minimum daily amounts for vitamins, minerals, and other nutrients such as fiber are set by the independent Institute of Medicine and the federal Food and Drug Agency (FDA).

◆ You can safely take more than the RDA or AI for almost all vitamins and minerals.

◆ Everyone's needs are different. Kids, older adults, and vegetarians have special nutritional needs.

◆ Almost everyone can benefit from taking a daily multivitamin/mineral supplement.

Part 2

The A to K of Vitamins

We could write this part of the book using just six letters: A, B, C, D, E, and K. These are the vitamins you absolutely, positively must have in very small amounts to live. No single vitamin is any more important than any other.

After you get beyond your basic needs, though, some vitamins may be more useful to you than others. But which ones? And how much? Here is where you need an understanding of how vitamins work and the effects they have on you.

Remember when you were a kid and had alphabet soup for lunch? You'd poke around in the bowl until you came up with the letters of your name. That's what the alphabet soup of vitamins is like—you can arrange those six letters to spell good health for yourself.

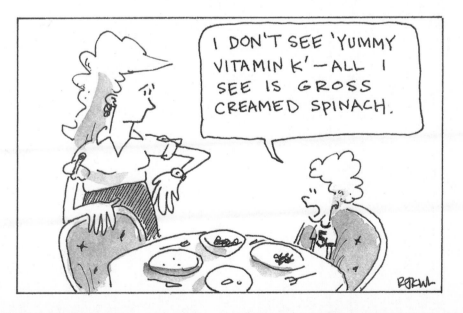

3

Vitamin A and Carotenes: Double-Barreled Health Protection

In This Chapter

- ◆ Needing Vitamin A and carotenes
- ◆ Finding foods that are high in Vitamin A and carotenes
- ◆ Choosing the right supplements
- ◆ Protecting your vision and boosting your immune system with Vitamin A
- ◆ Protecting against the free radicals that can cause cancer and heart disease

Vitamin A was the first vitamin to be discovered, back in 1913. But the importance of Vitamin A was already well-known to the ancient Greeks. Back then, Hippocrates, the father of modern medicine, told patients with failing eyesight to eat beef liver. When they did, they were able to see much better, especially at night. Hippocrates didn't know why liver helped so much, but today we know that animal liver is a rich source of Vitamin A—and we know that our eyes need plenty of Vitamin A to work properly in the dark.

Today we know a lot more than Hippocrates about the importance of Vitamin A for a wide range of body functions—from keeping your skin smooth to warding off cancer. We also know that Vitamin A is only half the story. Health researchers are very excited about carotenes, the natural plant forms of Vitamin A. Your body converts some of the carotenes in plant foods into the Vitamin A you need and uses the leftovers to help you fight off the free radicals that can cause cancer, heart disease, and other problems.

Why You Need Vitamin A

When Vitamin A was first discovered, it was called the *anti-infective agent.* Lab animals that were fed a diet low in animal foods, vegetables, and fruits soon got eye infections—infections that cleared up as soon as these foods were put back into their diet. The mysterious "agent" in the foods turned out to be a fat-soluble substance that was dubbed Vitamin A.

To fend off infections and illnesses, Vitamin A helps you put up strong frontline barriers to infection. How? By helping your body's *epithelial tissues*—the cells that make up your skin and line your eyes, mouth, nose, throat, lungs, digestive tract, and urinary tract—grow and repair themselves. These tissues line your body's external and internal surfaces and keep out trespassers. Without enough Vitamin A, these cells become stiff, dry, and much more likely to let down their guard. When that happens, germs can easily pass through them and into your body. Even if your body has plenty of Vitamin A, those nasty germs still sometimes get through your outer defenses. When that happens, Vitamin A helps your immune system come riding to the rescue.

Vitamin A is essential for healthy eyes—an important subject we'll talk a lot about later in this chapter. Children and teens need plenty of Vitamin A to help them grow properly and build strong bones and teeth. Your need for Vitamin A doesn't stop then, though. Even after you're fully grown, your body constantly replaces old, worn-out cells with new ones. You need Vitamin A to produce healthy replacement cells and to keep your bones and teeth strong.

def•i•ni•tion

Your **epithelial tissues** cover the internal and external surfaces of your body. Because your skin covers the outside, for example, it's one giant external epithelial tissue. Epithelial tissue also lines your nose and your eyes. Your entire digestive tract, from start to finish, is lined with epithelial tissue. So are your lungs and your urinary and reproductive tracts.

Why You Need Carotenes Even More

Now that you know why you need Vitamin A, we're going to confuse you by explaining why you need carotenes even more. Bear with us as we journey back into vitamin history to explain why.

After Vitamin A was discovered, researchers believed that the only way to get this was by eating animal foods such as eggs or liver that naturally contain *retinoids*, or *preformed* Vitamin A. Your body can use this Vitamin A as-is just as soon as you eat it.

def•i•ni•tion

The Vitamin A found in animal foods such as egg yolks, is **preformed**—meaning that your body can use it immediately. Actually, there are three kinds of preformed Vitamin A: *retinol, retinaldehyde,* and *retinoic acid.* These names refer to your retina, the light-sensitive layer of cells at the back of your eye. One of the first signs of Vitamin A deficiency is trouble seeing at night, because your retina needs Vitamin A to function properly.

In 1928, researchers discovered the other way to get your As: by eating plant foods that contain *carotenes*—the orange, red, and yellow substances that give plant foods their colors. The most abundant of the carotenes in plant foods is beta carotene. Your body easily converts beta carotene to Vitamin A in your small intestine, where special enzymes split one molecule of beta carotene in half to make two molecules of Vitamin A.

def•i•ni•tion

Carotenes are natural pigments in red, orange, and yellow plant foods (such as cantaloupes, carrots, and tomatoes). Carotenes are also found in potatoes and dark-green, leafy vegetables. The name comes from carrots. Because your body has to change the carotenes into Vitamin A before you can use them, carotenes are sometimes called *precursor* (meaning something that precedes or goes before) *Vitamin A* or *provitamin A* (where *pro* means "before").

If you don't happen to need any Vitamin A when you eat a food containing carotenes, you don't convert the beta carotene. Instead, a lot of it circulates in your blood and enters into your cells; the rest gets stored in your fatty tissues. Whenever you need some extra As, your liver quickly converts the stored beta carotene.

Carotenes are just one small group of plant substances in the much larger *carotenoid* family. In this chapter we focus on the two main carotenes that are converted to Vitamin A: *alpha carotene* (sometimes written α-carotene) and *beta carotene* (sometimes written β-carotene). (A few other carotenes have some Vitamin A activity, but it's so minor we don't really need to discuss them.)

Why is it better to convert your As from the carotenes in plant foods rather than getting them straight from animal foods or supplements? There are some very good reasons:

◆ **The antioxidant *power* of carotenes.** About 40 percent of the carotenes you eat are converted to Vitamin A in your liver and small intestine as you need it. The rest act as powerful antioxidants. Beta carotene is especially good at quenching singlet oxygen. (Remember that destructive little molecule from Chapter 1?) Alpha carotene is an even better antioxidant—it may be 10 times as effective for mopping up free radicals.

◆ **The safety of carotenes.** Large doses of supplemental Vitamin A can be toxic—and some people show overdose symptoms even at lower doses. Your body converts carotenes to Vitamin A only as needed, however, so it's almost impossible to overdose. Also, beta carotene is nontoxic—even if you store so much in your fatty tissues that you turn yellow, it's harmless.

◆ **The health benefits of fruits and vegetables.** Carotenes are found in almost every fruit and vegetable. Five servings a day will give you all the Vitamin A you need, along with plenty of other vitamins, minerals, antioxidants, and fiber. What you won't get are calories and the cholesterol found in animal sources of preformed Vitamin A, such as beef liver (and let's not even discuss the yucky taste).

def•i•ni•tion

The **carotenoids** are a large family of red, orange, and yellow plant substances found in many fruits and vegetables. Your body can convert two related carotenoids, **alpha carotene** and **beta carotene,** into Vitamin A. The two carotenes are similar, but beta carotene is much more abundant in foods and accounts for most of the Vitamin A you make from plant foods.

The RDA for Vitamin A

If you eat a typical diet, you'll get some of your Vitamin A the preformed way from milk, eggs, and meat. You'll get the rest in the form of carotenes (mostly beta) from the fruits and vegetables you eat. That means the RDA for Vitamin A assumes that you get some of your As from animal foods and some from plant foods. But that leads to a problem. How can you measure how much Vitamin A you're actually making from the beta carotene you eat in plant foods?

Measuring Vitamin A

Up until 1980, the RDA for Vitamin A was given in *International Units* (*IUs*). One IU was defined as 0.3 mcg of retinol (the most common type of preformed Vitamin A) or 0.6 mcg of beta carotene. After 1980, the measurement unit for Vitamin A was changed. International Units didn't take into account the difference in absorption between preformed Vitamin A and beta carotene. About 80 percent of the preformed Vitamin A you take in gets absorbed into your body; but only about 40 percent of the beta carotene does, so you need more beta carotene to make the same amount of Vitamin A. After much deliberation (the idea was first proposed in 1967), the measurement unit was changed to give a more accurate idea of how much Vitamin A is really in a food or supplement. The new unit was called a *Retinol Equivalent* (*RE*). In 2001, the Retinol Equivalent measurement was changed to the more accurate term Retinol Activity Equivalent (RAE). One mcg of preformed Vitamin A in the form of retinol equals one Retinol Activity Equivalent. You need 12 mcg of beta carotene to make one RAE; you need 24 mcg of alpha carotene to make one RAE.

def•i•ni•tion

Two ways to measure Vitamin A are currently in use: **International Units** (**IU**) and **Retinol Activity Equivalents** (**RAE**). One IU equals 0.3 mcg of Vitamin A in the form of retinol or 0.6 mcg of beta carotene. One RAE equals 1 mcg of retinol or 12 mcg of beta carotene. IUs continue to be used as a standard measurement on vitamin labels, but researchers today prefer the more accurate RAE.

Are you with us so far? There's one more complicating fact: most vitamin manufacturers still list the Vitamin A and beta carotene content on the label in IUs. To convert from IUs to RAEs, divide by 3.3 (in other words, 2,640 IUs is equal to 800 RAEs). To help you figure out what's in your vitamins, we list the amounts in the RDA charts in both RAEs and IUs.

The RDA for Vitamin A

Age/Sex	RAE	IU
Infants		
0 to 6 months	400	1,300
7 to 12 months	500	1,700
Children		
1 to 3 years	300	1,000
4 to 6	400	1,300
7 to 8	500	1,650
9 to 13	600	1,200
Adults		
Men 14+ years	900	3,000
Women 14+	700	2,300
Pregnant women	770	2,600
Nursing women	1,300	4,300

Vitamin A is an essential nutrient, so it's got an established RDA. Beta carotene, although it's certainly important, isn't considered essential, so it doesn't have an RDA. How can you decide how much to take? The U.S. Department of Agriculture and the National Cancer Institute suggest a daily dose of 6 mg, but many nutritionists feel this is too low. Some think you should take as much as 30 mg a day. A good compromise might be 15 mg a day—roughly the equivalent of 16,500 IU (5,000 RAE) of Vitamin A. That's about six times the RDA for Vitamin A, but without the toxic side effects.

Studies show that most people get the RDA for Vitamin A every day, but only a few get anywhere near the suggested 6 mg of beta carotene. Most people eat only about 1.5 mg of beta carotene daily. On an average day, only about 20 percent of the population eat any fruits and vegetables rich in beta carotene.

Vitamin A Cautions

Taking supplements that contain the RDA for Vitamin A is generally safe for everyone, but use caution. Vitamin A in large doses can be toxic, causing a condition called *hypervitaminosis A*. Symptoms of A overload include blurred vision, bone pain, headaches, diarrhea, loss of appetite, skin scaling and peeling, and muscular weakness.

Vitamin A toxicity doesn't usually occur until you've been taking really large doses (more than 25,000 IU daily) for a long time, but don't take any chances—stick to the RDA.

Babies and children can reach toxic Vitamin A levels at much smaller doses. Most multi-vitamin supplements contain only the RDA, but some contain more. Read labels carefully and talk to your doctor before giving vitamins to babies and children. Fortunately, most symptoms of Vitamin A toxicity gradually go away without lasting damage when you stop taking it.

Be very careful about Vitamin A supplements if you are or might become pregnant. Too much Vitamin A (more than 3,000 IU or 1,000 RAE) can cause birth defects, especially if taken in the first seven weeks of pregnancy—when you might not even realize you're pregnant. Today many doctors suggest that women of childbearing age take beta carotene instead of Vitamin A supplements.

> **Warning**
>
> Excess Vitamin A during pregnancy can cause birth defects! If you are a woman of childbearing age, talk to your doctor about taking beta carotene supplements instead of Vitamin A.
>
> Vitamin A can cause serious problems for people with kidney disease. If you have kidney disease, talk to your doctor about taking Vitamin A or beta carotene supplements.

Beta Carotene Cautions

There's an easy way to avoid any possible problems from taking Vitamin A supplements: take beta carotene supplements instead. You'll safely get all the Vitamin A you need, along with the bonus of powerful antioxidant protection. It's almost impossible to take too much beta carotene. If you do, the only side effect is that you might turn yellow. Extra beta carotene builds up in the fat under your skin, giving your fat an orange-yellow color that shows through your skin—technically, *hypercarotenodermia*. You may look a little odd, but the color is harmless and goes away in a few weeks when you cut back your dosage.

Carotenes and CARET

In 1996 a major study that was supposed to prove the positive effects of beta carotene against lung cancer turned out to suggest just the opposite. The Beta Carotene and Retinol Efficacy Trial (better known as CARET) studied the effects of beta carotene and Vitamin A supplements on people who had been or still were heavy smokers. The researchers expected that the people who took the supplements would have lower rates of lung cancer. In fact, they ended up with higher rates. The researchers were so upset by the results that they stopped the study nearly two years early.

Does all this mean that the excitement about beta carotene is just so much hype? Not at all—numerous other studies show over and over that people with high beta carotene levels are generally healthier. The one thing the CARET study suggests for sure is that people who smoke shouldn't take beta carotene supplements. As we'll discuss later in this chapter, there are a lot of other studies showing the benefits of beta carotene.

Are You Deficient?

Generally speaking, a real Vitamin A deficiency is rare in the Western world because so many common foods, including milk and breakfast cereals, are fortified with it.

Almost everyone gets the RDA or pretty close to it, but some people are at high risk of a Vitamin A deficiency. If you fall into any of these categories, you may need more Vitamin A than you're actually getting:

- **You're a strict vegetarian or vegan.** Be sure to eat plenty of orange and dark-green vegetables.

- **You have liver disease, cystic fibrosis, or chronic diarrhea.** These problems can reduce the amount of Vitamin A you absorb or store.

- **You abuse alcohol.** Alcohol reduces the Vitamin A and beta carotene stored in your liver. In addition, animal studies suggest that beta carotene combined with alcohol is a one-two punch that could do a lot of damage to your liver.

- **You smoke.** People who smoke cigarettes have low beta carotene levels. But if you smoke, don't take beta carotene or Vitamin A supplements—they could do more harm than good. Talk to your doctor about vitamin supplements and how to get help with quitting smoking.

- **You take birth-control pills.** The Pill raises the amount of Vitamin A in your blood but reduces the amount you store in your liver. (This doesn't happen with beta carotene.)

- **You're sick or have a chronic infection.** Being sick makes you produce extra free radicals, which lowers your Vitamin A level.

◆ **You're under a great deal of stress—physical or psychological.** Overwork, fatigue, and too much exercise all create free radicals, which lower your Vitamin A level. Also, when you're too busy or tired to eat right, you don't get enough beta carotene.

◆ **You're pregnant or breastfeeding.** You're passing a lot of your Vitamin A on to your baby. You need some extra for yourself—but talk to your doctor first. Too much Vitamin A during pregnancy can cause birth defects.

◆ **You take a bile-sequestering drug such as Colestid, Locholest, Questran, or Welchol to lower your cholesterol.** These drugs can keep you from absorbing fat-soluble vitamins such as Vitamin A correctly. If you take these drugs, your doctor will probably recommend vitamin supplements and tell you to take them at a different time than the medicine. Discuss any other supplements with your doctor before you try them.

◆ **You take the drug methotrexate (known as Rheumatrex or Trexall) to treat arthritis, psoriasis, or cancer.** This drug affects your intestines, making it harder to absorb Vitamin A and beta carotene. Discuss supplements with your doctor before you try them.

After several weeks without much Vitamin A in your diet, you'd start to have some signs of deficiency. One of the earliest is night blindness and other eye problems (we'll talk about these later). Another sign of Vitamin A deficiency is a condition called *follicular hyperkeratosis*. When this happens, your epithelial tissues, especially your skin, start to make too much of a hard protein called keratin. You start to get little deposits of keratin that look like goosebumps around your hair follicles and your skin feels rough and dry. Vitamin A deficiency can also cause reproductive problems for both men and women. A shortage of Vitamin A can also make you more likely to get respiratory infections, sore throats, sinus infections, and ear infections.

Eating Your As

The RDA assumes that you'll be getting most of your Vitamin A from animal sources such as eggs, liver, poultry, milk, and dairy products. That's a pretty good assumption, because most people don't eat that many fruits and vegetables and don't get much beta carotene from their diet. Animal foods that are high in Vitamin A, however, also tend to be high in calories and cholesterol.

Nutritionists today strongly recommend getting your As the beta carotene way, through five daily servings of fresh fruits and vegetables. One medium carrot contains more than 8,000 IU of beta carotene—with no toxic side effects, no fat, and only 35 calories. Plus, you'll be getting the antioxidant protection carotenes provide. How many of these foods do you regularly eat?

The Vitamin A in Food

Food Equivalent	Amount	Vitamin A in Retinol Activity
American cheese	1 oz.	82
Beef liver	3 oz.	9,000
Butter	1 tsp.	35
Cheddar cheese	1 oz.	86
Chicken leg, with skin	1	45
Chicken liver	3½ oz.	4,913
Egg	1 large	97
Ice cream, vanilla	1 cup	133
Milk, skim	1 cup	149
Salmon	3 oz.	11
Sole	3 oz.	10
Swiss cheese	1 oz.	72
Swordfish	3 oz.	35
Yogurt, low-fat	8 oz.	36

The old saying "Have a lot of color on your plate" is the best advice for eating your carotenes. Remember, carotenes are the substances that give foods such as carrots, tomatoes, sweet potatoes, and apricots their vivid color. Actually, carotenes are found in practically all vegetables and fruits, including dark-green, leafy vegetables such as spinach and broccoli. The carotenes are there—you just can't see the bright reddish colors because they're disguised by the green.

Traditional food tables from standard sources treat beta carotene and Vitamin A as if they were interchangeable. The beta carotene contents of plant foods vary quite a bit, even within the same food. Farmers grow different carrot varieties, for example, depending on which kind does best on their land. Any listing of beta carotene content is approximate. In general, though, the listings are accurate enough to give you a good idea of how much beta carotene is in the foods you eat. Check the beta carotene content in your favorite fruits and veggies.

The Beta Carotene in Food

Food	Amount	Beta Carotene in IU
Apple	1	120
Apricots, fresh	3	2,890
Asparagus, cooked	1 cup	1,220
Banana	1	230
Beet greens	½ cup	3,700
Broccoli, cooked	½ cup	1,940
Brussels sprouts	½ cup	405
Cabbage	½ cup	90
Cantaloupe	1 cup	2,720
Carrot, raw	1 medium	8,100
Cauliflower	1 cup	80
Collard greens, cooked	½ cup	7,410
Corn kernels	½ cup	330
Grapefruit	½ medium	80
Green beans, cooked	½ cup	340
Kale, cooked	½ cup	4,560
Orange	1 medium	400
Peach	1 large	2,030
Peas	½ cup	430
Pepper, green	½ cup	210
Pepper, sweet red	½ cup	2,225
Prunes, stewed	½ cup	1,065
Spinach, cooked	½ cup	7,290
Squash, winter	½ cup	6,560
Sweet potato, cooked	1 medium	9,230
Tomato	1 medium	1,110
Tomato juice	6 oz.	1,460
Turnip greens, cooked	½ cup	4,570
Watermelon, cubed	1 cup	940
Zucchini	½ cup	270

Now You're Cooking

Cooking destroys some of the carotenes in vegetables, but also releases others by breaking down tough cell membranes. On the whole, you absorb more carotenes from cooked veggies. But don't overdo it, or you'll lose the other vitamins in the vegetables. Cook vegetables lightly in as little water as possible—steaming or stir-frying is a great way to preserve nutrients. Baking or grilling also gently releases the beta carotene.

Getting the Most from Vitamin A and Carotenes

Vitamin A and beta carotene are fat-soluble, which means you store them in your liver and in the fatty tissues of your body. To avoid any chance of a toxic buildup, we suggest you stick to the Vitamin A in your daily multivitamin supplement and skip any additional A supplements.

But if you're having one of those frantic days where eating right is way down on your priority list, taking a mixed carotenoid supplement can help make up for that skipped breakfast, fast-food lunch, and takeout dinner. These supplements contain beta carotene, lycopene, lutein, and other carotenoids. (We'll talk about these more when we get to Chapter 25.)

To get the most out of your Vitamin A and beta carotene, be sure to also get at least the RDA for Vitamin E, zinc, and selenium. You need Vitamin E to help Vitamin A work more effectively; you also need extra Vitamin E if you take large doses (more than 15 g daily) of beta carotene supplements (see Chapter 15 for more information on Vitamin E). You need zinc to help transport Vitamin A around your body, and you need selenium to help beta carotene work more effectively (see Chapter 21 for more information on zinc and selenium).

Thumbs Up/Thumbs Down

Vitamin A and Beta Carotene Work Better If You Also Take ...	
All other vitamins and minerals	Selenium
Vitamin E	Zinc

Vitamin A and Beta Carotene Are Blocked By ...	
Alcohol	Cigarette smoke
Birth-control pills	Methotrexate, a drug used to treat arthritis, psoriasis, and cancer
Bile-sequestering cholesterol drugs	

Which Type Should I Take?

Vitamin A supplements usually come in soft gelcaps in retinyl acetate or retinyl palmitate form. Either is fine, but retinyl palmitate is best for people with intestinal problems. An old-fashioned way to get your As is by taking cod-liver oil. Aside from the fact that it's truly horrible tasting—even the cherry-flavored kind is awful—cod-liver oil isn't a good choice. It's high in calories and often causes digestive upsets. Don't overdo it on the Vitamin A supplements—more than 3,300 IU (1,000 RAE) a day can be harmful. To avoid possible problems, we suggest taking mixed carotenes instead—you'll get your As along with extra antioxidant protection.

Today most Vitamin A supplements actually contain only beta carotene or a mixture of half beta carotene and half retinyl acetate or retinyl palmitate. The beta carotene generally comes from palm oil or vegetable sources; some supplements are made from a type of algae called *Dunaliella salina*. You can also purchase supplements that contain mixed carotenoids, including beta carotene, alpha carotene, and others. Which form is best? We suggest mixed carotenoids, because that way you'll be getting the potential benefits of them all—and avoiding any potential problems from too much Vitamin A. To be sure you're getting a good product, choose mixed carotenoids that contain beta carotene along with at least 20 percent alpha carotene and also xanthophylls and lycopene. No matter which form you buy, store it away from light.

Bugs Bunny Had Great Eyesight

Elmer Fudd never catches that pesky wabbit because Bugs always sees him coming. Why does Bugs have such great eyesight? It's all those carrots. What's good for Bugs is good for you, too. Vitamin A and beta carotene are essential for your eyesight. The following sections discuss three reasons why.

Quack, Quack
Some manufacturers offer micellized or emulsified Vitamin A, which means the Vitamin A is broken up into very tiny droplets. The manufacturers claim that this improves absorption. In fact, you absorb about 80 to 90 percent of plain old Vitamin A. If you buy the micellized or emulsified brands, you'll be spending a lot more, but you won't really be absorbing much more.

Preventing Night Blindness

Vitamin A helps you see well in the dark. Your retina (the layer of light-sensitive cells at the back of your eye) contains large amounts of Vitamin A, especially in the tiny structures called rods that are used for night vision. If you don't get enough Vitamin A, you develop night blindness—you can't see well in the dark or in dim light. We all lose a little of our night vision as we grow older, but Vitamin A can help slow or even prevent the loss. If you've noticed that you don't see as well at night as you used to, see your eye doctor to rule out other eye problems. If your eyes are okay otherwise, extra Vitamin A or beta carotene might help. Discuss the right amount with your doctor before you try it.

Preventing Cataracts

A cataract forms when the lens of your eye becomes cloudy, reducing or even completely blocking the amount of light that enters your eye. At one time, cataracts were a leading cause of blindness, but today simple outpatient surgery can fix the problem. But wouldn't it be better if a cataract never developed in the first place? There's solid evidence that a diet rich in carotenoids, especially beta carotene, helps prevent cataracts by mopping up free radicals before they can damage the lens.

Preserving Eyesight

Vitamin A helps prevent age-related macular degeneration (AMD). Your macula is a tiny cluster of very sensitive cells in the center of your retina. It's essential for sharp vision. As you grow older, your macula may start to degenerate, causing vision loss and eventual blindness. AMD is the leading cause of blindness in people older than 65, and about 30 percent of Americans aged 75 or older suffer from it. What about the other 70 percent? It's likely they eat more foods that are high in beta carotene. According to one study, eating just one serving a day of a food high in beta carotene could reduce your chances of AMD by 40 percent. Helpful as beta carotene is for preventing AMD, other carotenoids such as lutein and zeaxanthin are even better—we'll talk about them more in Chapter 25.

Warning!

Millions of grateful teenagers treat their severe acne with prescription drugs such as Accutane (isotretinoin) and Retin-A (tretinoin), which are derived from Vitamin A. Another drug, Tegison (etretinate), helps severe psoriasis. Taking large doses of Vitamin A will not have the same effect as taking these drugs! Large doses of Vitamin A are toxic!

A as in Aging Skin

The cells of your skin grow very rapidly—your outer skin turns over completely in about four weeks. All rapidly growing cells, including those in your skin, need plenty of Vitamin A. An early symptom of Vitamin A deficiency is skin that is rough, dry, and scaly. To help keep your skin smooth and supple, make sure to get the RDA for Vitamin A. This is especially important as you get older and your risk of skin cancer rises. One recent study shows that taking Vitamin A could cut your chances of getting basal cell carcinoma, the most common type of skin cancer, by 70 percent.

Down to the Bones

Too much Vitamin A—but not beta carotene—can interfere with the formation of new bone and could increase your risk of a fracture. In 2002, researchers published results from the long-running Nurses' Health Study suggesting that older women who took large doses of supplemental Vitamin A (at least 3,000 mg, which is the upper limit considered safe by the Institute of Medicine) were at higher risk of hip fracture. In 2003, a study in Sweden found that men aged 49 to 51 with high levels of Vitamin A in their blood were more likely to break a bone than men with lower levels. Again, there was no link between blood levels of beta carotene and fracture risk. What these studies tell us is that the best way to be sure you're getting enough Vitamin A is to get it in the form of beta carotene, preferably from your diet.

To Beta or Not to Beta ...

... that is the cancer question. There's a lot of controversy about beta carotene and cancer. Does it prevent cancer or not? Yes—or maybe not. Let's try to sort out the issues here.

Study after study shows that if you have a high beta carotene level because you eat a lot of foods that contain carotenoids, you're less likely to get cancer. In one important study, for example, 8,000 men were followed for 5 years. The ones who had the lowest intake of beta carotene had the highest risk of lung cancer. A 1999 study of Swedish women reported that those who ate the most beta carotene foods over the longest time had the lowest risk of breast cancer. A 2005 study of nearly 60,000 French women found that among those who had never smoked, a diet containing moderate amounts of beta carotene cut their risk of tobacco-related cancer (from second-hand smoke) by up to 28 percent. The women who took beta carotene supplements cut their risk by 56 percent.

Almost all researchers today agree that beta carotene *foods* play a major role in preventing cancer, especially cancer of the lung, stomach, prostate, and cervix. The real question is, do beta carotene *supplements* prevent cancer? Here's where the evidence is growing that they don't.

Three important studies come down hard against beta carotene supplements: the CARET study we talked about earlier, the Alpha-tocopherol Beta-carotene Cancer Prevention Study Group (the ABC study), and the Physicians' Health Study. As with the CARET study, the ABC study found that people taking beta carotene supplements had an *increased* risk of lung cancer. The Physicians' Health Study has had some mixed results. Initially the researchers reported that beta carotene supplements had no effect on cancer or heart disease rates. But in 1997, they reported that participants who took beta carotene supplements had a reduced risk of prostate cancer. So what do these studies prove? Only that beta carotene supplements may have a bad effect on people who are already at high risk for lung cancer. The people in the CARET and ABC studies all smoked cigarettes and drank alcohol. Among the people in the Physicians' Health Study, about 11 percent were smokers. In the bigger picture, the studies suggest two things. First, beta carotene supplements alone can't overcome a lifetime of smoking, drinking, and eating a diet low in the valuable nutrients found in fruits and vegetables. Second, people who eat foods high in beta carotene are also eating lots of other carotenoids—and you need a range of carotenoids, not just beta carotene, to help ward off cancer.

Colorectal Cancer

The ABC study we mentioned in the previous section also found that for people who smoke, drink alcohol, or do both, beta carotene supplements increased the risk of colorectal cancer. But in 2003, results from the Antioxidant Polyp Prevention Study (APPS) showed that if you don't smoke or drink, taking beta carotene supplements could reduce your risk of colon cancer. The 864 participants in the APPS study all had previous adenomas, benign polyps that can lead to colorectal cancer. They took a variety of antioxidants, including Vitamin C and beta carotene, to see if they would prevent tumor recurrence. The nonsmoking, nondrinking beta carotene group reduced their risk of polyp recurrence by 44 percent; the smoking group saw their risk increase by 36 percent.

Preventing Prostate Cancer

Every year more than 300,000 men are diagnosed with prostate cancer; it's the second-leading cause of cancer death in men. Given those scary statistics, let's look more closely at how beta carotene can help.

In 1997, results from the ongoing Physicians' Health Study at Harvard University showed that beta carotene supplements can sharply reduce the risk of prostate cancer among men who have low levels of beta carotene in their blood. The 22,000 men in the study were divided into two groups: half got a placebo and half took 50 mg of beta carotene every other day. Their blood levels of beta carotene were measured at the start of the study. Over the next 12 years, the doctors with the lowest levels of beta carotene, presumably because they didn't eat many fruits or vegetables, were one third more likely to develop prostate cancer. But among that group, the ones who took beta carotene supplements were 36 percent less likely to develop prostate cancer. The supplements made up for the lack of beta carotene in their diets.

Warning!

If you smoke, don't take beta carotene or Vitamin A supplements!

Researchers have focused on beta carotene because it's easy to measure in your blood, but perhaps now it's time to look further. In the meantime, get your beta carotene from your food whenever possible. If you want to take supplements, take mixed carotenoids, not beta carotene alone.

Carotenes and Cardiac Cases

As with cancer, so with heart disease: people who eat foods high in beta carotene definitely have fewer heart attacks and strokes. In one major study of women nurses, for example, the ones who ate the most beta carotene foods had 22 percent fewer heart attacks than those who ate the least. The biggest beta carotene eaters did even better when it came to strokes—they had 40 percent fewer. A study of older adults showed that the higher their beta carotene intake from food, the lower their risk of a heart attack. Again, though, just taking beta carotene supplements doesn't necessarily give you the same protection. In the Physicians' Health Study, for example, people who took beta carotene supplements didn't really have any less heart disease than people who didn't. The message? You need *all* the carotenoids, not just beta carotene. The best way to get them all is to eat plenty of fruits and vegetables. If you want to take supplements, take mixed carotenoids.

Dodging Diabetes

Can carotenes help prevent Type 2 diabetes? Maybe—the evidence is mixed. On the one hand, those cooperative doctors from the Physicians' Health Study didn't show any decrease in their risk of Type 2 diabetes from taking beta carotene supplements. On the other hand, several smaller recent studies show that people with high levels of carotenoids from their diet do have a lower risk of diabetes, and that people with prediabetes and diabetes tend to have lower levels. The problem is it's hard to know which comes first—the low levels or the diabetes. What we can say is that carotenoid levels in the blood are a marker of fruit and vegetable consumption. The lower your levels, the poorer your diet—and a poor diet low in fruits and veggies is a major risk factor for diabetes. Eating better helps lower your risk while almost automatically raising your carotenoid levels.

Boosting Your Immunity with Vitamin A

The anti-infective powers of Vitamin A have been known ever since the vitamin was discovered. Today Vitamin A is being used to help boost immunity in some cases—and some very exciting research suggests more uses in the future. Here's the current rundown:

   ◆ **Treating measles and respiratory infections.** Extra Vitamin A has been shown to help children get over the measles faster and with fewer complications. It also seems to help babies with respiratory infections. Talk to your doctor before you give Vitamin A supplements to babies or children.

   ◆ **Treating viral infections.** If you're low on Vitamin A, you're more susceptible to illness, especially viral infections. If you're sick with a virus, extra Vitamin A in the form of beta carotene could help you fight it off.

   ◆ **Boosting immune cells.** Large doses of beta carotene may help increase the number of infection-fighting cells in your immune system. This could be very beneficial for AIDS patients and anyone whose immune system is depressed.

Research continues on the benefits of Vitamin A and beta carotene for your immune system. We believe that the future will bring solid evidence that these nutrients can help not only immunity, but many other health problems as well.

The Least You Need to Know

◆ You need Vitamin A for healthy eyes, cell growth, and a strong immune system.

◆ Your body converts the beta carotene found in many fruits and vegetables into Vitamin A as needed.

◆ Beta carotene is also a powerful antioxidant that can help protect you against cancer and heart disease.

◆ The adult RDA for Vitamin A is between 700 and 3,000 RAE (2,300–3,000 IU). There is no RDA for beta carotene, but 15 mg is often recommended.

◆ Vitamin A can be toxic in large amounts—don't exceed the RDA. Beta carotene is safe even in very large doses.

◆ Foods high in Vitamin A include eggs, milk, liver, and meat.

◆ Foods high in beta carotene include orange, yellow, and red fruits and vegetables such as cantaloupes, tomatoes, carrots, and butternut squash. Potatoes and dark-green, leafy vegetables are also high in beta carotene.

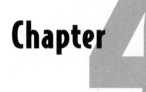

Meet the B Family

In This Chapter

◆ Why you need the entire B family of vitamins

◆ What the B vitamin foods are

◆ How to choose the right supplements

◆ How the B family protects your heart, gives you energy, boosts your immune system, and keeps you mentally alert

What big brood of vitamins is basic for keeping your brains, your blood, and a broad bunch of body functions in balance? Are you baffled? It's the B complex—that bunch of vitamins with the little numbers underneath and the weird names.

The B family members pull together to keep you healthy. You need each and every one of them—two doses of B_6 don't equal one of B_{12}. The range of jobs the Bs do is pretty amazing. You need all the Bs to help your cells grow and reproduce properly. You also need them all to send messages back and forth from your brain along your nerves. Another big chore done by most of the Bs is helping you produce energy by breaking down the foods you eat into fuel your body can use. And we're just starting to realize that three different Bs—folic acid, cobalamin, and pyridoxine—work together to do another very important job: keep your heart healthy. On their own, each

B vitamin also has special jobs to do, such as keeping your red blood cells healthy and preventing birth defects.

One Big Happy Family

The vitamins in the B family are all closely related. You could think of them as eight siblings and four cousins. We'll discuss all the siblings in later chapters, but for now, here are the main branches of the family tree:

- **Thiamin, or Vitamin B_1.** You need thiamin to keep all your body's cells, but especially your nerves, working right. Thiamin is important for mental functions, especially memory. You also need it to convert food to energy.

- **Riboflavin, or Vitamin B_2.** Riboflavin is really important for releasing energy from food. It's also vital for normal growth and development, for normal red blood cells, and for making many of your body's hormones.

- **Niacin, or Vitamin B_3.** More than 50 body processes, from releasing energy from food to making hormones to detoxifying chemicals, depend on niacin.

- **Pantothenic acid, or Vitamin B_5.** This vitamin works closely with several of the other Bs in the breakdown of fats, proteins, and carbohydrates into energy. You also need it to make Vitamin D, some hormones, and red blood cells.

- **Pyridoxine, or Vitamin B_6.** The main job of pyridoxine is shuffling around your amino acids to make the 50,000-plus proteins your body needs to run properly. It's also involved in making more than 60 different enzymes.

- **Biotin, or Vitamin B_7.** Biotin is needed for a lot of body processes that break down fats, proteins, and carbohydrates into fuel you can use. Biotin is sometimes called Vitamin H.

- **Folic acid, or Vitamin B_9.** The main job for folic acid is helping your cells grow and divide properly—it's important for preventing birth defects. You also need it for making the natural chemicals that control your mood, your appetite, and how well you sleep. And folic acid is vital for keeping your arteries open and lowering your chances of a heart attack or stroke.

- **Cobalamin, or Vitamin B_{12}.** You need cobalamin to process the carbohydrates, proteins, and fats in your food into energy. It also forms the protective covering of your nerve cells, keeps your red blood cells healthy, and helps prevent heart disease.

When you have plenty of all the Bs in your body, they work together to keep your body running efficiently, producing the energy and the many complicated chemicals your body needs to function normally. But just as no one but Aunt Rose can make her famous potato salad, and just as it wouldn't be a family barbecue without it, each member of the B family has its own essential role to play. You need them all—if you're low on any one B vitamin, the others can't do their jobs.

What the Little Numbers Mean

Why do most of the B vitamins have those little numbers underneath? And what happened to B_4, B_8, B_{10}, and B_{11}? The first B vitamin to be discovered was called water-soluble B. That meant only that it was the second vitamin ever identified (the first was fat-soluble A). Riboflavin was discovered next, so water-soluble B became B_1 and riboflavin became B_2. The system began to get confusing in 1926, when researchers realized that Vitamin B_1 was actually two vitamins, thiamin and niacin. Thiamin kept the B_1 name. B_2 was already taken, so niacin got B_3. As vitamin research continued, scientists found a number of substances they thought at first were new B vitamins. Some turned out to be the same as Bs that had already been discovered, while others turned out not to be vitamins at all. These phantom Bs are the missing numbers. To avoid confusion, scientists now prefer to use the B vitamin names instead of the numbers.

The Bs at a Glance

B Vitamin	Function
Thiamin (Vitamin B_1)	Helps regulate nerve growth, mental functions, and memory. Helps convert food to energy.
Riboflavin (Vitamin B_2)	Releases energy, aids in growth and development; needed for normal red blood cells and hormones.
Niacin (Vitamin B_3)	Needed for more than 50 body processes. Releases energy, makes hormones, removes toxins, and helps keep cholesterol normal.
Pantothenic acid (Vitamin B_5)	Releases energy from food. Necessary to make Vitamin D, hormones, and red blood cells.
Pyridoxine (Vitamin B_6)	Needed to make proteins, hormones, and enzymes. Helps prevent heart disease.
Biotin (Vitamin B_7)	Releases energy from food.
Folic acid (Vitamin B_9)	Aids cell growth and division. Prevents birth defects and heart disease.
Cobalamin (Vitamin B_{12})	Releases energy from food. Necessary for healthy red blood cells. Helps prevent heart disease.

The B Minors

The four cousins of the main B family are sometimes called the "unofficial" B vitamins because they're important for your health but don't have RDAs. Choline has an Adequate Intake, but the others don't because technically they're not vitamins—you make them in your body from other substances. We'll talk more about choline, inositol, and PABA in Chapter 12. We'll also talk a lot about lipoic acid in Chapter 24. For now, these are the twigs that come off the main B branch:

- ◆ **Choline.** Your brain uses choline to help store memories. It's also sometimes helpful for treating depression and may be useful for treating hepatitis.

- ◆ **Inositol.** You need inositol to make healthy cell membranes and messenger chemicals. It's also sometimes helpful for relieving nerve damage from diabetes.

- ◆ **PABA.** The initials stand for Para-aminobenzoic acid. This powerful antioxidant protects your skin from sun damage and is found in many sunscreen lotions and creams.

- ◆ **Lipoic acid.** A helper for the B vitamins, lipoic acid works closely with thiamin, riboflavin, niacin, and pantothenic acid to convert carbohydrates, fats, and proteins in your food into energy. Lipoic acid is also a powerful antioxidant and helps recycle Vitamins C and E.

DRIs for B Vitamins

The DRIs for the B vitamins are a little controversial these days. That's because several of the RDAs, which are one part of the DRIs, were lowered in the 1989 recommendations and then changed again in the new DRIs issued in 1998. At that time, the amount for folic acid was raised a little and some of the other B recommendations were increased a touch. Overall, however, the new RDAs within the DRIs were a disappointment to the many nutritionists and researchers who believe that higher amounts of all the Bs, but especially of folic acid, could do a lot to improve everyone's health. Also, many doctors are starting to realize that their older patients show subtle signs of B vitamin deficiencies, even though they're getting the RDA. Another major role for the Bs is cell growth and division. Growing children and teens need plenty of Bs, and their needs go up as they enter their young-adult years. Women who are pregnant or breastfeeding also need extra Bs because they are passing a lot of their vitamins on to their babies.

We'll discuss the latest RDAs further when we get to each B in the upcoming chapters. In the meantime, check out the charts to see the RDAs for the six major B vitamins and the Adequate Intakes for choline, biotin, and pantothenic acid.

RDAs for the B Vitamins

Age in Years/Sex	Thiamin	Riboflavin	Niacin	Pyridoxine	Folic Acid	Cobalamin
Infants						
0 to 0.5	0.2 mg	0.3 mg	2.0 mg	0.1 mg	65 mcg	0.4 mcg
0.5 to 1	0.3 mg	0.4 mg	4.0 mg	0.3 mg	80 mcg	0.5 mcg
Children						
1 to 3	0.5 mg	0.5 mg	6.0 mg	0.5 mg	150 mcg	0.9 mcg
4 to 8	0.6 mg	0.6 mg	8.0 mg	0.6 mg	200 mcg	1.2 mcg
9 to 13	0.9 mg	0.9 mg	12.0 mg	1.0 mg	300 mcg	1.8 mcg
Men						
14 to 18	1.2 mg	1.3 mg	16.0 mg	1.3 mg	400 mcg	2.4 mcg
19 to 30	1.2 mg	1.3 mg	16.0 mg	1.3 mg	400 mcg	2.4 mcg
31 to 50	1.2 mg	1.3 mg	16.0 mg	1.3 mg	400 mcg	2.4 mcg
50+	1.2 mg	1.3 mg	16.0 mg	1.7 mg	400 mcg	2.4 mcg
Women						
14 to 18	1.0 mg	1.0 mg	14.0 mg	1.2 mg	400 mcg	2.4 mcg
19 to 30	1.1 mg	1.1 mg	14.0 mg	1.3 mg	400 mcg	2.4 mcg
31 to 50	1.1 mg	1.1 mg	14.0 mg	1.3 mg	400 mcg	2.4 mcg
50+	1.1 mg	1.1 mg	14.0 mg	1.5 mg	400 mcg	2.4 mcg
Pregnant	1.4 mg	1.4 mg	18.0 mg	1.9 mg	600 mcg	2.6 mcg
Nursing	1.4 mg	1.6 mg	17.0 mg	2.0 mg	500 mcg	2.8 mcg

Three B vitamins—choline, pantothenic acid, and biotin—work closely with the other Bs to help convert your food into energy. Pantothenic acid is also needed for making Vitamin D and normal red blood cells. Because choline, pantothenic acid, and biotin are found so widely in foods, nobody is ever deficient. For that reason, these vitamins don't have RDAs—instead, researchers have figured out Adequate Intakes.

Adequate Intakes for Choline, Biotin, and Pantothenic Acid

Age in Years/Sex	Choline	Pantothenic Acid	Biotin
Infants			
0 to 0.5	125 mg	1.7 mg	5 mcg
0.5 to 1	150 mg	1.8 mg	6 mcg
Children			
1 to 3	200 mg	2 mg	8 mcg
4 to 8	250 mg	3 mg	12 mcg
9 to 13	375 mg	4 mg	20 mcg
Men			
14 to 18	550 mg	5 mg	25 mcg
19+	550 mg	5 mg	30 mcg
Women			
14 to 18	400 mg	5 mg	25 mcg
19+	425 mg	5 mg	30 mcg
Pregnant	450 mg	6 mg	30 mcg
Nursing	550 mg	7 mg	35 mcg

Are You Deficient?

The B vitamins are found in many different foods; they're also added to a lot of foods such as bread and breakfast cereals. Almost everybody gets enough to cover the RDA and then some. If your diet is poor or you have a digestive problem, though, you might be deficient in Bs. Some people are especially at risk, such as the following:

- **Alcohol abusers.** Alcohol blocks your ability to absorb B vitamins and also makes you excrete them faster. Alcoholics are most likely to be deficient in thiamin, riboflavin, pyridoxine, and folic acid.

- **The elderly.** You absorb less of some of the Bs as you age. Also, elderly people who live alone or in nursing homes often don't eat properly and don't get enough Bs from their food.

- **Smokers.** Tobacco smoke decreases your absorption of B vitamins across the board.

- **People with chronic digestive problems.** These people may not be absorbing enough B vitamins through their intestines.

- **People on strict diets.** Vegetarians and vegans (vegetarians who don't eat any animal foods such as milk or eggs) may not get enough B vitamins. Vegetarian children and people following macrobiotic diets are especially at risk.

The B vitamins all pull together to do the larger jobs of producing energy, making body chemicals such as hormones, and controlling how your cells grow and divide. When it comes to releasing energy, for example, niacin, riboflavin, folic acid, pantothenic acid, and biotin all work together. A shortage of any one of these Bs can throw off the entire process. And because the Bs are found in many of the same foods, if you're deficient in one you're likely to be deficient in the others, too. Because the Bs work together so often, sometimes a shortage of one covers up a shortage of another. A good example is that a shortage of folic acid can mask a shortage of cobalamin. Other vitamin shortages also affect your B levels. If you're low on Vitamin C, you're probably also low on folic acid—and vice versa.

Eating Your Bs

Some or all of the B vitamins are found in just about every food you're likely to eat: milk, meat, fish, oranges, peanut butter, bread, breakfast cereal, eggs, yogurt, and a lot more. Here's a rundown of the best foods for each B:

- **Thiamin:** Pork, liver, fish, oranges, peas, peanut butter, wheat germ, beans, and whole grains.

- **Riboflavin:** Milk; dairy products; meat; beans; nuts; green, leafy vegetables; and avocados.

- **Niacin:** Meat, chicken, fish, beans, peas, peanut butter, milk, dairy products, and nuts.

- **Pantothenic acid:** Liver, meat, fish, chicken, whole grains, and beans.

- **Pyridoxine:** Meat, fish, chicken, peanuts, beans, peas, bananas, avocados, and potatoes.

- **Biotin:** Liver, oatmeal, eggs, peanut butter, milk, salmon, clams, and bananas.

- **Folic acid:** Dark-green, leafy vegetables; liver; orange juice; beans; avocados; and beets.

- **Cobalamin:** Meat, chicken, fish, milk, yogurt, cheese, and eggs.

Light can actually destroy some of the Bs, especially riboflavin. To preserve the Bs, store foods out of the light. Pyridoxine is easily destroyed by freezing. Use fresh meats and vegetables whenever you can.

Getting the Most from B Vitamins

The B vitamins are all water-soluble, which means that you need daily doses to keep your levels high. It also means that your body excretes what you don't absorb. For most of the Bs, there are no toxic effects even with very large doses—but there are two important exceptions:

Warning!

B vitamins can interfere with medicines for some conditions such as Parkinson's disease and epilepsy. If you take medicine for these or any other chronic condition, discuss B supplements with your doctor before you try them.

- **Niacin.** Large doses of niacin (more than 1,000 mg) in the form of nicotinic acid can give you a niacin "flush." The sensation is sort of like blushing badly: your face turns red and feels hot or tingly. The flush goes away fairly soon with no lasting harm. To avoid this problem, choose a no-flush product containing niacin in the form of inositol hexaniacinate. Super-large doses of niacin (more than 3 g a day) could cause liver problems. Three grams are thousands of times more than the RDA—few people would have any reason for taking so much.

- **Pyridoxine.** The one B vitamin that might do real damage in megadoses is pyridoxine. If you take more than 2,000 mg a day for a long time, you might get a tingling sensation in your neck and feet, lose coordination, and have permanent nerve damage. In a few cases, people who took 200 mg a day for a number of years also had these symptoms. The adult RDA for pyridoxine is only 1.0 to 2.0 mg a day, though, so you're not likely to have problems unless you take nearly a hundred times more than that.

Any good multivitamin supplement contains all the extra B vitamins you need. Pick one that has at least 400 mcg of folic acid (we'll tell you why in Chapter 9). You can also buy each B in separate supplements or in assorted combinations. In general, you don't need to bother with these if you take a good multivitamin every day. If you feel you need more Bs, look for a complete B formula to get them all. B-50 complex formulas generally contain 400 mcg of folic acid and 50 mg or mcg of all the other Bs. B-100 complex formulas generally have 400 mcg of folic acid and 100 mg or mcg of all the other Bs. If you have a cobalamin deficiency, your doctor will probably recommend shots every 2 weeks (see Chapter 10 to learn why).

Choline is found in most good multivitamins, but the amount is usually only 10 or 20 percent of the Adequate Intake (AI). To get more choline than that, you'll need to take a separate supplement—but there's virtually never any reason to. To get extra lipoic acid or inositol, you'll have to buy separate supplements. Lipoic acid supplements can be helpful for diabetics (see Chapter 24 for more information). Inositol supplements won't do anything for you—skip them.

The best use for PABA is in sunscreen products. It's available as a supplement, but we don't recommend it. As we'll explain in Chapter 12, PABA pills won't do anything positive for you and they could be harmful.

The Three Bs and Homocysteine

Homocysteine in your blood is a natural byproduct created by metabolizing the essential amino acid methionine. Three Bs—folic acid, pyridoxine, and cobalamin—break down homocysteine and remove it from the blood. Since the 1960s, researchers have known that there's a connection between homocysteine levels and levels of the three Bs; they've also known that people with high homocysteine levels are at greater risk of heart disease and stroke. What's been controversial ever since, however, is whether lowering homocysteine by taking more of the three Bs lowers the risk of heart disease and stroke.

A major study in the prestigious *New England Journal of Medicine* in 1995 showed that people with high blood levels of homocysteine were much more likely to have clogged arteries, which means they were more likely to have a heart attack. The people in the study with the highest B levels cut their risk of a heart attack *in half*. Two thirds of the people with dangerously high homocysteine had inadequate levels of the three vital Bs.

Since the 1995 study, there have been several more that point to the importance of B vitamins for lowering homocysteine levels to prevent not just heart attacks, but also strokes. On the other hand, studies in 2005 and 2006 suggest that while high homocysteine is connected to heart disease, it's not the cause—it may simply be a marker of something else instead, just as a fever is a marker for infection. Giving B vitamins to people at high risk of heart disease or stroke does lower their homocysteine level, but doesn't seem to help prevent heart attacks or strokes. We'll talk about all this in more detail in Chapter 9 because folic acid seems to be the most important of the three Bs that lower homocysteine.

Staying on the B-all

It's possible that lowering homocysteine levels with the same three Bs—folic acid, pyridoxine, and cobalamin—may help slow the progression of Alzheimer's disease (AD). People with AD are known to have higher homocysteine levels than people the same age without the disease. An encouraging preliminary study in 2006 from Georgetown University Medical Center's Memory Disorders Program showed that high doses of the three Bs safely lowered homocysteine in people with AD. The next phase of the study will look at whether lowering homocysteine helps slow the disease.

Boning Up with Bs

People who have had a stroke are two to four times more likely to fall and break a hip. A 2006 study in the *Journal of the American Medical Association* showed that older stroke patients who took folic acid and cobalamin supplements had a much lower rate of hip fractures. The reason is that the supplements lowered their homocysteine levels by 38 percent—enough to strengthen their bones and prevent fractures.

Niacin for High Cholesterol

In the days before statin drugs such as Lipitor, niacin was often recommended as a way to lower cholesterol. It's still used for that purpose—in fact, a prescription drug called Advicor contains both niacin and a statin drug called Lovastatin. We'll talk more about this in Chapter 7.

Aging and the B Vitamins

You may have noticed that your elderly grandmother has started to get a little forgetful and confused, even depressed. Well, you think, that's normal for someone who's in her 80s. But is it? Not necessarily. There are lots of medical problems that can make an elderly person seem senile, but bad nutrition can also play a big role—especially for someone who falls into the risk categories we talked about in Chapter 1.

Studies show that many elderly people are low in B vitamins, particularly cobalamin. Part of the reason is that as you age, you just don't absorb as many Bs from your food. Because some of the Bs aren't absorbed all that well in the first place, older people can easily start to be deficient. Then the deficiency makes them a little depressed, so they eat less and get even fewer Bs, which makes them more depressed or so forgetful that they eat even less, which makes them so forgetful, confused, and depressed that they end up in a nursing home. The food there might not help—institutional food often has most of its vitamins processed or cooked away.

Other studies show that a large number of elderly people have overall B vitamin shortages that affect their health and their mental abilities. For example, many elderly people are low on thiamin, folic acid, choline, and cobalamin. The statistics here are disturbing—about a third of the elderly are low on pyridoxine, and thiamin deficiency may affect nearly half of all elderly people sent to hospitals. B shortages in older people are enough to cause depression, confusion, and memory problems, even though the usual blood tests show normal levels. Instead, the doctor and the family think poor old Grandma has just gotten senile. What she may really need are some extra Bs.

Warning!

Low levels of B vitamins are common among the elderly. That's because our bodies naturally absorb fewer B vitamins as we age. The problem is worsened if you don't eat a healthy diet or don't eat large enough portions. If you're older than 60, discuss taking a complete B-vitamin supplement with your doctor.

Don't Worry, B Happy

If you're seriously low on any of the B vitamins, depression is one of the earliest symptoms. In fact, studies show that at least one in four of all people hospitalized for depression is deficient in pyridoxine and cobalamin; another study suggests that more than three quarters of all depressed patients have a pyridoxine deficiency. Giving these patients even small doses of pyridoxine improves their depression. Folic acid supplements have been shown to help elderly patients who are depressed.

People who take lithium to control bipolar disorder (manic depression) sometimes benefit from taking additional choline. If you take lithium, read the information in Chapter 12 and discuss choline supplements with your doctor before you try them.

Boosting Your Immune System

When your body comes under attack from germs, your immune system swings into action. To launch an effective counterattack, your body needs to quickly produce a bunch of complicated proteins and the enzymes that help them work better and faster. And for that, you need all your B vitamins, because the Bs are all closely involved with moving amino acids around to make proteins, hormones, and enzymes.

Pyridoxine, folic acid, and cobalamin are especially important for your immune system. You need pyridoxine to help regulate and maintain your immune system. Folic acid keeps your frontline defenses against infection—your skin, your lungs, your intestines—strong. And without enough folic acid and cobalamin, you can't produce enough infection-fighting white blood cells.

Although low levels of B vitamins make you more likely to get sick, taking extra Bs won't help you get better faster. Your best bet: keep your B levels high to help avoid illness and infection.

The Least You Need to Know

- The B family contains eight vitamins and four related substances that work closely with each other—you need them all.

- If you have a shortage of one B vitamin, you probably have a shortage of the others as well.

- Foods rich in B vitamins include meat; chicken; fish; milk and dairy products; nuts; beans; peas; and dark-green, leafy vegetables.

- Most people get all the Bs they need from their food. Strict vegetarians, the elderly, and alcohol abusers may not get enough.

- High levels of folic acid, pyridoxine, and cobalamin help protect you from heart disease.

- The B family helps keep your immune system working at peak efficiency.

Chapter 5

Thiamin: The Basic B

In This Chapter

- ◆ Learning why you need thiamin (Vitamin B_1)
- ◆ Discovering the foods that are high in thiamin
- ◆ Having thiamin helps give you energy
- ◆ Protecting your heart muscles and nerve cells with thiamin

Thiamin's special job on the B team is to help you convert carbohydrates in your food into energy your body can use. All you have to do is give yourself a reliable daily supply and your thiamin will chug along, day in and day out, nourishing your brain and nervous system and keeping your heart pumping smoothly.

Why You Need Thiamin

Your body goes through an amazingly complex series of steps to turn the food you eat into energy. All the B vitamins are involved in every one of those steps, alone or working together; but let's focus on thiamin here. One particular step in the process needs an enzyme called *thiamin pyrophosphate*, or *TPP*, to work. Without thiamin, you can't make the enzyme—and without the enzyme, the whole process grinds to a halt.

You also need thiamin to keep your brain and nervous system fueled. Your brain runs on glucose, a type of sugar that's made from the carbohydrates you eat. Thiamin helps your brain and nervous system absorb enough glucose. Without it, they take in only half of what they really need. And when your brain doesn't get enough fuel, you start to get forgetful, depressed, tired, and apathetic.

Thiamin helps keep your heart muscles elastic and working smoothly, which keeps your heart pumping strongly and evenly, with just the right number of beats.

The RDA for Thiamin

The amount of thiamin you need daily for good health is very small—the RDA for an adult male is only 1.2 mg. That's based on the mythical average man, because the RDA is calculated on the basis of how much you eat. Figure on 0.5 mg of thiamin for every 1,000 calories you eat. If you take in fewer than 2,000 calories a day, though, make sure you still get at least 1.0 mg of thiamin. Check the following table to make sure you're getting your daily requirement.

The RDA for Thiamin

Age in Years/Sex	Thiamin in mg
Infants	
0 to 0.5	0.2
0.5 to 1	0.3
Children	
1 to 3	0.5
4 to 8	0.6
9 to 13	0.9
Adults	
Men 14 to 18	1.2
Men 19 to 30	1.2
Men 31 to 50	1.2
Men 50+	1.2
Women 14 to 18	1.0
Women 19 to 30	1.1

Age in Years/Sex	Thiamin in mg
Women 30+	1.1
Pregnant women	1.4
Nursing women	1.4

Are You Deficient?

Starting in the early 1800s, rice mills in Asia began removing the brown outer covering of the rice grains. Polishing, as it was called, produced white rice that cooked quickly and tasted good. People who ate a lot of white rice and little else, however, developed a disease called beriberi. Millions of people across Asia lost muscle strength, had leg spasms or paralysis, and became mentally confused. For a long time, people thought some sort of germ in the white rice was making them sick. It was only in the late 1890s that researchers realized people who ate mostly *brown* rice didn't get beriberi. Something in the brown rice husk was clearly important to human health, but it wasn't until 1911 that *thiamin* was isolated.

def•i•ni•tion

The word **thiamin** (sometimes spelled *thiamine*) combines the prefix *thio-* with the word "vitamin." The *thio-* part comes from the Greek word for sulfur. Thiamin gets its name because the complicated molecule for this vitamin contains an atom of sulfur.

Today beriberi still occurs in the less-developed world, but it's extremely rare in our modern society. You need so little thiamin, and it's so easily found in the typical diet, that few people are seriously deficient.

There's one very big exception to that last statement: people who abuse alcohol. In fact, so many people in the developed world abuse alcohol that thiamin deficiency may be the most common vitamin deficiency of all. Alcoholics tend to eat poorly, so their vitamin intake in general is very low. They don't eat enough thiamin, and the alcohol destroys most of what little they do take in. Alcohol also makes them excrete more thiamin. Chronic alcoholics need large amounts of thiamin supplements—anywhere from 10 to 100 mg per day.

Eventually, thiamin deficiency from alcoholism causes a type of nerve damage called *Wernicke-Korsakoff syndrome*. The symptoms can usually be helped by giving up alcohol and eating a good diet, but the syndrome only worsens and leads to death if alcohol abuse continues.

def•i•ni•tion

After years of heavy drinking, an alcoholic's thiamin levels can drop so low that **Wernicke-Korsakoff syndrome**—nerve damage from thiamin deficiency—develops. The symptoms include immediate memory loss, jerky eye movements, disorientation, and a staggering gait. The symptoms go away or at least get better if the alcoholic stops drinking and starts eating right. If not, there's permanent damage that leads to psychosis and finally death.

Too many elderly people are deficient in thiamin. Often it's because elderly people don't eat well and don't get enough thiamin in their diets. In fact, nearly half of all elderly people sent to hospitals may be deficient in thiamin. It's entirely possible that many complaints of the elderly, such as irritability, confusion, poor sleep, and generally just not feeling well are due simply to a mild thiamin deficiency.

Some other people, especially those with special health problems, may become deficient in thiamin. Mild thiamin deficiency generally causes tiredness, muscle weakness, a pins-and-needles feeling in the legs, depression, and constipation. You could be deficient if ...

◆ **You're pregnant or breastfeeding.** You're passing a lot of thiamin on to your baby, so you need about 0.5 mg extra every day.

◆ **You diet a lot.** If you eat fewer than 1,500 calories a day, or if you eat only a few different foods, you're probably not getting enough thiamin.

◆ **You fast frequently.** You need thiamin every day for good health.

◆ **You have diabetes.** You could be excreting too much thiamin in your urine.

◆ **You have kidney disease and are on dialysis.** Talk to your doctor about all vitamin supplements before you try them.

◆ **You're sick with something, such as a chronic infection, that causes frequent fevers.** Fever makes your body run faster, so you need more thiamin.

Eating Your Thiamin

What do bagels and brown rice have in common? They're both good sources of thiamin. Actually, thiamin is found in lots of different foods; it's also added to flour, breads, pasta, and breakfast cereals. Because you need fewer than 2 mg to meet the RDA, most people get enough from their diet. Even someone who eats mostly burgers and fries will get enough thiamin, although just barely.

Wheat germ, sunflower seeds, whole grains, and all kinds of nuts are excellent food sources of thiamin. Beans and peas are also good sources. Some other good sources are oranges, raisins, asparagus, cauliflower, potatoes, milk, and whole-wheat bread. Oatmeal, whole wheat, and brown rice are grains that are high in thiamin. Among meats, pork and beef liver are high in thiamin; there's some in all beef and chicken. How many of these thiamin-rich foods do you eat regularly?

The Thiamin in Food

Food	Amount	Thiamin in mg
Asparagus, steamed	1 cup	0.12
Bagel	1	0.21
Beans, black	½ cup	0.21
Beans, kidney	½ cup	0.14
Beef, lean	3 oz.	0.05
Beef liver	3 oz.	0.23
Bread, whole-wheat	1 slice	0.09
Cashews	3 oz.	0.18
Chicken, roasted	3 oz.	0.06
Corn	½ cup	0.18
Green peas	½ cup	0.21
Ham	3 oz.	0.82
Milk, nonfat	1 cup	0.09
Oatmeal	1 cup	0.26
Orange	1	0.13
Peanuts	3 oz.	0.36
Pecans	3 oz.	0.27

continues

The Thiamin in Food   (continued)

Food	Amount	Thiamin in mg
Pork, roasted	3 oz.	0.52
Potato	1 medium	0.22
Raisins	1 cup	0.21
Rice, brown	1 cup	0.20
Sunflower seeds	3 oz.	1.95
Wheat germ	¼ cup	0.55

What you drink with your food affects how much thiamin you get. Alcohol and the tannins found in tea destroy thiamin. To get the most thiamin from your food, skip these beverages during your meal and have them afterward instead.

Getting the Most from Thiamin

Most people don't really need to take a thiamin supplement. The amount in your diet, along with any you take in a daily multivitamin, is fine. Your body doesn't store thiamin because it's water-soluble, so you need to get some every day. There's no known toxicity from taking thiamin supplements—people have taken more than 300 mg a day (more than 200 times the RDA) with no bad effects. There's no reason to take that much, but it is safe.

The B vitamins work together to convert the foods you eat into energy you can use. You need all of them. Fortunately, they're all found in many of the same foods, so eating foods high in thiamin will also give you riboflavin, niacin, pyridoxine, biotin, and pantothenic acid.

Thumbs Up/Thumbs Down

Thiamin Is Helped By ...	Thiamin Is Hurt By ...
All other B vitamins	Alcohol
Magnesium	A shortage of other B vitamins

Protecting Your Heart

Thiamin helps your heart beat strongly and regularly. It also keeps your heart muscles elastic and lets them bounce back quickly from each beat. If you're low on thiamin, your heart muscles won't be elastic enough, which could lead to abnormal heartbeats.

A study in 2006 showed that among patients hospitalized with congestive heart failure, about one in three had thiamin levels that were too low. Heart failure can increase your body's need for some nutrients, including thiamin, to the point where even eating a good diet doesn't provide enough—and many heart failure patients have difficulty eating enough to maintain good nutrition. Also, the diuretic medications often prescribed to treat heart failure can increase the normal loss of thiamin. Does this mean that thiamin supplements can help prevent congestive heart failure? No, but it's possible that thiamin can help the symptoms. Talk to your doctor about the importance of maintaining good nutrition if you have congestive heart failure.

Although too little thiamin definitely causes heart problems, it's not clear that taking more thiamin than the RDA will help heart problems. Some researchers are looking into using thiamin to treat heart attacks, but it's too soon to say whether it will be really valuable. In the meantime, if you have a heart problem, talk to your doctor about thiamin supplements before you try them.

Thiamin and Diabetes

Because thiamin is involved in glucose production, one symptom of thiamin deficiency is that you don't use glucose normally. That's similar to the problem people with diabetes have, but unfortunately, the similarity ends there. A diabetic who is deficient in thiamin—and some are—will use glucose better after the deficiency is fixed, but then after that, there won't be any improvement. Diabetics with normal thiamin levels aren't helped by taking thiamin supplements, and thiamin won't help control blood-sugar levels.

Thiamin and Canker Sores

If you're low on thiamin, you're much more likely to get frequent canker sores (aphthous stomatitis)—painful, crater-like sores in your mouth. Interestingly, a recent study showed that taking extra thiamin after the sores have started doesn't help them go away. If you often get canker sores, your best bet is probably prevention. Try getting more thiamin in your diet.

The Least You Need to Know

◆ Thiamin (Vitamin B_1) is a water-soluble vitamin.

◆ Thiamin works closely with all the other B vitamins.

◆ You need thiamin to help convert your food to energy and to keep your brain, nervous system, and heart running well.

◆ The RDA for thiamin is small—adults need only between 1.1 and 1.2 mg a day.

◆ Thiamin is found in many different foods, including meat, whole grains, and nuts, and is usually added to rice, pasta, breads, and breakfast cereals.

◆ Most people get the RDA from their diet and don't need supplements. Older adults, however, may need extra thiamin.

Chapter 6

B Energetic: Riboflavin

In This Chapter

- ◆ Why you need riboflavin (Vitamin B_2)
- ◆ What the foods are that are high in riboflavin
- ◆ How riboflavin gives you energy
- ◆ Why athletes need riboflavin
- ◆ How riboflavin can prevent migraine headaches

Does anybody ever complain about having too much energy? Of course not—most of us go around wishing for more, enough to get through a busy day of work and family with a little bit left over for ourselves. Some sort of sub-space energy-transference beam would be nice, but until that happens, you'll just have to settle for riboflavin. Your cells need riboflavin to make energy, so you need to be sure you're getting enough of this vital member of the B family.

Riboflavin does lots of other good things for you as well, mostly by working with the other Bs to keep your body's systems, such as your immune system, running smoothly. Riboflavin works especially closely with niacin and pyridoxine—in fact, without riboflavin, these two B siblings can't do their main jobs at all.

Why You Need Riboflavin

Riboflavin gives you energy at the most basic level—inside your cells. You need it to make two of the enzymes that are absolutely vital for releasing energy from the fats, carbohydrates, and proteins you eat. To make a complicated story short, riboflavin keeps you alive.

Aside from that little chore, riboflavin also does a bunch of other things in your body, either by itself or along with the other members of the B team (especially pyridoxine and niacin). Riboflavin regulates cell growth and reproduction and helps you make healthy red blood cells. It helps your immune system by keeping the mucous membranes that line your respiratory and digestive systems in good shape. If invading germs still sneak in, riboflavin helps you make antibodies for fighting them off. Your eyes, nerves, skin, nails, and hair all need riboflavin to stay healthy. It might even help your memory—older people with high levels of riboflavin do better on memory tests.

The RDA for Riboflavin

As important as riboflavin is, you don't really need a lot of it for good health—less than 2 mg a day is enough. Riboflavin is found naturally in many foods, especially meat; milk products; and dark-green, leafy vegetables. It's also added to flour, bread, and most breakfast cereals.

The RDA for riboflavin is based on your caloric intake—the more you eat, the more you need. The basic formula is approximately 0.6 mg for every 1,000 calories. Your daily intake should be at least 1.1 mg if you're a woman and 1.3 mg if you're a man, even if you eat fewer than 2,000 calories. Check the table to see how much you need per day.

The RDA for Riboflavin

Age in Years/Sex	Riboflavin in mg
Infants	
0 to 0.5	0.3
0.5 to 1	0.4

Age in Years/Sex	Riboflavin in mg
Children	
1 to 3	0.5
4 to 8	0.6
9 to 13	0.9
Adults	
Men 14 to 18	1.3
Men 19 to 30	1.3
Men 31+	1.3
Women 14 to 18	1.0
Women 19 to 30	1.1
Women 31+	1.1
Pregnant women	1.4
Nursing women	1.6

Are You Deficient?

Riboflavin is an exception to the water-soluble rule, because you store small amounts of it in your kidneys and liver. Because of that, riboflavin deficiency can take as long as 3 or 4 months to show up.

True riboflavin deficiency is quite rare. Most people get plenty of riboflavin in their food. When deficiency symptoms do occur, they're usually related to a shortage of all the Bs. You need riboflavin to help niacin and pyridoxine work correctly. In fact, if you're short on riboflavin, you might have deficiency symptoms for one of the other vitamins. Usually, though, riboflavin deficiency shows up as problems with the mucous membranes, skin, eyes, and blood. An early and clear sign are sores and cracks on the lips, especially at the corners. Scaly skin, reddened eyes, and anemia are other deficiency signs. Some people are at special risk for riboflavin deficiency:

◆ **Athletes.** You need extra riboflavin if you exercise a lot—we'll talk more about this later in this chapter.

◆ **Diabetics.** You may be excreting a lot of your riboflavin in your urine. Talk to your doctor about vitamin supplements before you try them.

◆ **Pregnant and breastfeeding women.** You're passing a lot of your riboflavin on to your baby, so you need about 0.5 mg more a day.

◆ **Elderly people.** About a third of all elderly people have a riboflavin deficiency, mostly from poor absorption or poor diet.

◆ **People who can't digest milk.** Milk and dairy products such as cottage cheese are important sources of riboflavin. If you can't digest these foods, you might not be getting enough riboflavin.

◆ **People who take tricyclic antidepressants.** Drugs such as amitriptyline (Elavil) can interfere with riboflavin. If you take a tricyclic antidepressant, talk to your doctor about vitamin supplements before you try them.

Eating Your Riboflavin

Large amounts of riboflavin are found in milk and other dairy foods. Good choices here include cheese, yogurt, and ice cream. Naturally, even this really good justification for indulging in chocolate butternut chip has guilt attached—the higher the fat, the less the riboflavin.

Meat, especially liver, is a good source of riboflavin, as is fish. Vegetable foods that are high in riboflavin include broccoli, spinach, avocados, mushrooms, and asparagus. Most breads, baked goods, and pasta are made with flour that has been enriched with riboflavin and other B vitamins; most breakfast cereals also have riboflavin and other Bs added to them.

The Riboflavin in Food

Food	Amount	Riboflavin in mg
Almonds, dry-roasted	1 oz.	0.22
Asparagus, cooked	½ cup	0.13
Avocado, California	1 medium	0.22
Beef, ground	3 oz.	0.20
Beef liver	3 oz.	3.60
Bread, whole-wheat	1 slice	0.05
Broccoli, cooked	½ cup	0.12
Brie cheese	1 oz.	0.15
Cheddar cheese	1 oz.	0.11

Food	Amount	Riboflavin in mg
Chicken breast	3 oz.	0.16
Chickpeas	1 cup	0.10
Cottage cheese, low-fat	1 cup	0.42
Egg	1 large	0.26
Ice cream, vanilla	½ cup	0.16
Kidney beans	1 cup	0.10
Milk, low-fat	1 cup	0.52
Mushrooms, cooked	½ cup	0.23
Peas	½ cup	0.12
Pork, roasted	3 oz.	0.30
Salmon, canned	3 oz.	0.16
Spinach, cooked	½ cup	0.21
Sweet potato, baked with skin	1 medium	0.15
Swiss cheese	1 oz.	0.10
Turkey breast	3 oz.	0.10
Wheat germ	¼ cup	0.23
Yogurt, low-fat	8 oz.	0.49

Getting the Most from Riboflavin

Most people get all the riboflavin they need from their food. Riboflavin is added to so many common foods, such as bread and pasta, that even someone with lousy eating habits will probably get enough. If you're a strict vegetarian or vegan or if you exercise a lot (or both), you might need extra riboflavin. You also might need extra if you fall into the other risk categories we talked about earlier. Most daily multivitamins contain the full RDA for riboflavin. If you think you need more, consider taking a complete B supplement. You need all the B vitamins for your riboflavin to work well—and vice versa.

If you want just extra riboflavin, these supplements come as tablets or capsules. They usually contain either 50 mg or 100 mg—either amount is more than the RDA. You absorb only about 15 percent of the riboflavin from supplements, especially if you take them on an empty stomach. To get the most from your riboflavin, take the supplements with meals. You can't really overdose on riboflavin, because even very large doses (more than 1,000 mg) are safe. There is one side effect from large doses, though: your urine will turn a bright, fluorescent yellow. It may be a little startling, but it's harmless.

Producing Energy

By itself, riboflavin's most important role is in cell respiration. Just as you breathe in oxygen and exhale the waste product carbon dioxide from your lungs, so does each and every cell in your body. Molecules of oxygen and food enter a cell and are carried into the *mitochondria*, the tiny structures within the cell that act like little power plants. Enzymes in the mitochondria release the energy from the oxygen and food. Two of those enzymes, *flavin mononucleotide* and *flavin adenine dinucleotide*, must work together as part of the process. As you can tell from the flavin part of their names, these enzymes contain riboflavin. Not enough riboflavin, not enough enzymes—and therefore not enough energy.

Serious athletes who train hard are making their mitochondria work super hard and super fast to provide enough energy. At the same time, they may not be taking in enough riboflavin from their food to make the flavin enzymes they need—especially if they are also watching their weight and avoiding meat and dairy foods. Some athletes and body builders claim that riboflavin supplements help them train harder and longer. They also say riboflavin helps them bounce back faster from training sessions and cuts the time they have to spend resting. Does this really work? Although it's true that exercising hard increases your need for riboflavin, there's no real evidence that taking supplements really improves athletic performance.

Preventing Migraines

No headache is quite as awful as a migraine. There's the terrible pain along with nausea, vomiting, and sensitivity to light. Because these headaches are so incapacitating, and because they affect some 11 to 18 million Americans every year, a lot of research goes into them. Despite all the studies, we still don't really know what causes migraines, though there are a lot of good theories. (We'll talk more about migraines in Chapters 18, 27, and 29.) One of the more interesting recent studies showed that high daily doses of riboflavin—400 mg a day—sharply reduced the number and severity of migraine attacks for more than half the participants. The researchers think it works because people who get migraines have low cellular energy reserves in their brains.

Riboflavin helps the cells use energy better, which seems to help prevent the migraines to begin with and make them less severe when they do happen. And unlike many other drugs used to treat migraines, riboflavin is cheap, safe, and has no side effects. The research is still in the early stages, however, so if you want to try high doses of riboflavin for your migraines, talk to your doctor first.

Riboflavin and Your Eyes

Whether riboflavin helps your eyes is open for debate. One good example is the cataract question. In theory, people with high levels of riboflavin should have fewer cataracts. Here's how the thinking runs: you need riboflavin to utilize glutathione, one of your body's main antioxidants, most effectively. (We'll talk a lot more about glutathione in Chapter 24.) Your eyes need a lot of glutathione to counteract the damaging ultraviolet rays in sunlight, so a shortage of riboflavin leads to a shortage of glutathione, which could lead to cataracts from free-radical damage. It's nice in theory, but it's never held up well in studies. Although about a third of the elderly are riboflavin-deficient, their cataract rate isn't any different from the rest of the population.

On the other hand, too much riboflavin could cause cataracts or make them worse if you already have them. The reason is similar: free-radical damage. Riboflavin is sensitive to light, so the riboflavin in the cells of your eyes breaks down when light hits it. Free radicals are released in the process, which then damage the lens and cause a cataract. The same free radicals could also damage the macula, the tiny area of super-sensitive cells in your retina, leading to macular degeneration. Older people who are low on riboflavin should definitely get their levels up, but only by a better diet and riboflavin in small doses—no more than 10 mg a day. If you have cataracts and low riboflavin, raise your level only by eating more riboflavin-rich foods.

The Least You Need to Know

♦ Riboflavin is also called Vitamin B_2. Riboflavin works closely with all the other B vitamins, especially niacin and pyridoxine.

♦ You need riboflavin to make energy within your cells, to keep your red blood cells healthy, and to help keep your immune system working well.

♦ Riboflavin is found in many different foods, including meat and dairy products, and is usually added to rice, pasta, breads, and breakfast cereals.

♦ Most people get the RDA for riboflavin from their diet and don't need supplements.

Chapter 7

Niacin: Cholesterol B Gone

In This Chapter

◆ Why you need niacin (Vitamin B₃)

◆ What the foods are containing high niacin

◆ How niacin can help lower your cholesterol

◆ How niacin can help diabetes

Suddenly it seems that everyone you know is worried about their cholesterol. They're talking about their LDL and HDL levels and cutting back on fat in their diets. Some are taking two different drugs to lower their cholesterol—maybe you are, too.

Are cholesterol drugs the price you have to pay for all those double cheeseburgers with bacon and a big side of fries? Not necessarily. Swap those buckets of fried chicken for green, leafy vegetables; give up cigarettes; get more exercise; lose some weight; and watch your cholesterol drop. Add some niacin—but only under your doctor's care—and watch it drop even more.

At the ordinary RDA level, niacin doesn't do anything very dramatic. But you do need it for some of the most important functions in your body, such as releasing energy in your cells, making hormones, and working with the other members of the B team to keep your body running smoothly.

Why You Need Niacin

Niacin is essential for more than 50 different processes in your body. What most of these processes boil down to is helping your body produce energy from the foods you eat. Niacin makes enzymes that help your cells turn carbohydrates into energy. As part of the energy end of things, niacin also helps control how much glucose (sugar) is in your blood, which in turn helps give you energy when you need it—when you exercise, for example.

def•i•ni•tion

Niacin, a water-soluble B vitamin, comes in two forms: *nicotinic acid* and *niacinamide* (also sometimes called nicotinamide). To avoid confusion with nicotine, the addictive substance in tobacco, the name nicotinamide isn't used very often (actually, niacin has nothing to do with nicotine). The word "niacin" is generally used to mean both forms. Niacinamide is the form usually found in supplements.

Niacin also acts as an antioxidant within your cells—every little bit helps when it comes to battling free radicals. However, niacin only works as an on-the-spot antioxidant for mopping up the free radicals made when it's being used to release energy. It's nowhere near as powerful as some other vitamins, such as Vitamin C, for battling free radicals in general.

Niacin works closely with all its B relatives, but it's especially close to riboflavin and pyridoxine. All three work together to keep you in overall good health. They're especially important for your skin, nervous system, and digestion. In very large amounts—much, much more than the RDA—niacin can be a valuable treatment for lowering high cholesterol. The research in this area is so exciting that we'll discuss it a lot more later in this chapter. We'll point out now, however, that taking a lot of niacin doesn't keep you from getting high cholesterol.

Another interesting new role for niacin may be in helping people with the severe form of diabetes called Type 1, or insulin-dependent diabetes mellitus (IDDM). Again, we'll talk about this in more depth later in the chapter.

The RDA for Niacin

The RDA for niacin is based mostly on how many calories you eat—but which foods those calories come from is also part of the picture. The calorie part is easy: at a bare minimum, you need 7 to 8 mg of niacin for every 1,000 calories you eat. This ratio assumes that you eat 2,000 calories a day and get at least 14 mg of niacin a day if you're a woman and 16 mg a day if you're a man. If you don't eat that much (say, you're dieting), you still need the same amount of niacin.

Here's where the food part comes in. You probably think your niacin comes straight from your food. Well, most of it does, but some is also made in your body from the proteins you eat. It works like this: when you eat animal or plant protein, your body breaks down the proteins into their building blocks—amino acids (and we'll spend all of Chapter 22 talking about them). One of those building blocks is the amino acid *tryptophan.*

Your body uses about half your tryptophan for making some of the 50,000-plus proteins you need. The other half gets converted to niacin. In fact, only about half your niacin comes directly from the foods you eat; the other half is converted from tryptophan. You need about 60 mg of tryptophan to make 1 mg of niacin. Because most people eat somewhere between 500 to 1,000 mg of tryptophan a day, they make about 8 to 17 mg of niacin.

The RDA chart ignores tryptophan and counts only the niacin you get as preformed niacin from your food. That's why, even though studies show that most Americans get only about 11 mg of niacin from their diet, very few people are actually deficient—they make up the rest of the RDA from tryptophan. To be on the safe side, though, try to get your full RDA from foods rich in niacin.

def•i•ni•tion

Tryptophan is one of the nine essential amino acids—you can get it only from your food. Your body uses half the tryptophan it gets to help make the thousands of complicated proteins that keep you running. The rest is converted to niacin. The best way to get your tryptophan is through the proteins in your food (see Chapter 22 for more on tryptophan).

The RDA for Niacin

Age in Years/Sex	Niacin in mg
Infants	
0 to 0.5	2.0
0.5 to 1	4.0
Children	
1 to 3	6.0
4 to 8	8.0
9 to 13	12.0

continues

The RDA for Niacin   (continued)

Age in Years/Sex	Niacin in mg
Adults	
Men	16.0
Women	14.0
Pregnant women	18.0
Nursing women	17.0

Are You Deficient?

Because you don't really need all that much niacin to begin with, and because you can make niacin from the tryptophan in protein, real niacin deficiency is very rare in the developed world today. That hasn't always been the case. Starting in the eighteenth century—when corn became a staple food for many poor people in Europe, Africa, and North America—pellagra, the deficiency disease caused by a lack of niacin, was a common problem. Corn is low in niacin and tryptophan. It wasn't until well into the 1940s that the cause of pellagra was fully understood. Today pellagra is almost unknown in the developed world, although it unfortunately still happens in impoverished areas of Asia and Africa. You are very unlikely to get pellagra or even be slightly deficient in niacin, unless ...

◆ **You abuse alcohol.** Alcohol blocks your uptake of all B vitamins, including niacin. Also, alcohol abusers eat very badly and don't get enough vitamins in general.

◆ **You're a strict vegetarian or a vegan.** If you don't eat a lot of high-quality protein (protein from animal sources such as eggs, milk, fish, and meat), you might be on the low side for niacin—this is especially true for kids. Vegetarian or vegan children should probably take niacin as part of an overall B-vitamin supplement.

Usually someone who's low on niacin is low on all the B vitamins. The reason is almost always poor diet. To solve the problem, eat more protein and take a supplement that includes all the B vitamins.

Eating Your Niacin

Niacin is found in lots of common foods, especially meat, fish, poultry, eggs, and whole grains. It's also added to breakfast cereals, rice, bread, and many baked goods. Tryptophan is found in just about every protein food, especially milk, dairy foods, and eggs. Most people can easily get their RDA for niacin and tryptophan from their diet. Strict vegetarians and vegans need to eat plenty of nuts and whole grains, such as oatmeal, to meet their RDAs. Check the charts to find the foods that give you the niacin and tryptophan you need.

The Niacin in Food

Food	Amount	Niacin in mg
Almonds, roasted	1 oz.	0.8
Asparagus	½ cup	1.0
Avocado	½ medium	1.5
Bagel	1	1.9
Beef, ground	3 oz.	4.0
Beef liver	3 oz.	10.0
Bread, whole-wheat	1 slice	1.0
Chicken breast	3 oz.	8.5
Chickpeas	1 cup	0.9
Corn, kernels	½ cup	1.2
Cottage cheese, low-fat	1 cup	0.3
Cream of wheat	¾ cup	1.1
Flounder	3 oz.	2.5
Kidney beans	1 cup	1.0
Milk, low-fat	1 cup	0.2
Mushrooms, cooked	½ cup	3.5
Navy beans	1 cup	1.0
Nectarine	1 medium	1.3
Peanut butter	2 TB.	3.8
Peanuts, dry-roasted	1 oz.	3.8

continues

The Niacin in Food   (continued)

Food	Amount	Niacin in mg
Peas	½ cup	1.6
Pork, roasted	3 oz.	5.5
Potato, baked	1 medium	3.3
Rice, brown	1 cup	3.0
Rice, white	1 cup	3.0
Rice, wild	1 cup	2.1
Salmon, canned	3 oz.	5.0
Spinach, cooked	½ cup	0.4
Sunflower seeds	1 oz.	1.1
Sweet potato	1 medium	0.7
Tomato	1 medium	0.8
Tuna, canned in water	3 oz.	11.3
Turkey breast	3 oz.	8.5
Wheat germ	¼ cup	2.0

Remember that about half the tryptophan you consume is converted into niacin. The rest of this amino acid is used to help make the proteins that keep you going.

Tryptophan in Food

Food	Amount	Tryptophan in mg
Avocado	1 medium	45
Banana	1 medium	14
Beef, ground	3 oz.	243
Beef liver	3 oz.	301
Black beans	1 cup	181
Cheddar cheese	1 oz.	91
Chicken breast	3 oz.	326
Corn	½ cup	19
Cottage cheese, low-fat	1 cup	312
Dates, dried	10	42
Egg	1 large	76

Food	Amount	Tryptophan in mg
Flounder	3 oz.	230
Milk	1 cup	113
Oatmeal	1 cup	84
Peanuts, dry-roasted	1 oz.	64
Pear	1 medium	17
Tuna, canned in water	3 oz.	243
Turkey, without skin	3 oz.	267

Getting the Most from Niacin

Although you might not get enough niacin in your diet to meet the RDA, the trypto-phan you eat will probably boost you over the top. Not too many people need supple-ments of niacin alone—if you're low on niacin, you're almost certainly low on the other B vitamins as well, and should take a complete B supplement.

If you really feel you need a niacin supplement due to inadequate diet, you can buy tablets or capsules containing 100 mg, 250 mg, or 500 mg. You'll have a choice of niacinamide or nicotinic acid. If you just want to supplement your niacin level, choose niacinamide in the smallest dose. Don't overdo it—even 100 mg of niacinamide can cause heartburn, nausea, and headaches for some people.

The only real reason to take nicotinic acid at all is to treat high blood cholesterol under a doctor's supervision. There are some nasty side effects from the large doses you need to take—and some very good reasons why some people shouldn't take it at all. We'll talk about this in detail later in this chapter.

Powering Your Cells

The members of the B team work together to turn the fats, carbohydrates, and proteins you eat into energy you can use. Niacin plays its role by being an essential part of two coenzymes: nicotinamide adenine dinucleotide (NAD) and nicotinamide adenine dinu-cleotide phosphate (NADP). You need both enzymes working in sync to use fats and sugar properly. Without them, your cells can't make enough energy to keep going.

Your body needs just enough niacin—20 mg a day, tops—and no more. Although you'll feel weak and tired if you don't get enough niacin, taking extra won't give you extra energy.

Warning! _____

Do not take any sort of niacin supplement if you also take medicine for high blood pressure! The niacin could make your blood pressure drop way too low!

If you have diabetes, niacin supplements could raise your blood sugar levels. If you have gout, niacin could raise your uric acid levels and cause an attack.

Lowering High Cholesterol

You can't open a newspaper or magazine today without seeing big ads that trumpet statin drugs to treat high cholesterol. The ads tell you how well the drugs work and how they help prevent heart attacks. If you look more closely at those ads, though, you'll see paragraph after paragraph of tiny type describing the side effects in scary detail.

The one thing that's not mentioned in the ads is the cost. These drugs are expensive. A month's supply of atorvastatin (Lipitor) costs about $80—and you'll probably be taking it for the rest of your life. The generic versions of statin drugs are less expensive, but the cost still adds up.

Warning! _____

Take large doses of nicotinic acid only under a doctor's supervision!

For some people, there's a better and cheaper way: niacin. Doctors have known for many years that large doses of nicotinic acid—between 2 and 3 g a day—lower LDL ("bad") cholesterol and triglycerides and raise HDL ("good") cholesterol (see Chapter 1 for more information about cholesterol).

Lowering your LDL cholesterol and triglycerides, and raising your HDL cholesterol, definitely decreases your risk of a heart attack. In fact, a major study that went on for 15 years showed not only that the group who took niacin had lower cholesterol and fewer heart attacks, but they also had fewer deaths for any reason.

Niacin works for high cholesterol pretty well by itself. Many people need a combination of drugs to really make a dent in their high cholesterol, though. Niacin can work well here too, especially when it's combined with drugs such as atorvastatin (Lipitor), lovastatin (Mevacor), pravastatin (Pravachol), or simvastatin (Zocor). The one-two punch can bring your cholesterol way down. In fact, there's a prescription drug called Advicor that combines extended-release niacin with lovastatin.

Do not try niacin supplements on your own to lower your cholesterol. The doses needed are so high that the niacin stops being a supplement and becomes a drug. You must work with your doctor and have your cholesterol and liver functions checked often. If you're already taking a cholesterol drug, don't stop taking it and switch to niacin. Also, don't keep taking your cholesterol drug and then also start taking niacin. Discuss your cholesterol and the drugs you take with your doctor before trying niacin.

Not everyone with high cholesterol should take niacin. If you have Type 2 diabetes, extra niacin could cause your blood sugar to go up, but as we'll discuss later in this chapter, the benefits may outweigh the risk. If you have gout, extra niacin could trigger an attack. If you take medicine for high blood pressure, niacin could make your blood pressure drop too low. And if you have liver disease or ulcers, niacin could make these problems worse.

 Warning!

If you have liver problems, diabetes, ulcers, gout, or take high blood pressure medication, niacin could make these problems worse. Always consult your doctor before taking anything.

Boy, Was My Face Red

Large (and even not-so-large) doses of nicotinic acid cause a nasty side effect called the niacin flush. About 15 to 30 minutes after you take it, your face and neck get really red and hot—you blush so badly it reminds you of being back in junior high. The flush can go on for half an hour or longer and then wears off.

You can build up a tolerance to niacin flushing by starting with smaller doses and gradually taking bigger ones. You can usually also prevent the flush by taking an aspirin about half an hour before you take the niacin. Taking the niacin on a full stomach also seems to help.

Another way to avoid flushing is to use the sustained-release (SR) form of nicotinic acid. SR nicotinic acid is good for lowering your LDL cholesterol and triglycerides, but it doesn't do much to raise your HDL level. Also, it can cause serious liver problems. Use it with caution.

The best way to avoid flushing is to avoid nicotinic acid and take niacin in the form of *inositol hexanicotinate* (*IHN*, also known as *inositol hexaniacinate*). IHN works on cholesterol just as well as nicotinic acid, but

def•i•ni•tion

Inositol hexaniacinate (IHN) is a form of nicotinic acid that also includes inositol, one of the unofficial B vitamins (see Chapter 12 for more on inositol). It works just as well or better than nicotinic acid, but doesn't cause flushing or other side effects.

without the side effects and without the possibility of liver damage. If you'd like to try IHN, talk to your doctor.

Niacin and Diabetes

A serious form of diabetes called Type 1 (also called insulin-dependent diabetes mellitus or IDDM) strikes children and young people. This disease is pretty mysterious, but we do know that something destroys the part of the pancreas that makes insulin, the hormone that controls your blood sugar. It's possible that the diabetic's own immune system has something to do with causing the destruction. Powerful drugs that suppress the immune system can sometimes slow down or stop the destruction in the pancreas.

Recently researchers have turned to niacinamide to try to stop Type 1 diabetes soon after it starts. The results of several trials have been encouraging, but there's still a long way to go before this becomes standard treatment.

Another approach is to use niacin in the form of nicotinamide to prevent Type 1 diabetes in kids who are at high risk for it because of family history. A major study in New Zealand in 1996 showed that among kids who already have some of the telltale antibodies in their blood, niacin supplements may reduce the number of cases by half or more. But in 2004, the results of the European Nicotinamide Diabetes Intervention Trial (ENDIT) were disappointing—among the at-risk young people who participated, there was no difference in the incidence of Type 1 diabetes between those who took niacin supplements for 5 years and those who took a placebo.

Niacin and Type 2 Diabetes

In Type 2 diabetes, also called adult-onset or noninsulin-dependent diabetes, the pancreas still produces insulin, but your cells become resistant to it. Instead of getting into your cells efficiently, glucose builds up in your bloodstream, causing hyperglycemia, or high blood sugar. People with Type 2 diabetes almost always also have high cholesterol and high triglycerides and are at serious risk of heart disease. In large doses, niacin can raise your blood sugar, so doctors have discouraged its use for lowering cholesterol in people with diabetes. New research, however, suggests that in lower doses—1,000 to 1,500 mg daily—the extended-release form of niacin helps lower cholesterol without raising blood sugar and is safe for most people with Type 2 diabetes. The dose works best when it's combined with a statin drug.

Other Problems Helped by Niacin

Niacin in the form of niacinamide seems to help several other common health problems. Talk to your doctor about niacin for the following:

♦ **Intermittent claudication.** This is a circulatory problem that makes your legs ache and your calf muscles cramp up when you walk. The reason is that your leg muscles aren't getting enough oxygen because your circulation is poor. Niacin makes your blood vessels widen, which brings more blood to your legs.

> **Quack, Quack**
>
> Some researchers claim that megadoses of niacin cure the devastating mental illness schizophrenia. Sadly, there's no evidence that niacin helps.

♦ **Dizziness (vertigo) and ringing in the ears (tinnitus).** Niacin helps these problems, although doctors aren't quite sure why.

♦ **PMS headaches.** B vitamins in general help some women with PMS. Niacin seems to help PMS headaches.

♦ **Alzheimer's disease.** High intake of niacin from food sources may reduce your risk of Alzheimer's disease and age-related mental decline. In one study of several thousand older adults in Chicago, the ones with the highest intake of niacin had an 80 percent reduction in risk compared to those with the lowest intake.

Niacin may not cure any of these problems, but it may be worth a try if nothing else is helping. Be sure to discuss niacin supplements with your doctor before you try them.

The Least You Need to Know

♦ Niacin, also called Vitamin B_3, works closely with all the other B vitamins, especially riboflavin and pyridoxine.

♦ You need niacin to release energy within your cells and for about 50 other body processes.

♦ Niacin is found in many different foods, especially meat, fish, poultry, eggs, nuts, and whole grains. It's also added to breakfast cereals, bread, and many baked goods.

♦ Your body makes some of the niacin it needs from the amino acid tryptophan.

◆ Niacin supplements can help lower high cholesterol—but talk to your doctor before you try it.

Chapter 8

Pyridoxine: Have a Healthy Heart

In This Chapter

- Why you need pyridoxine (Vitamin B₆)
- Which foods are high in pyridoxine
- How pyridoxine helps prevent heart disease
- How pyridoxine helps asthma
- How pyridoxine boosts your immune system
- Why pyridoxine is important for people with diabetes

It's hard to believe that fewer than 2 mg a day of anything could make a big difference to your health—but that's all the pyridoxine you need to make more than 60 different enzymes, help your immune system stay in top gear, keep your red blood cells red, and help your nerves communicate with the rest of you. All that, and we haven't even gotten to what a little *extra* pyridoxine could do for you.

When pyridoxine teams up with folic acid and cobalamin, your risk of heart disease drops. You don't need a lot of extra pyridoxine to get the benefit.

Just doubling your pyridoxine intake—to a whopping 3.6 mg—could make a big difference. Not only will your heart be healthier, you might also help some other health problems. People with asthma and diabetes often benefit from pyridoxine, and it may also help high blood pressure and PMS.

Why You Need Pyridoxine

The Institute of Medicine (the people who bring you the DRI) says you need pyridoxine as a coenzyme in the transamination process, for the decarboxylation and racemization of amino acids, and as the essential coenzyme for glycogen phosphorylase. Just in case you've forgotten your advanced organic biochemistry, we'll simplify: you need pyridoxine to turn the proteins you eat into the proteins your body needs, and you need it to convert carbohydrates from the form you store them in into the form you can use for energy.

What sort of proteins does your body need? For starters, hemoglobin—the stuff that carries oxygen in your red blood cells. Pyridoxine is needed to make lots of other proteins including hormones, neurotransmitters, and enzymes. You also need it to make prostaglandins, hormone-like substances that regulate things such as your blood pressure.

Pyridoxine is crucial for converting the foods you eat into carbohydrates or fat your body can store—and for turning the stored forms into forms you can use when you need extra energy.

Normal amounts of pyridoxine keep your body working normally. What do extra amounts of pyridoxine do? A lot, especially for your heart and immune system, and for asthma and diabetes. You need to be cautious here, though—pyridoxine can be toxic in very large doses.

The RDA for Pyridoxine

You need pyridoxine to turn your amino acids into all the other proteins your body needs. If you eat a lot of protein, however, you don't really need any extra pyridoxine, and you still need the RDA even if you don't eat much protein. Check the following table to see how much you need each day.

The RDA for Pyridoxine

Age in Years/Sex	Pyridoxine in mg
Infants	
0 to 0.5	0.1
0.5 to 1	0.3
Children	
1 to 3	0.5
4 to 8	0.6
9 to 13	1.0
Adults	
Men 14 to 18	1.3
Men 19 to 50	1.3
Men 50+	1.7
Women 14 to 18	1.2
Women 19 to 50	1.3
Women 50+	1.5
Pregnant women	1.9
Nursing women	2.0

Are You Deficient?

Like the other B vitamins, pyridoxine is found in many common foods, especially high-protein foods such as meat, fish, milk, and eggs. It's also added to flour, breakfast cereals, and many baked goods. You get so much from your food that it's not likely you're deficient.

If you're low on pyridoxine, you're probably also low on the other Bs, usually from poor diet. More than 40 different prescription drugs affect your pyridoxine levels, though, and there are some other reasons for being low on pyridoxine:

◆ **You're pregnant or breastfeeding.** Your baby is taking up a lot of your pyridoxine, so you need about 0.7 mg extra every day.

◆ **You're a strict vegetarian or vegan.** Milk and dairy products are relatively poor sources of pyridoxine. Most fruits and vegetables have little or no pyridoxine, so vegans have to get theirs mostly from nuts and whole grains. Kids who don't eat any animal products are especially at risk.

◆ **You take birth-control pills.** Your pyridoxine level could be 15 to 20 percent below normal. Talk to your doctor about taking a complete B supplement.

◆ **You abuse alcohol.** About a third of all alcoholics are deficient in pyridoxine.

◆ **You smoke.** Tobacco blocks your use of pyridoxine.

◆ **You take certain prescription drugs that make you excrete more pyridoxine.** These include hydralazine (Apresoline), used to treat high blood pressure; isoniazid (Laniazid), used to treat tuberculosis; and penicillamine (Cuprimine), used to treat rheumatoid arthritis. Talk to your doctor about taking a complete B supplement.

◆ **You take theophylline to treat asthma or another respiratory problem.** We'll discuss this drug more in the section on asthma a little later in this chapter.

> **Now You're Cooking**
>
> Large amounts of pyridoxine are lost when grains are milled into flour. To compensate, pyridoxine and other B vitamins are added back to flour, cornmeal, and other grain products. Freezing can destroy up to 70 percent of the pyridoxine in food. A lot of pyridoxine also ends up in the cooking water. Use the freshest foods you can and cook them in as little liquid as possible.

Pyridoxine is needed for a lot of different roles in your body, but the first place a deficiency shows up is usually your immune system—you get sick more. That might be blamed on a lot of things, but the next common symptom, *anemia*, or red blood cells that aren't carrying enough oxygen, is the clincher. There are different kinds of anemia (and we'll tell you more about them in Chapter 10), but your doctor can tell from a blood test if yours is caused by pyridoxine deficiency. The cure? Supplements and a better diet with more protein.

Eating Your Pyridoxine

The best source of pyridoxine in your food is high-quality protein: chicken, pork, beef, fish, milk, dairy products, and eggs. Milk, dairy products, and eggs have less pyridoxine than fish and other meats, but they're still good sources. Also, pyridoxine is added to flour, cornmeal, breakfast cereals, and many baked goods.

Here's a rare case where we can't tell you to eat more fresh fruits and vegetables: most of them don't have much or any pyridoxine. Even broccoli, our old standby, has only 0.15 mg in a half cup. The best plant choices are avocados, bananas, mangos, and potatoes. Whole grains are also good: a 3-ounce serving of oatmeal has 0.74 mg. Look at the food chart to find other good sources of pyridoxine.

The Pyridoxine in Food

Food	Amount	Pyridoxine in mg
Apricots, dried	10 halves	0.06
Avocado	½ medium	0.40
Banana	1 medium	0.66
Beef, ground	3 oz.	0.17
Beef liver	3 oz.	0.78
Black beans	1 cup	0.12
Cheddar cheese	1 oz.	0.02
Chicken breast	3 oz.	0.34
Chickpeas	1 cup	0.23
Corn, kernels	½ cup	0.26
Cottage cheese, low-fat	1 cup	0.15
Flounder	3 oz.	0.20
Kidney beans	1 cup	0.21
Lentils	1 cup	0.35
Mango	1 medium	0.28
Milk, low-fat	1 cup	0.10
Navy beans	1 cup	0.30
Pork, roasted	3 oz.	0.39
Potato, baked with skin	1 medium	0.70
Prunes, dried	10	0.22
Raisins, golden	⅔ cup	0.32
Rice, brown	1 cup	0.28
Rice, white	1 cup	0.19
Sweet potato, baked with skin	1 medium	0.28

continues

The Pyridoxine in Food (continued)

Food	Amount	Pyridoxine in mg
Tuna, canned in water	3 oz.	0.30
Turkey breast, with skin	3 oz.	0.28
Wheat germ	¼ cup	0.38
Yogurt, low-fat	8 oz.	0.11

Warning!

Large doses of pyridoxine can make the drug phenytoin (Dilantin), which helps control epilepsy and seizures, break down too quickly in your system. If you take this drug, talk to your doctor about taking any vitamin supplements before you try them.

Getting the Most from Pyridoxine

The RDA for pyridoxine is in most multivitamin supplements; it's also in B-vitamin formulas, usually in amounts anywhere from 10 to 50 mg. Supplements of pyridoxine alone come in tablets or capsules in sizes ranging from 25 to 500 mg.

Be very, very cautious about taking pyridoxine supplements. This is one of the few water-soluble supplements that you can actually overdose on. Too much pyridoxine causes neurological problems such as numbness or tingling in the hands and feet and trouble walking. The symptoms usually go away if you cut back on the dose, but sometimes they're permanent.

Neurological symptoms usually happen only when you're taking really big doses of more than 2,000 mg a day. Most people can take up to 500 mg a day without any problems, but even 200 mg a day could cause trouble. To be on the safe side, take no more than 50 mg a day of pyridoxine.

You need to have good levels of magnesium—at least the RDA—for pyridoxine to work properly (see Chapter 18 for more information).

Thumbs Up/Thumbs Down

Pyridoxine Is Helped By ...	Pyridoxine Is Hurt By ...
Riboflavin	Alcohol
Vitamin C	Birth-control pills
Magnesium, selenium	Some prescription drugs for asthma, tuberculosis, high blood pressure, and rheumatoid arthritis

Help for Heart Disease

Coming up in Chapter 9 we'll talk a lot about how folic acid combines with pyridoxine and cobalamin to help fight heart disease by breaking down homocysteine. You need all three working together for the maximum effect.

On its own, pyridoxine plays some other roles that also help prevent heart disease. One of the most important is keeping your red blood cells from getting "sticky" and clumping together, or aggregating. When that happens, the cells release powerful chemicals that eventually cause atherosclerosis—deposits that clog up your arteries and can lead to a heart attack or stroke. (Check back to Chapter 2 for more information about atherosclerosis.)

If enough cells clump together, they form a clot that blocks an artery. Again, the result is a heart attack or stroke. If you're at risk for atherosclerosis or already have it, taking pyridoxine supplements could slow down the process. Talk to your doctor before you try it, however.

Here's another interesting fact: people who have just had heart attacks have low levels of pyridoxine. Is this a cause or an effect? Nobody knows, but researchers are looking into it.

Pyridoxine supplements in fairly high doses—about 500 mg a day—can lower your blood pressure. It's cheaper than prescription drugs and doesn't have their side effects, but you do have to worry about the possible side effects of the large dose. Don't try this on your own, especially if you already take medicine to lower your blood pressure. If you want to try pyridoxine, talk to your doctor first.

Preventing Colorectal Cancer

An intriguing 2005 study of nearly 67,000 Swedish women suggests that a high dietary intake of pyridoxine can significantly reduce the risk of colorectal cancer. The study, which looked at women aged 40 to 75, also found that the protective effect is greatest among women who drink moderate to large amounts of alcohol. In that group, those who had the highest pyridoxine intake reduced their risk by 70 percent.

Immune Booster

You need all the B vitamins for your immune system to work correctly, but pyridoxine is the key. Without it, you can't produce enough of the special infection-fighting cells that fend off illness. People with low immunity—alcoholics, the elderly, cancer patients, and others—also usually have low pyridoxine levels.

Elderly people are very vulnerable to illness—and up to a third of all elderly people have low pyridoxine levels. In part, that's because you just absorb less of the Bs from your food as you grow older. It's also because many elderly people don't eat well, especially if they live alone or in a nursing home. The lack of pyridoxine makes them more likely to get sick and also makes them take longer to get better. If you're aged 60 or older or if your immune system isn't working well for some reason, be sure to get plenty of Bs in your diet every day. To be sure you're getting enough, take a good daily multivitamin as well.

Helping Asthma

Some people with asthma benefit from pyridoxine supplements, possibly because their bodies don't use it properly to begin with. Taking extra may bring their pyridoxine level closer to normal, which reduces their wheezing and cuts back on how often they have attacks.

A drug called theophylline is sometimes prescribed for asthma—and also for bronchitis and emphysema. It's an effective treatment, but it has a lot of bad side effects, including headaches, nausea, irritability, tremors, sleeping problems, and even seizures. The side effects are caused because theophylline blocks the way your body uses pyridoxine. Even if you're taking in enough through your food, the drug is keeping you from using it. Pyridoxine supplements have been shown to reduce the side effects of theophylline, especially tremor. If you're taking this drug, talk to your doctor about pyridoxine supplements before you try them.

Preventing Diabetic Complications

People with diabetes sometimes get diabetic neuropathy, a painful nerve condition. The symptoms are similar to the symptoms you would get with severe pyridoxine deficiency—and many diabetics are low on pyridoxine. Is there a connection? Some researchers say yes. They feel diabetic neuropathy could be prevented by taking 150 mg of pyridoxine daily.

If you have diabetes and want to try pyridoxine to treat or prevent diabetic neuropathy, talk to your doctor first (and also see Chapter 24 for information about lipoic acid).

Relief for Carpal Tunnel Syndrome

Your wrist is a marvel of engineering. To make this joint flexible, bones, ligaments, and muscles all come tightly together, leaving only a narrow passage—the carpal tunnel—for the nerves leading to your hand. If anything swells up in your wrist, even a little, it presses on the passage and squeezes the nerves. The result? Carpal tunnel syndrome (CTS), a painful problem that is becoming very common. Symptoms include pain, numbness, and tingling in the fingers, wrist, or hand. Women seem to get CTS more often than men.

A lot of people claim that pyridoxine supplements help or even "cure" CTS. Is there any evidence for this? Not a lot. The most careful studies show that hardly anyone with CTS is deficient or even low in pyridoxine. The studies also show no real benefit from treating CTS just with large doses of pyridoxine—and as we discussed earlier, large doses could be dangerous. It's possible that pyridoxine can help, however, if it's taken in moderate doses (150 mg a day) along with other treatments, such as physical therapy and drugs to relieve the swelling.

Pyridoxine for PMS

Researchers have been looking into pyridoxine for treating PMS since the early 1970s. There have been more than a dozen serious studies, and none of them have proven that pyridoxine does much one way or the other. In the studies, women who took pyridoxine felt that their symptoms—including depression, irritability, headaches, and fluid retention—got better. The problem is that the women who thought they were taking pyridoxine, but were actually taking sugar pills, also felt their symptoms got better.

So should you take pyridoxine for PMS? In a 2006 review of nine earlier studies, researchers concluded that doses of pyridoxine up to 100 mg a day are likely to be of benefit. Studies aside, many of Dr. Pressman's patients really have benefited from this, so we suggest you try taking 50 to 100 mg a day in the days before your period. It won't hurt and there's a good chance it might help.

Other Problems and Pyridoxine

Depending on who you ask, a long list of ailments, from autism to vomiting, is helped by pyridoxine. Not all these claims hold up, but here are a few that do:

◆ **Depression.** Some people hospitalized for depression have low pyridoxine levels and seem to get better if they take supplements. The supplements don't help if their pyridoxine is normal to begin with.

◆ **Kidney stones.** If you get the calcium oxalate type of kidney stone, pyridoxine could keep the stones from coming back. In 2006, results from the ongoing Nurses' Health Study showed that a high dietary intake of pyridoxine worked to lower the risk of kidney stones in women—but results from their counterparts in the all-male Physicians' Health Study showed pyridoxine didn't help men. Talk to your doctor before you try pyridoxine supplements for kidney stones.

◆ **Cancer drug toxicity.** The nasty side effects of some cancer drugs, such as vincristine, may be reduced by extra pyridoxine.

◆ **Morning sickness.** A small daily dose of pyridoxine (25 mg) seems to work for about one out of three women. If nothing else is helping your morning sickness, talk to your doctor about trying pyridoxine.

The Least You Need to Know

◆ Pyridoxine, also called Vitamin B_6, works closely with all the other B vitamins, especially niacin, folic acid, and cobalamin.

◆ You need pyridoxine to convert amino acids into proteins and for turning stored sugar into energy.

◆ Pyridoxine is vital for your immune system and can help prevent heart disease.

◆ The RDA for pyridoxine is 1.3 mg a day for adult men and women. Adults older than age 50 need slightly more.

◆ Pyridoxine is found in high-protein foods such as eggs, fish, poultry, and meat. It's also added to breakfast cereals, bread, and many baked goods.

◆ Pyridoxine supplements in large doses can be toxic.

Chapter 9

Folic Acid: Healthy Babies, Healthy Hearts

In This Chapter

◆ Why you need folic acid (Vitamin B_9)

◆ What foods have high folic acid

◆ How folic acid can help prevent birth defects

◆ How to help your heart with folic acid

◆ How folic acid can help prevent cancer, especially colon cancer

Popeye the Sailor Man always eats his spinach so he'll be strong to the finish. Why does Popeye eat spinach instead of one of those other green, leafy vegetables we keep talking about, such as collard greens, or maybe Swiss chard? Aside from the fact that those vegetables don't rhyme with finish, they don't have anywhere near as much *folic acid*—and you need folic acid to build muscles and to keep your body strong and in good repair.

Spinach gives Popeye lots of muscles and energy. Does it do the same for Olive Oyl? It sure does—and it helped little Swee'pea, too, because folic acid helps prevent birth defects. Folic acid could even help that big bully

Bluto. He's a prime candidate for a heart attack—and the latest research shows that folic acid can help prevent heart disease.

Why You Need Folic Acid

You may not realize it, but your body is constantly making new cells to replace old ones that wear out. Your red blood cells are a good example—every day, you make *millions* of new ones to replace old ones that are too beat up to work well anymore. All those new cells are why you need a good supply of folic acid. Without it, you can't make enough new cells fast enough or well enough. And folic acid is especially important for cells that wear out and divide rapidly, such as red blood cells, skin cells, and the cells that line your small intestine. What it all comes down to is that you need folic acid for the normal growth and maintenance of every cell in your body.

def•i•ni•tion

Researchers in the early 1940s found an interesting substance in spinach leaves. They called it **folic acid** (or folate or folacin) from the Latin word for leaf—*folium*. Folic acid is the synthetic form, whereas folate is the natural form found in foods. For practical purposes, they're the same. If you hang out with organic chemists and want to show off, you can call it *pteroylglutamic acid* or *pteroylmonoglutamate*.

Folic acid does some other amazing things for your health. In the past few years we've learned that folic acid prevents birth defects, helps prevent heart disease, and may even help prevent cancer. The evidence is so convincing that, since 1998, many common grain products, including bread, breakfast cereal, pasta, and rice, have been fortified with extra folic acid by order of the FDA. The amount that's added is 140 mcg per 100 g of grain. An unexpected side benefit of fortification is that it reduces your risk of having a stroke—we'll talk about that more later in this chapter.

The RDA for Folic Acid

In 1989, the RDA for folic acid was lowered by about half. The earlier RDA for adult males, for example, was 400 mcg; this was reduced to 200 mcg. The RDA for women of childbearing age was also cut in half, from 800 mcg to 400 mcg. Studies in the 1980s showed that although the average folic acid intake for all age groups was considerably below the RDA, few people showed any signs of deficiency. So the reasoning went, the RDA should be lowered to the amount taken in on average by most healthy people, because they all seemed to be okay.

The lowered basic amount is a really good example of how the old RDAs gave you just the bare minimum needed to prevent deficiency, and not the amount that leads to good health. At the time, many doctors and nutritionists believed that the RDA was way, way too low. They recommended that *everyone* get at least 400 mcg of folic acid every day, and most said that 800 mcg would be even better. When the new DRIs for B vitamins were issued in the spring of 1998, the RDA for adults was raised back up to 400 mcg—and the RDA for pregnant women was raised to 600 mcg.

The RDA for Folic Acid

Age in Years/Sex	Folic Acid in mcg
Infants	
0 to 0.5	65
0.5 to 1	80
Children	
1 to 3	150
4 to 8	200
9 to 13	300
Adults	
Men 14+	400
Women 14+	400
Pregnant women	600
Nursing women	500

Are You Deficient?

Even after the RDA for folic acid was lowered, studies show that the average American diet contains only about 200 mcg a day—a far cry from the 400 mcg now recommended. Not surprisingly, a shortage of folic acid is one of the most common vitamin deficiencies, especially among women. You could be deficient in folic acid if …

◆ **You're pregnant.** Because your unborn baby is growing fast, he or she is taking a lot of your folic acid. If you're pregnant, your doctor will probably prescribe folic acid supplements. And if you're a woman of childbearing age (between 15 and 47), keep reading—in a little while we'll tell you why you need extra folic acid even if you're not pregnant.

◆ **You're breastfeeding.** You're passing a lot of your folic acid on to your baby, so you need some extra for yourself. And if you don't get enough, your baby may not get enough either.

◆ **You abuse alcohol.** Alcoholics have bad nutrition and don't get enough B vitamins in general. Also, alcohol seems to block your absorption of folic acid.

◆ **You smoke cigarettes.** Smokers are low on all the B vitamins, including folic acid.

◆ **You take birth-control pills.** If you're on the Pill, you could be low on all the B vitamins, but especially folic acid. Talk to your doctor about taking supplements. And even though you're not interested in babies right now, read the "Folic Acid for Healthy Babies" section later in this chapter.

◆ **You take drugs such as phenytoin (Dilantin) for seizures, sulfasalazine (Azulfidine) for inflammatory bowel disease, or trimethoprim (Proloprim) for urinary-tract infections.** Many drugs keep you from absorbing enough folic acid (see the chart for a longer list).

◆ **You take methotrexate (Folex or Rheumatrex) for rheumatoid arthritis, psoriasis, or inflammatory bowel disease.** This drug blocks your uptake of folic acid. Recent studies have proven that folic acid supplements help you tolerate the drug better. If you take this medicine, talk to your doctor about folic acid supplements.

◆ **You're older than 65.** Many elderly people, especially if they live alone or in a nursing home, don't get enough folic acid from their food. That's partly because their ability to absorb folic acid has dropped, and partly because they tend to eat foods low in folic acid to begin with.

If you suddenly become deficient in folic acid, it could be an indication that you have cancer. The rapidly growing cancer cells are using up your folic acid to fuel their uncontrolled division.

Drugs That Block Folic Acid

Drug	Used For
Anticonvulsants	Preventing seizures
Chloramphenicol	Bacterial infections
Cortisone drugs	Severe inflammation, arthritis
Methotrexate	Rheumatoid arthritis

Drug	Used For
Oral contraceptives	Preventing pregnancy
Pyrimethamine	Intestinal parasites
Quinine	Malaria
Sulfasalazine	Ulcerative colitis
Sulfa drugs	Infection
Trimethoprim	Urinary-tract infections

Folic acid deficiency affects the growth and repair of your body's tissues. The tissues that have the fastest rate of cell replacement are the first ones to be affected, so your blood and digestive tract are where the signs of deficiency will most likely first appear. If you're deficient in folic acid, you might have some of these symptoms:

◆ Anemia

◆ Nausea and loss of appetite

◆ Diarrhea

◆ Malnutrition from poor nutrient absorption

◆ Weight loss

◆ Weakness

◆ Sore tongue

◆ Headaches

◆ Irritability and mood swings

◆ Heart palpitations

Hardly anyone in today's society will be seriously deficient in folic acid just from eating too much junk food. It's much more likely that deficiency symptoms such as anemia, malnutrition, and heart palpitations will appear in someone who is an alcoholic or has some other severe health problem that keeps them from eating or digesting properly.

> **Now You're Cooking**
>
> Beans are an excellent natural source of folic acid—but there is that embarrassing little problem: beans produce gas. To reduce the problem, soak dried beans in nine cups of water for every cup of beans. Drain the beans and change the water at least twice during the 24-hour soaking period. Drain and rinse well before using. If you're using canned beans, drain and rinse well before using.

Mild deficiencies are likely for people who eat only institutional food—nursing-home residents, for example. That's because the folic acid in food is easily destroyed by processing, overcooking, or reheating.

In general, if you're deficient in folic acid, you're likely to be deficient in the other B vitamins as well. It's almost always from poor diet or poor absorption, so eating better and taking supplements if needed will usually solve the problem.

Eating Your Folic Acid

As you can see from the chart, folic acid isn't found in that many animal foods. The only good animal sources are chicken liver and beef liver; there's hardly any in milk and other dairy foods. Beans of all kinds are a great way to get your folic acid. Other good plant sources are spinach and asparagus. On the whole, most fruits don't contain much folic acid. The best choices are bananas, oranges, and cantaloupe.

The Folic Acid in Food

Food	Amount	Folic Acid in mcg
Asparagus, cooked	½ cup	132
Avocado	½ medium	56
Banana	1 medium	22
Beets, cooked	½ cup	45
Black beans	1 cup	256
Black-eyed peas	1 cup	123
Bread, whole-wheat	1 slice	14
Broccoli, cooked	½ cup	39
Brussels sprouts, cooked	½ cup	47
Cantaloupe	1 cup	27
Chickpeas	1 cup	282
Collard greens, cooked	½ cup	65
Corn, kernels	1 cup	38
Endive, raw	½ cup	36
Kidney beans	1 cup	229
Lentils	1 cup	358
Lima beans, baby	1 cup	273
Liver, beef	3 oz.	200

Food	Amount	Folic Acid in mcg
Liver, chicken	3 oz.	660
Navy beans	1 cup	255
Orange	1 medium	47
Peanuts, dry-roasted	1 oz.	41
Romaine lettuce	½ cup	38
Spinach, raw	½ cup	54
Spinach, cooked	½ cup	131
Wheat germ	¼ cup	82

Even if you regularly eat lots of beans and fresh vegetables, it's hard to get enough folic acid through your diet alone. That's because you absorb only about half of the folic acid you eat. Also, a lot of it is lost in processing and cooking. Cook fresh veggies lightly in as little water as possible to preserve the folic acid.

Is It Working?

Because most Americans don't begin to eat enough beans and fresh vegetables, as of 1998 the FDA began to require folic acid fortification of breads, flours, cornmeal, rice, noodles, pasta, and other grain products, with the goal of making sure everyone gets at least 400 mcg a day from their food. Is it working? According to an important study in *The New England Journal of Medicine* in 1999, yes. After flour fortification was instituted, the folic acid levels of a study population went up 117 percent, and the percentage of individuals with low folic acid levels dropped by 92 percent. Average folic acid levels doubled between 1998 and 2000, and folic acid deficiency went from 16 percent of the population to 0.5 percent. Most significant of all, a study by the Centers for Disease Control and Prevention found that between 1995 and 2002, there were significant decreases in the prevalence of spina bifida and anencephaly. We'll talk more about these two neural tube birth defects a little later in this chapter.

Getting the Most from Folic Acid

Like the other B vitamins, folic acid is water-soluble. That means your body can't really store it, so it's important to get enough every day.

Folic acid works closely with the other B vitamins, especially pyridoxine, cobalamin, and choline. If you're low on any of the Bs, you're probably low on folic acid as well— and vice versa. You may need to take a complete B supplement.

Vitamin C prevents folic acid from being broken down too quickly in your body. Most nutritionists today strongly recommend getting at least 500 mg of Vitamin C every day. Virtually all multivitamin supplements, especially those formulated for women, contain 400 mcg of folic acid.

It's almost impossible to overdose on folic acid. Any excess just comes out harmlessly in your urine—although if you take a lot, your urine will have a bright-yellow color.

Most doctors recommend taking no more than 1 mg a day in supplements. The reasoning is that taking larger amounts could mask the serious type of anemia caused by a deficiency of cobalamin. If the deficiency isn't discovered in time, you could have permanent nerve damage. It's a good point, but it may be too cautious. Anemia from cobalamin deficiency is actually fairly rare, and it almost always occurs in older adults. Overall, your chances of getting heart disease or colon cancer are much higher—and as we'll see, folic acid could really lower those odds.

Thumbs Up/Thumbs Down

Folic Acid Is Helped By ...	Folic Acid Is Hurt By ...
All other B vitamins	Alcohol
Vitamin C	Anticonvulsant drugs, especially phenytoin (Dilantin)
	Birth-control pills
	Many other prescription drugs

Folic Acid for Healthy Babies

Recent studies have conclusively shown that taking 400 mcg of folic acid each day *before* getting pregnant can prevent between 50 and 75 percent of all neural tube defects (NTD), especially the crippling defect spina bifida, or "open spine," which occurs when the vertebrae don't form a complete ring to protect the spine. Sometimes the brain never develops at all, a rare and always fatal condition called anencephaly. In 1992, the U.S. Public Health Service recommended that *all* women of childbearing age consume 400 mcg of folic acid daily. Every agency and organization concerned with birth defects, from the FDA to the March of Dimes, strongly endorsed this recommendation. And in 1998, the RDA was raised to 600 mcg a day for pregnant women. Why the jump?

Your unborn baby needs folic acid the most during the first month of pregnancy, when the neural tube is formed—but you might not realize you're pregnant during that critical time, even if you've been trying to have a baby. Also, some recent studies in the Netherlands suggest that women with high folic-acid levels have fewer miscarriages. It's vitally important for every woman to get enough folic acid. If you're a woman between the ages of 15 and 47, the time to start taking folic-acid supplements is *now*.

Since the FDA began mandating folic acid fortification of grain-based foods in 1998, the number of severe brain and spinal birth defects has dropped 27 percent overall. Spina bifida cases dropped 31 percent, and anenecephaly cases dropped 16 percent. A 2005 study in Utah showed that in that state, overall neural tube birth defects dropped 50 percent between 1992 and 2003, simply because of folic acid fortification and supplements for pregnant women.

Other studies have shown some unexpected side benefits of folic acid fortification and supplementation. A diet rich in folic acid may cut the risk of having a baby with a cleft palate or low birth weight. The benefits of maternal folic acid may help the child even after birth. A study in Canada showed that the incidence of neuroblastoma, a deadly childhood brain cancer, has dropped 60 percent since Canada began requiring folic acid fortification in 1997.

Two myths about folic acid and pregnancy need to be debunked. First, folic acid fortification and supplementation does not increase the likelihood of having twins. Second, folic acid fortification and supplementation does not increase the likelihood of having a miscarriage—but having low folic acid levels does, by nearly 50 percent.

Folic Acid and Heart Disease

Like most health-conscious people, you already know that high cholesterol is a warning sign of possible heart disease. The cholesterol clogs your arteries and can eventually lead to a heart attack. So you've been watching your diet and cutting back on how much fat you eat—and at your last checkup, your cholesterol level was well within the normal range. "That's good," you thought, "at least I don't have to worry about having a heart attack."

We hate to break the news to you, but you still have to worry. The fact is, most people who have a first heart attack have *normal* cholesterol levels—but their arteries are still clogged. If cholesterol isn't causing the problem, what is?

The answer could be high blood levels of *homocysteine*, an amino acid found naturally in your body as a byproduct of metabolizing the essential amino acid methionine.

Researchers theorize that homocysteine damages the lining of your arteries. The next question is, what causes the homocysteine to build up to high levels? The answer is not enough folic acid. Working with pyridoxine and cobalamin, folic acid quickly breaks down the homocysteine and removes it from your body. Today we've come to realize that high homocysteine levels by themselves are a warning sign of possible heart trouble—and also indicate a raised risk of having a stroke. But does lowering your homocysteine level reduce the risk? That's an extremely controversial question that has been debated for years. The answer, based on three major studies published in 2006, seems to be probably not. In all three studies, patients at high risk of heart disease or stroke were given supplements of folic acid, pyridoxine, and cobalamin or a placebo. In all three studies, the patients taking the B vitamins saw a drop in their homocysteine levels—but they had just as many heart attacks and strokes as the people taking the placebo. The researchers concluded that homocysteine isn't damaging in itself, but that it is a marker for heart disease and stroke, just as fever is a marker for infection.

def•i•ni•tion

Homocysteine is an amino acid formed when other amino acids in your blood are broken down by normal body processes. Folic acid breaks down the homocysteine into methionine and prevents a buildup.

All the people in the studies were already at risk—they had diabetes or documented heart disease, or had already had a heart attack or stroke. What the studies still don't tell us is whether people who start taking the supplements before they have health problems will reduce their long-term risk of heart disease or stroke. All in all, making sure you get at least the RDA for folic acid is good insurance for heart health.

Folic Acid and Blood Pressure

Another unexpected side benefit of folic acid fortification could be preventing high blood pressure. Again, the obliging women of the Nurses' Health Study show how. Researchers looked at nearly 94,000 participants ages 27 to 44 and found that those who took in at least 1,000 mcg a day of total folic acid, from food and supplements, decreased their risk of high blood pressure by 46 percent compared to the women who took in only 200 mcg or less a day. Among a second group of more than 62,000 women aged 43 to 70, those with the highest folic acid intake had a 13 percent reduced risk of high blood pressure. None of the women had high blood pressure when the study started. Interestingly, the women in the study who got their folic acid only from food and didn't take supplements saw no decrease in their risk of high blood pressure—a clear example of the value of supplements.

Why does folic acid help? Researchers theorize that it relaxes the lining of the blood vessels, which lowers blood pressure. They think it's also possible that lowering homocysteine helps.

Folic Acid and Stroke

In 2002, a study in the journal *Stroke* reported that a diet rich in folic acid may reduce the risk of stroke. The researchers followed nearly 10,000 men and women aged 25 to 74 for 20 years. In that time, the people who consumed at least 300 mcg of dietary folic acid daily had a 20 percent lower risk of stroke.

A 2006 study in *Circulation*, the journal of the American Heart Association, reported that deaths from strokes in the United States and Canada dropped sharply after folic acid fortification of food became law in 1998. Deaths from stroke had been dropping by about 0.3 percent a year before fortification began. After 1998, however, the death rate began to drop by 2.9 percent. Similar rates weren't seen in countries without fortification, such as England.

Why does folic acid have such a dramatic effect on stroke risk? Researchers believe that a reduction in homocysteine could be the reason. The studies only show an association, however, not cause and effect. Even so, this is another example of why it's so important to get at least 400 mcg of folic acid every day.

> **Warning!**
>
> Folic acid keeps the drug vitamin phenytoin (Dilantin) and most other anticonvulsant drugs from working properly. Do not take folic acid supplements if you take these drugs. Discuss all vitamin supplements with your doctor before you try them.

Preventing Cancer with Folic Acid

For a long time, cancer researchers were so focused on the powerful antioxidant Vitamins A, C, and E that they sort of forgot about the B vitamins. Recently, though, folic acid has been getting a lot of attention for its role in preventing cancer of the colon, cervix, and breast—and maybe for preventing other cancers as well.

Folic Acid Helps Prevent Colon Cancer

Recent studies show that people with low folic acid levels are more likely to get colon cancer. If you're a woman and get a lot of folic acid in your diet, for instance, your chances of colon cancer are sharply lower—by as much as 60 percent. (For some reason, this doesn't work as well for men.)

If you have a family history of colon cancer (a parent or sibling with the disease), folic acid could sharply lower your risk of getting it yourself. Again, the women of the Nurses' Health Study provided the clues to researchers. First they looked at the health histories of nearly 89,000 participants to find those with a family history of colon cancer. They then compared the diets of those women to those of the rest to see what behaviors were related to the risk of getting colon cancer. They found that among the women with a family history of colon cancer, those who ate diets high in folic acid and limited their intake of alcohol had a risk of colon cancer that was the same as women with no family history. The women with a family history who had a low folic acid intake and drank more alcohol were 2.5 times more likely to develop colon cancer than the women with no family history.

The study was only of women, but it's likely that men can benefit as well. If colorectal cancer runs in your family, a diet rich in folic acid and low in alcohol may help reduce your risk. Discuss your risk with your doctor. Diet can help, but it's also important to have regular colonoscopies to detect polyps and any cancer early on.

People with ulcerative colitis (UC), a serious chronic disease of the large intestine, have an increased risk of getting colon cancer—and they also often have low folic acid levels. For many patients, the reason is that the drug sulfasalazine (Azulfidin), which is used to treat UC, also blocks their uptake of folic acid. Recent studies show that UC patients who take 1 mg a day of extra folic acid cut their chances of colon cancer nearly in half. If you have ulcerative colitis, discuss folic acid supplements with your doctor before you try them.

Preventing Cervical Cancer

Women with cervical dysplasia may later develop cancer of the cervix, especially if the problem isn't detected and treated early on. Many women infected with human papillomavirus (HPV) have cervical dysplasia. Women who smoke are more likely to have cervical dysplasia, probably because smokers have low folic acid levels.

Recent studies have shown that women with HPV *and* low folic acid levels were five times more likely to have cervical dysplasia. Other studies suggest that minor cervical dysplasia can be effectively treated with large doses (more than 5 mg daily) of folic acid. This is not something you should do on your own, however. If you have cervical dysplasia, discuss all your treatment options with your doctor.

Preventing Breast Cancer

Regularly drinking alcohol (one drink or more a day) is known to increase a woman's risk of breast cancer, especially after menopause. A study in 2001 showed that women who drink more than half a glass of alcohol daily and also have low intakes of folic acid are 59 percent more likely to develop breast cancer. The study also showed that the risk from alcohol can be lowered by taking 400 mcg of supplemental folic acid every day. Another study in 2003 backed this up, showing that among women who had at least one alcoholic drink a day, those with the highest levels of folic acid were 89 percent less likely to get breast cancer than those with the lowest levels.

Alcohol interferes with your body's absorption of folic acid and also makes you excrete more folic acid through the kidneys. You need folic acid to keep your DNA functioning normally, so it's possible that low levels may cause breast cancer by damaging your genetic material. If you drink alcohol—and even if you don't—be sure to get your 400 mcg of folic acid every day.

Folic Acid and Other Cancers

The research is still preliminary in many cases, but high levels of folic acid are linked to lower rates of some other cancers as well:

◆ **Childhood leukemia.** The children of mothers who take folic acid supplements during pregnancy are less likely to get acute lymphoblastic leukemia, the most common childhood cancer in industrialized countries.

◆ **Ovarian cancer.** A 2004 study in Sweden found that women who got at least 200 mcg daily of dietary folic acid had a reduced risk of developing this dangerous cancer. Among women who also drank alcohol, the risk was reduced even more.

◆ **Pancreatic cancer.** Another study from Sweden in 2006 found that folic acid from food may help prevent this deadly cancer. Participants who took in 350 mcg a day were 75 percent less likely to develop pancreatic cancer compared to participants who took in under 200 mcg a day.

◆ **Prostate cancer.** Getting a lot of folic acid in your diet doesn't seem to reduce the risk of getting prostate cancer, but it does seem to slow it down a bit.

Folic Acid and Depression

Could it be that eating more dark-green, leafy vegetables can lift your mood? Quite possibly. A study of depressed outpatients at Massachusetts General Hospital showed that low folic acid levels are linked to depression. The most depressed patients in the study had the lowest levels of folic acid—and were the least likely to benefit from antidepressant drugs. Studies in Finland and Denmark in 2004 showed similar results, although they didn't look at the effect of antidepressants.

The Least You Need to Know

- Folic acid, also called folate or folacin, is a B vitamin.

- Foods high in folic acid include chicken liver and all kinds of beans, spinach, and asparagus.

- The adult RDA for folic acid is 400 mcg for adult men and women and 600 mcg for pregnant women.

- All women of childbearing age should get at least 400 mcg of folic acid (through daily supplements if necessary) to prevent birth defects.

- Folic acid may help stroke and high blood pressure.

- Folic acid may help prevent cancer, especially cancer of the cervix, breast, and colon.

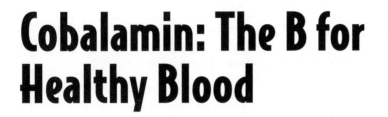
Cobalamin: The B for Healthy Blood

In This Chapter

- ◆ Why you need cobalamin (Vitamin B_{12})
- ◆ Where to find foods high in cobalamin
- ◆ How cobalamin prevents and treats anemia
- ◆ Why you need more cobalamin as you get older

Until recently, doctors and nutritionists didn't pay much attention to cobalamin. Sure, we know you need it to keep your red blood cells healthy, but as long as you didn't actually have anemia, we figured you were getting enough. After all, the amount you need is the tiniest of any vitamin—just a few mcg a day.

Well, we were wrong. Even that tiny amount is essential—not just for your blood, but for a lot of other things, including preventing heart disease, keeping your mind sharp as you grow older, and keeping your immune system working in top gear. And because so little has to do so much, you need to be absolutely, positively sure you're getting enough.

Why You Need Cobalamin

Cobalamin does plenty for you, but let's start with its most important role: making healthy red blood cells. If you eat enough cobalamin, and if your body can use it properly, you make millions of nice, round, healthy red blood cells every day. If you don't eat enough, or you can't use it properly, you can't make enough red blood cells, and the ones you do make are too large and fragile to work well. When you don't have enough red blood cells to carry oxygen and nutrients around your body, you develop anemia (we'll talk about this a lot more in a little while).

def•i•ni•tion

Vitamin B$_{12}$ is called **cobalamin** because it contains the trace element cobalt. The form of Vitamin B$_{12}$ used in vitamin pills is *cyanocobalamin*. The *cyano-* part comes from *cyanide*, which is also in this vitamin—but don't worry, the amounts are very, very small, far too tiny to harm you.

All your cells, not just your red blood cells, need cobalamin to grow and divide properly. For example, you need it to make all the different cells in your immune system, including white blood cells.

Cobalamin's next big role is in making the protective fatty layer, or sheath, that coats your nerve cells—sort of like insulation on electric wires. If the sheath is damaged because you don't have enough cobalamin, you start getting the equivalent of static on the line. Really bad static can interfere with your mental function—so much that people think you're senile.

Cobalamin is a team player. Working with the other B vitamins, but especially with pyridoxine and folic acid, it helps you turn the carbs, fats, and proteins in your food into energy in your cells.

The RDA for Cobalamin

Important as cobalamin is, you need only very small amounts of it. That's why the RDA for an adult is less than 3 mcg. But there's a big problem with that RDA. It doesn't take into account the fact that you absorb less cobalamin as you get older. We'll talk more about why that's so and what to do about it later in this chapter. For now, let's just say that many doctors and nutritionists feel that people older than age 50 need a lot more cobalamin. Doctors usually recommend daily supplements containing 500 to 1,000 mcg. It's a safe and inexpensive form of health insurance. At the least, check the RDA chart to be sure you're getting the minimum.

The RDA for Cobalamin

Age in Years/Sex	Cobalamin in mcg
Infants	
0 to 0.5	0.4
0.5 to 1	0.5
Children	
1 to 3	0.9
4 to 8	1.2
9 to 13	1.8
Adults	
14+	2.4
Pregnant women	2.6
Nursing women	2.8

Are You Deficient?

That's an important question, because it can be hard to tell. To understand why, we'll have to explain how cobalamin gets into your body. Cobalamin is found only in animal foods such as liver, eggs, fish, and meat—and only in very small amounts that are hard to take in. To get even the small amount of cobalamin you need, your body needs to be really good at absorbing it. In fact, you make a special substance in your stomach, called *intrinsic factor*, just to help you do that—and even that lets you absorb only about half the cobalamin you eat. Fortunately, most people take in more than twice the RDA through their diet, so they usually get enough.

def•i•ni•tion

To absorb cobalamin from your food, your stomach naturally secretes a special substance called **intrinsic factor**. Without it, you can't absorb cobalamin.

On the other hand, recent studies suggest that cobalamin deficiency might be more common than we think. For example, middle-aged and older women who get the RDA every day can still show signs of mild cobalamin deficiency. The problem goes away when they raise their daily intake to 6 mcg. Another study suggests that 39 percent of the population have low-normal levels of cobalamin and 17 percent have levels low enough to be deficient. Some researchers believe that the adult RDA should be raised to 6 mcg to prevent deficiency across the board, not just in older people.

Although cobalamin is a water-soluble vitamin, you still store some of it in your liver and kidneys. Also, your body is really good at recycling cobalamin, so you don't use up your body stores very quickly.

def•i•ni•tion

Anemia is a general term meaning your red blood cells either don't have enough *hemoglobin* (the stuff that carries oxygen) or you have a below-normal number of them. **Megaloblastic anemia** (sometimes called *macrocytic anemia*) happens when you don't get enough cobalamin in your diet. **Pernicious anemia** happens when your stomach, for reasons nobody really understands, stops making intrinsic factor and you are unable to absorb cobalamin from your food.

What we're leading up to here is that if you don't get much cobalamin in your diet, it could take a long time—4 or 5 years—for deficiency symptoms to start showing up. Sometimes people slowly stop making intrinsic factor, but here, too, it could take several years for real deficiency symptoms to appear.

The most obvious symptom of cobalamin deficiency is *anemia*—in this case, because you don't have enough healthy red blood cells. When the anemia comes from a shortage of cobalamin in the diet, it's called *megaloblastic anemia*. When it comes from a lack of intrinsic factor, it's called *pernicious anemia*. The causes are different, but the result is the same: you don't have enough red blood cells, and the ones you do have are too big and fragile to survive long in your circulation.

Who's at Risk?

On the whole, most people younger than 50 get enough cobalamin from their diet, but older people and some others are at real risk for a deficiency. You might be in that category if …

◆ **You're a strict vegetarian or vegan.** Because cobalamin is found naturally only in animal foods, people who don't eat these foods can be deficient if they don't take supplements. Kids are especially at risk. (If you don't eat animal foods, be sure to read the section on eating cobalamin later in this chapter.)

◆ **You're older than age 50.** As you get older, you naturally make less intrinsic factor and absorb less cobalamin. Sometimes you stop making intrinsic factor completely. You also make less stomach acid, which means less cobalamin gets released from your food while it's in your stomach.

◆ **You're breastfeeding.** Your growing baby is taking a lot of your cobalamin. You need to get extra in your food or through supplements.

◆ **You smoke cigarettes.** Smokers have low blood levels of cobalamin and all the other B vitamins.

◆ **You regularly take the drug omeprazole (Prilosec), famotidine (Pepcid), ranitidine (Zantac), or similar acid-reducing drugs to treat severe heartburn or ulcers.** These drugs interfere with your absorption of cobalamin—talk to your doctor about supplements.

◆ **You take the drug metformin (Glucophage) to treat high blood sugar or Type 2 diabetes.** This drug causes reduced absorption of cobalamin. Talk to your doctor about supplements.

◆ **You've been taking prescription potassium supplements for a long time.** These drugs can interfere with your absorption of cobalamin—talk to your doctor about supplements.

◆ **You've had part of your stomach surgically removed or have had gastric bypass surgery.** You might not be making enough intrinsic factor in what's left of your stomach. Discuss supplements with your doctor.

Long before you actually get anemic, you could be having other cobalamin deficiency symptoms, especially if you're an older adult. Early symptoms often show up in your nervous system, such as the following:

◆ Tingling or a "pins-and-needles" feeling in the hands and feet

◆ Numbness in the hands or feet

◆ Moodiness and depression

◆ Trouble sleeping

◆ Memory loss

◆ Dizziness and loss of balance

◆ Dementia

> **Now You're Cooking**
>
> People who don't eat animal foods often rely on soybean foods such as tempeh, miso, and soy milk for their cobalamin. However, many soy products contain very little cobalamin, even when the labels say otherwise. Plant foods such as spirulina, sea vegetables, shiitake mushrooms, and brewer's yeast don't have cobalamin in a form your body can use. To be on the safe side, take cobalamin supplements.

These symptoms can slowly develop even when blood tests show that your cobalamin level is "normal." If you're elderly, they might be mistaken for dementia—except

Great-Grandpa might be getting depressed, forgetful, and shaky on his legs not from old age but from a simple vitamin deficiency. That's bad enough, but what's worse is that the damage could be permanent if the deficiency isn't fixed soon.

Cobalamin deficiency in the elderly has other serious effects. Recent research shows that being short on cobalamin is associated with a twofold risk of severe depression in older women. And another very interesting result shows that elderly women with hearing loss are low on cobalamin compared to women the same age with normal hearing.

By the time your cobalamin deficiency shows up on a blood test, you're not doing very well. You're getting sick more often because you're making fewer infection-fighting white blood cells. You can't replace the cells that line your intestines quickly enough, so you have diarrhea, appetite loss, and vomiting. Finally, you have anemia symptoms. This is unmistakable, because you'll be unbelievably tired and weak. You'll also be very pale and bruise easily. If you start getting more cobalamin, though, your symptoms will quickly disappear.

Eating Your Cobalamin

Only animal foods such as meat, fish, and eggs naturally have cobalamin in them (it's added to some breakfast cereals). As you can see from the chart, even then they don't have much—but on the other hand, you don't need much, so most people get enough from their diet.

The big exceptions are people who are strict vegetarians or vegans, or follow a macro-biotic diet. Because they eat no meat and sometimes no animal foods at all, they have to get their cobalamin from some other source. That source is usually soybean foods, but these probably don't provide enough, especially for children. If you don't eat meat or animal foods, we strongly suggest that you take cobalamin supplements. Which foods in the following list do you eat regularly?

The Cobalamin in Foods

Food	Amount	Cobalamin in mcg
Beef, ground	3 oz.	2.1
Beef liver	3 oz.	68.0
Cheddar cheese	1 oz.	0.23
Chicken leg	1 medium	0.35
Chicken liver	3 oz.	16.6

Food	Amount	Cobalamin in mcg
Clams, steamed	3 oz.	84.06
Cottage cheese, low-fat	1 cup	1.43
Egg	1 large	0.56
Flounder	3 oz.	2.13
Liverwurst	1 slice	2.42
Milk, low-fat	8 oz.	0.90
Pâté de foie gras	1 oz.	2.66
Swiss cheese	1 oz.	0.48
Tuna, light, in water	3 oz.	2.54
Yogurt, low-fat	8 oz.	1.28

Getting the Most from Cobalamin

Generally speaking, people who are deficient in cobalamin are eating enough of it—the problem is that they're not absorbing it because they don't have enough intrinsic factor.

In the 1920s, researchers found that if people with pernicious anemia ate a pound of raw beef liver every day, they got better. Until 1948, when cobalamin was finally isolated, choking down a hefty daily dose of raw liver was the only treatment.

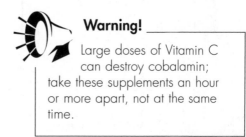

Warning!

Large doses of Vitamin C can destroy cobalamin; take these supplements an hour or more apart, not at the same time.

Fortunately, today you can take cobalamin supplements as tablets or capsules. (If you actually *like* the disgusting taste of slimy raw liver, go right ahead and get it that way instead.) The supplements usually have anywhere from 100 to 500 mcg. Even 100 mcg is a lot more than the RDA, but it's virtually impossible to overdose on cobalamin—any excess is just excreted.

If you're taking supplements because your diet is low in cobalamin, you may also be low in the other B vitamins. Folic acid needs cobalamin to work properly, so it's important to be sure you're getting all your Bs.

Food for Thought _____

Some people prefer to take cobalamin supplements sublingually—that is, under the tongue. Sublingual cobalamin supplements are usually flavored lozenges containing 1,000 mcg or more. You put one under your tongue and let it slowly dissolve; the cobalamin is absorbed straight into your bloodstream. If you have pernicious anemia, talk to your doctor about sublingual cobalamin supplements before you try them. When you're first diagnosed with the problem, you may need eight weekly shots or so to raise your cobalamin level back to normal.

If you're taking cobalamin because you don't make enough intrinsic factor to absorb it from your food, will you be able to absorb it from a pill? Good question. A lot of doctors would say no and make you come in for shots instead. But in fact, if the supplement dose is big enough (1,000 to 2,000 mcg), you will absorb enough from it, even if you don't make any intrinsic factor at all. If you have pernicious or megaloblastic anemia, discuss oral cobalamin supplements with your doctor before you try them.

Thumbs Up/Thumbs Down

Cobalamin Is Helped By ...	Cobalamin Is Hurt By ...
All other B vitamins	Folic acid deficiency
Calcium	Iron deficiency
	Large doses of Vitamin C
	Vitamin E deficiency

The Least You Need to Know

◆ Cobalamin, also called Vitamin B_{12}, is a water-soluble B vitamin.

◆ You need cobalamin for healthy red blood cells, to make the outer coverings of your nerves, and for a healthy immune system.

◆ Cobalamin is found only in animal foods such as liver, eggs, fish, and meat.

◆ The adult RDA for cobalamin is just 2.4 mcg—most people get more than enough from their food.

◆ As you get older, your ability to absorb cobalamin decreases.

Pantothenic Acid: It's Everywhere

In This Chapter

◆ Why you need pantothenic acid (Vitamin B$_5$)

◆ Which foods are high in pantothenic acid

◆ How pantothenic acid produces energy

◆ Why athletes need pantothenic acid

It's kind of nice to know that there's one vitamin you won't ever be deficient in—pantothenic acid. At least some pantothenic acid is found in every single food you eat, so there's no way you can't get enough. That's good, because you need pantothenic acid for turning those foods into energy.

Important as pantothenic acid is, it's one of those quiet types that just does its job without much fanfare. The noise about pantothenic acid comes from people who make a lot of claims for it. Do you need it to make hormones and healthy red blood cells? Definitely yes. Does it boost athletic performance, fix high cholesterol, and stop your hair from turning gray? Definitely maybe.

Why You Need Pantothenic Acid

The fats and carbohydrates you eat get turned into energy you can use with the vital help of *pantothenic acid.* To be exact, you need pantothenic acid to make two crucial coenzymes: coenzyme A (CoA) and acyl carrier protein (ACP). These enzymes help you use fats and carbs to make energy; you also need them for making some important hormones, for making healthy red blood cells, and for making Vitamin D (we'll talk about that more in Chapter 14). They're so important that just about all the pantothenic acid you get from your food is immediately turned into CoA and ACP—there's not really any left over to do anything else.

def•i•ni•tion

Pantothenic acid gets its name from the Greek word *pantothen,* meaning "from all sides." That's because pantothenic acid is found in every food.

Pantethine, a byproduct produced when your body metabolizes pantothenic acid, is also available in supplements. Although pantethine is derived from pantothenic acid, the two aren't interchangeable. Pantethine is more active in the production of CoA.

Adequate Intake

Most vitamins and minerals have established RDAs, guidelines that tell you the amount you need for basic good health. Pantothenic acid is an exception. It's the first (but not the last) supplement without an RDA that we'll discuss in this book.

Why isn't there an RDA for pantothenic acid? The Institute of Medicine scientists (the people who decide these things) have found that the average American gets between 4 and 10 mg of pantothenic acid every day. That must be enough to keep you healthy, because nobody's ever been deficient in it. And if nobody's deficient, why bother figuring out an RDA? Instead, pantothenic acid has an Adequate Intake, as you can see from the chart.

Adequate Intake for Pantothenic Acid

Age in Years/Sex	Pantothenic Acid in mg
Infants	
0 to 0.5	1.7
0.5 to 1	1.8

Age in Years/Sex	Pantothenic Acid in mg
Children	
1 to 3	2.0
4 to 8	3.0
9 to 13	4.0
Adults	
14+	5.0
Pregnant women	6.0
Nursing women	7.0

Are You Deficient?

You'd have to deliberately work at it to be deficient in pantothenic acid. It's never been reported in humans, except for test subjects. In fact, there isn't even a lab test for detecting it. The only people really at risk for a deficiency are long-term alcoholics. Anyone else who's a little low also is almost certainly low on the other Bs as well.

Eating Your Pantothenic Acid

Some pantothenic acid is found in just about every food you eat, animal or vegetable—the chart gives a sample but is by no means comprehensive. Organ meats, salmon, eggs, beans, milk, and whole grains are the best sources. As with the other B vitamins, a lot of pantothenic acid is lost when grains are milled into flour. Although the other Bs are added back, pantothenic acid isn't, so processed grain foods such as bread, pasta, rice, breakfast cereal, and baked goods aren't good sources.

The Pantothenic Acid in Food

Food	Amount	Pantothenic Acid in mg
Beef, ground	3 oz.	0.23
Beef liver	3 oz.	3.9
Black beans	1 cup	0.42

continues

The Pantothenic Acid in Food   (continued)

Food	Amount	Pantothenic Acid in mg
Broccoli, cooked	½ cup	0.40
Chicken leg, with skin	1 medium	1.32
Chicken liver	3 oz.	4.63
Chickpeas	1 cup	0.72
Corn	½ cup	0.72
Egg	1 large	0.70
Lentils	1 cup	1.26
Lima beans	1 cup	0.79
Milk	1 cup	0.77
Mushrooms, cooked	½ cup	1.69
Oatmeal	1 cup	0.47
Potato, baked with skin	1 medium	1.12
Sweet potato	1 medium	0.74
Tomato	1 medium	0.30
Tuna, canned in water	3 oz.	0.18
Wheat germ	¼ cup	0.66
Yogurt, low-fat	1 cup	1.34

Getting the Most from Pantothenic Acid

Pantothenic acid is one of the lesser-known members of the B team. It works best when you also have plenty of the other Bs, especially thiamin, riboflavin, niacin, pyridoxine, and biotin.

Warning!

If you take the drug levodopa for Parkinson's disease, do not take pantothenic acid supplements! They will interfere with the proper activity of the drug. Your doctor will explain the best way to take levodopa.

Pantothenic acid is sometimes called the "anti-stress" vitamin. That's because you make more of some hormones that need pantothenic acid, such as adrenaline, when you're under a lot of stress. If that's the case for you, some nutritionists suggest taking extra pantothenic acid. It can't hurt, but we don't think it will really help.

Pantothenic acid supplements usually contain calcium pantothenate in tablets or capsules. Just as there's no

RDA for pantothenic acid, there's no real overdose level. People who take very large doses (10 to 20 g a day) may get diarrhea, but there are no other known side effects. Any excess is excreted in your urine.

Pantethine supplements are also very safe, with no known side effects or overdose level. They're expensive, though, and so far there really aren't any good reasons to take them.

Another form of pantothenic acid called *panthoderm* is available in skin creams and lotions. It's useful for soothing cuts, scrapes, and mild burns.

Helping High Cholesterol

Pantothenic acid doesn't do a thing for high cholesterol, but it's possible that pantethine does. The research is still in the early stages, but it seems that pantethine may help lower your overall cholesterol and triglycerides—if your levels are high to begin with. It may also help raise your HDL ("good") cholesterol level. The research is promising, because even really large doses of pantethine have no side effects, but we're a long way from being able to recommend it.

Pantothenic Acid for Pentathletes

If you're already an athlete in really good shape—and we mean ready for the Olympics—pantothenic acid might improve your performance just a little bit. Bodybuilders, long-distance runners, and other serious athletes claim that pantothenic acid helps them train harder. There's only one serious study to back them up, but that one showed that long-distance runners who took 2 g a day out-performed those who didn't, though not by a lot. If you're just an ordinary weekend warrior, taking pantothenic acid won't help at all.

Quack, Quack, QUACK!

We usually have only one or two examples of real quackery for a particular supplement, but there are so many silly claims for pantothenic acid that we need a whole section.

◆ **Boosts immunity.** Actually, there might be something to this for pantethine, but it's still way too soon to tell.

◆ **Stops balding and gray hair.** Pantothenic acid deficiency in lab rats causes gray hair and hair loss. Based on that shaky connection, some hair products now contain a form of pantothenic acid called *pantothenyl alcohol,* or *panthenol.* Will putting this stuff on your hair stop you from balding or turning gray? Maybe—if you're a lab rat.

◆ **Stops aging.** In a study many years ago, lab mice were given megadoses of pantothenic acid and supposedly lived 20 percent longer. Since then, some people have claimed that pantothenic acid megadoses can slow aging in humans by "re-energizing" your cells. It's total quackery (or should we say squeakery?).

◆ **Helps arthritis.** The evidence here is pretty thin—just one study of people with a very severe form of arthritis. Skip it.

◆ **Cures allergies.** Some patients claim this works, but there's no evidence one way or the other. Skip it.

◆ **Improves brain function.** You're smart enough to know better about this claim.

The Least You Need to Know

◆ Pantothenic acid, also called Vitamin B_5, is a water-soluble vitamin.

◆ You need pantothenic acid to turn carbohydrates and fats in your food into energy and to make a number of hormones.

◆ There's no RDA for pantothenic acid. The Adequate Intake is between 4 and 5 mg a day for adults.

◆ Some pantothenic acid is found in almost every food. Good sources are organ meats, salmon, eggs, beans, milk, and whole grains.

The Key of B Minor

In This Chapter

- ◆ Why you need biotin, choline, inositol, and PABA
- ◆ How to find foods that are high in the unofficial Bs
- ◆ How biotin and PABA help your skin and hair
- ◆ How inositol and choline use fats and protect your liver
- ◆ Why you need inositol and choline for your nervous system

More B vitamins? Yes, sort of. Technically speaking, biotin and choline are full members of the B family, but inositol and PABA are more like first cousins. They're important, but you don't absolutely have to have them in your diet. You make all you need in your body and also get some from your food.

The good thing about the unofficial Bs is that you don't have to worry about them. You can't really be deficient in them—in fact, they don't even have RDAs.

When Is a B Not a B?

All the B vitamins work together, in complicated ways, to help you turn your food into energy and to make the vast array of chemical substances your body needs to work properly. They're also important for helping your cells grow and divide properly. The only way you can get your official B vitamins is by eating them—you can't make them in your body.

Inositol and choline do things that are similar to what B vitamins do, but you can get them from your food and also by assembling them in your body from other foods. So even though they act like B vitamins, technically speaking, they're not, because you don't have to get them from your food. You still need them, though, and sometimes there are good reasons for taking them in supplements.

Biotin: The B from Your Body

Biotin is definitely a full-fledged member of the B family, but with a twist. You need it to properly use fats and amino acids from your foods. Like any good member of the family, biotin works closely with other Bs, especially folic acid, pantothenic acid, and cobalamin. You don't necessarily have to eat biotin, though. That's because all the biotin you need is made for you in your intestines by the billions of friendly bacteria that live there. It's like having your own little vitamin factory—without having to meet the payroll or even go to the office.

Food for Thought

Biotin was "discovered" a number of times. In 1901, researchers found a substance in animal cells they called *bios*, from the Greek word for life. They didn't know what it did, though, and they quickly lost interest in it. Decades later, other researchers found the same substance but called it "coenzyme R"; still other researchers also "discovered" it and called it "protective factor X" or "Vitamin H" (they couldn't make up their minds about whether it was really a vitamin). Science isn't as straightforward as you might think, so it took a while to sort out the confusion. Finally, everyone realized that they had all "discovered" the same thing: a type of B vitamin they agreed to call "biotin."

Getting Your Biotin

There's no RDA for biotin, mostly because rarely is anybody ever deficient in it—your intestinal bacteria make pretty much all you need. In fact, most people excrete more biotin than they take in through their diet. In other words, your intestinal bacteria actually make more than you need, so you excrete not only the biotin you eat but also some that you make. You don't really need to worry about how much biotin you get, but we'll give you the Adequate Intake chart anyway.

Adequate Intake for Biotin

Age in Years/Sex	Biotin in mcg
Infants	
0 to 0.5	5
0.5 to 1	6
Children	
1 to 3	8
4 to 8	12
9 to 13	20
Adults	
14 to 18	25
19+	30
Pregnant women	30
Nursing women	35

Are You Deficient?

Biotin deficiency is very, very, rare, but there are some special cases:

◆ **Very low-calorie diets.** If you go on a really low-calorie diet for a long time, you can become deficient in biotin. You'll know, because your hair starts to fall out.

◆ **Raw eggs.** If, for some really strange reason, you ate a whole lot of raw eggs— such as 15 or 20 a day—for a long time, you might become deficient. A substance in the egg white binds with the biotin and keeps you from absorbing it. Cooked eggs don't have the same effect.

◆ **Antibiotics.** People who have to take antibiotics such as tetracycline or sulfa for a long time might become deficient because the antibiotics kill all bacteria, including the beneficial ones that make biotin.

Biotin supplements are available, but few people really need them. You can't overdose on them—large doses of biotin have no known toxic effects.

Eating Your Biotin

Biotin is found in many foods, but the best sources are beef liver and brewer's yeast. Egg yolks, nuts, and whole grains are also good sources. Check the chart to see every-day foods you consume that contain biotin.

The Biotin in Food

Food	Amount	Biotin in mcg
Banana	1 medium	6
Beef liver	3 oz.	82
Brewer's yeast	3 oz.	73
Eggs	1 large	10
Oatmeal, cooked	1 cup	9
Peanut butter	2 TB.	12
Rice, brown	½ cup	9
Rice, white	½ cup	2

Biotin for Your Hair and Nails

Some hair-care products now contain biotin, claiming that it helps make healthy hair and prevent balding and graying. It's true that you need biotin for healthy hair and that severe biotin deficiency causes hair loss. The biotin in a shampoo or conditioner isn't likely to do much for you, though. Hair lost from biotin deficiency grows back when you fix the problem, but hair lost from natural balding is gone for good.

> **Quack, Quack**
>
> Sadly, there's no cure for male pattern baldness. That doesn't stop some unscrupulous marketers, though, who sell biotin supplements as a way to stop your hairline from receding or to restore lost hair. Save your money for a toupee instead.

Horse breeders have known for decades that biotin helps make hooves harder. Does it also make human fingernails stronger? Possibly. You need a large dose—between 1,000 and 3,000 mcg a day—and it may not work. If you have brittle nails, it might be worth a try, because you can't overdose on biotin.

Biotin is also sometimes suggested for newborns who have cradle cap, an inflammation of the skin on the scalp. The logic is that infants don't yet have the bacteria to make biotin, so they need supplements. Talk to your pediatrician about biotin before you try it.

Choline: Brain Food

Choline isn't exactly a B vitamin, because you can make it in your body. On the other hand, it isn't exactly *not* a B vitamin, because you have to have it and it works in complicated ways with folic acid and cobalamin. You especially need it to make the neurotransmitter *acetylcholine*, which is crucial for brain functions—and to make *phosphatidylcholine* (*PC*), which is crucial for making the membranes of your cells. Recent evidence shows that choline is extremely important for proper cognitive development in newborns. All pregnant and nursing women especially need plenty of choline.

Choline also moves fats from your liver and keeps them from building up there. Because you make cholesterol in your liver, some people claim that choline lowers high cholesterol. There's some evidence that it might help.

def•i•ni•tion

Choline is vital for making the neurotransmitter **acetylcholine**, which you need to send messages about your emotions and behavior from one brain cell to another. Acetylcholine may also be involved in storing and retrieving memories. **Phosphatidylcholine** (**PC**) is a fatty substance you need to make the walls of your cells. Your body can use it as a source of choline.

There's no RDA for choline, and you can't really be deficient in it. Most people get anywhere from 300 to 1,000 mg a day from their diet. In 1998, the Institute of Medicine decided that choline is an essential nutrient for humans (in other words, it really is a B vitamin) and set an Adequate Intake for it.

Adequate Intake for Choline

Age in Years/Sex	Choline in mg
Infants	
0 to 0.5	125
0.5 to 1	150

continues

Adequate Intake for Choline   (continued)

Age in Years/Sex	Choline in mg
Children	
1 to 3	200
4 to 8	250
9 to 13	375
Men	
14+	550
Women	
14 to 18	400
19+	425
Pregnant	450
Nursing	550

Eating Your Choline

Boy, does this get complicated! You get choline in your diet from foods that contain *lecithin*. What's lecithin? Chemically, it contains phosphatidylcholine, which is in turn about 15 percent choline. When you eat lecithin, your body breaks it down into the choline and other stuff, then uses the choline to make more phosphatidylcholine and also acetylcholine as you need it.

Some choline is found in all animal and plant foods. The best sources are foods that contain lecithin—but some lecithin is found in all animal and plant foods, too! The best animal sources are eggs, red meat, liver, and caviar. Good vegetable sources are cabbage, cauliflower, soybeans, chickpeas, lentils, and rice.

Choline for Your Liver

You need choline to metabolize fats properly. Without it, the fats can get trapped in your liver. You also need phosphatidylcholine to make your cell membranes—and the densely packed cells of your liver have more than 39,000 square yards of them. Doctors in Germany are allowed to prescribe phosphatidylcholine to treat liver problems such as hepatitis or liver damage from toxins. Similar supplements are available at health-food stores, but talk to your doctor before you try them.

Drinking alcohol makes you metabolize choline much more quickly; alcoholics need more choline than normal and may become deficient.

Help for Alzheimer's Disease?

People with Alzheimer's disease usually have low levels of acetylcholine in their brains. Can choline or phosphatidylcholine supplements help? There's been a lot of research into this, and so far the answer is maybe yes, in some cases. Some researchers think that choline could help *prevent* Alzheimer's, but the evidence is pretty thin—it probably can't. (We'll go into this a little more in Chapter 30.)

> **Now You're Cooking**
>
> Picking the right choline supplement can be a little tricky. For the best results, choose a high-quality supplement that is at least 90 percent phosphatidylcholine.

Choosing a Choline Supplement

Hardly anybody ever really needs a choline supplement, but if you want extra you have a few options. You can buy choline capsules or tablets; you can also get a more pure form of phosphatidylcholine called PC-55. There's also a supplement called DMAE that's chemically very similar to choline; it's said to cross into your brain faster than choline. The traditional source of choline is lecithin granules made from soybean oil. These contain anywhere from 10 to 20 percent phosphatidylcholine. They go rancid quickly—store the container in the refrigerator.

You can't overdose on choline, but very large doses—more than 10 g—give you an unpleasant, fishy body odor. It's harmless, but you may find cats following you down the street. Stick to doses in the 500 to 1,500 mg range.

Inositol: Choline's Close Cousin

Inositol and choline work together very closely to make neurotransmitters and the fatty substances in your cell membranes; they also combine to move fats out of your liver. There's no DRI for inositol, so there's no RDA or AI. Most people get about 1,000 mg a day from their food. Doses as high as 50 g have no side effects.

You get inositol from your food in two ways. Phytic acid, a substance found in the fiber of plant foods, gets turned into inositol when bacteria in your intestines digest it. You also get it directly from most foods in the form of myo-inositol. Literally, *myo-* means "muscle," but it's found in both plant and animal foods. Good sources include organ meats, citrus fruits, nuts, beans, and whole grains. Some manufacturers make supplements that contain myo-inositol or myo-inositol and choline.

Inositol is said to help liver problems, diabetic neuropathy, depression, panic attacks, and even Alzheimer's disease. We can't make any recommendations—there just isn't enough evidence to back them up.

PABA: Protecting Your Skin

A lot of extravagant claims have been made for PABA. When you read them, it's like reading about the fountain of youth: PABA is said to extend your life, cure arthritis, and even turn gray hair back to its original color. Does it really do any of these things? Only in the catalogs of the less-scrupulous vitamin makers and health-food stores.

PABA is actually part of the folic acid molecule, but taking it by itself doesn't boost your folic acid levels. It's found naturally in some foods, including liver, wheat germ, brown rice, and whole grains. PABA supplements are available, but we don't recommend them. Aside from the fact that they don't do anything for you, they are potentially dangerous. Large doses of 1 g or more can nauseate you and give you diarrhea, a fever, or a skin rash; they might also damage your liver. If you're taking an antibiotic containing sulfa, PABA will keep it from working.

The one thing PABA does for sure is block ultraviolet radiation from sunlight. That's why it's an ingredient in sunscreens—it works well without clogging your pores.

The Least You Need to Know

◆ Biotin, choline, and inositol work closely with other B vitamins to turn the foods you eat into energy you can use.

◆ Biotin is a B vitamin made in your body by bacteria in your intestines.

◆ Choline, inositol, and PABA are similar to B vitamins but are made in your body from other building blocks.

◆ Choline and inositol work together closely to make your cell membranes and some brain chemicals.

◆ PABA blocks ultraviolet rays in sunlight and is an important ingredient in sunscreens.

Chapter 13

Vitamin C: The Champion

In This Chapter

- ◆ Why you need Vitamin C
- ◆ Which foods are high in Vitamin C
- ◆ How to choose the right supplement for you
- ◆ How Vitamin C can help prevent heart disease and stroke
- ◆ How Vitamin C can help other health problems such as asthma and the common cold

Nearly half of all American adults take extra Vitamin C. Can 50 million people be wrong? Not in this case, anyway. Those people know that a daily dose of Vitamin C helps keep them healthy—and they also know that when they're sick, Vitamin C can help them feel better faster. It may even help them live longer. A recent study shows that men who take Vitamin C supplements live, on average, 6 years longer than those who don't.

Is Vitamin C really that magical? Well, yes. Vitamin C really does help protect you against heart disease, stroke, cataracts, diabetes, asthma, and other serious health problems. Doctors once scoffed at the health claims for Vitamin C. Now many advise their patients to take Vitamin C supplements.

Why You Need Vitamin C

There's not much Vitamin C *doesn't* do for you. You need it for more than 300 different purposes in your body. Just for starters, Vitamin C is needed to make *collagen*, the strong connective tissue that holds your skeleton together, attaches your muscles to your bones, builds strong blood vessels, and keeps your organs and skin in place. Collagen is the glue that holds your body together—and you can't make it unless you have enough Vitamin C. (The next time someone tells you to pull yourself together, maybe you should reach for the C supplements!)

def•i•ni•tion

The connective tissue that holds your cells together and makes up your bones, tendons, muscles, teeth, skin, blood vessels, and every other part of you is made from a protein called **collagen**.

Because you need collagen to fix damage to your body, it stands to reason that Vitamin C helps heal wounds of all sorts. Broken bones, sprained joints, cuts, and other injuries all heal a lot faster if your body gets plenty of Vitamin C.

Vitamin C is your body's top antioxidant. Not only does it mop up those nasty free radicals, it helps many of your body's other antioxidants do their work better. And without Vitamin C, you can't use some other vitamins and minerals, such as folic acid and iron, properly.

Your immune system needs a lot of Vitamin C to run at peak levels. If you don't get enough, you're likely to get sick more often and stay sick longer. You also need Vitamin C to manufacture many of your body's hormones.

Vitamin C also does things—such as curing some types of male infertility and helping diabetics—that makes it seem more like a miracle drug than a plain old vitamin. People with high levels of Vitamin C have lower blood pressure, which makes them less likely to have a stroke or heart attack. And although Vitamin C can't cure heart disease or cancer, it could help keep you from getting them in the first place.

What about the common cold? Not even Vitamin C prevents or cures that. If you do catch a cold, though, Vitamin C may help you feel better sooner.

The RDA for Vitamin C

Humans, unlike almost all other animals, can't manufacture Vitamin C in their bodies. Because Vitamin C is water-soluble, you also can't store it in your body for very long. Both these facts mean that you need to have a new supply on a daily basis through the foods you eat and the supplements you take.

The old RDA for Vitamin C, set in 1980, was quite low (far too low in the opinion of many nutritionists), mostly because it was based on a compromise. On the one hand, you need only about 10 mg a day to prevent scurvy, a deficiency disease caused by a lack of Vitamin C. On the other hand, if you take in more than 200 mg at a time, you pass the rest out of your body in your urine within a few hours. Because the spread between the minimum dose needed and the maximum you can handle is fairly large, the Institute of Medicine came down in the middle for a long time. It decided that the RDA should be set at an amount that would keep you from getting scurvy if, for some strange reason, you suddenly got absolutely no Vitamin C for several weeks.

def•i•ni•tion

Scurvy is a deficiency disease caused by a prolonged lack of Vitamin C in the diet. Among the symptoms are sore and bleeding gums, loose teeth, fatigue, bruising, sore joints, slow wound healing, and anemia. Another name for Vitamin C is *ascorbic acid,* which literally means "acid that prevents scurvy."

In 2000, the Institute of Medicine issued a new DRI for Vitamin C. To the disappointment of many, the RDA was raised only slightly, from 60 mg daily for all adults to 75 mg daily for an adult woman and 90 mg daily for an adult man. Many researchers today believe that the amount should be much higher. A study by the National Institutes of Health (NIH) in 1996 found that 200 mg of Vitamin C a day—more than twice the RDA—is optimal. Many other researchers believe that even 200 mg a day is too low. These amounts prevent disease, but they don't do much to promote health. Decades of research plainly show that people who take large amounts of Vitamin C on a regular basis are healthier than those who don't. The research also clearly shows that large doses of Vitamin C help many health problems, such as asthma, as well as or better than strong prescription drugs—at less cost and without nasty side effects. Finally, extensive research shows that large doses of several thousand mg a day (or even more) are perfectly safe for almost everyone. Not surprisingly, today many doctors suggest taking at least 500 mg daily.

The major argument against larger Vitamin C doses is that you excrete anything beyond 200 mg a day. By that logic, taking more means you flush away the cost of the supplements. This isn't quite true. In fact, a healthy person's body contains about 5,000 mg of Vitamin C. You'll start excreting the excess only after you reach this saturation point—and only if you're in perfectly good health. Any sort of stress or illness increases your need for Vitamin C. During illness or stress, your body draws down its reserves and needs a refill quickly. Aside from that, many of Vitamin C's beneficial effects, such as blocking heart disease, seem to occur only at levels above 200 mg a day. Find the RDA for your age and sex in the following table.

Food for Thought

Scurvy is the oldest known vitamin-deficiency disease. For centuries, scurvy was a big problem for sailors on ocean voyages, who often had to go for many weeks with no fresh fruits or vegetables. In 1753, Dr. James Lind, the chief doctor for the British Navy, proved that lime juice prevented and cured the problem—although he didn't know why. After that, British sailors were given lime juice every day to prevent scurvy, which is why they have the nickname "limeys."

The RDAs for Vitamin C

Age in Years/Sex	Vitamin C in mg
Infants	
0 to 0.5	40
0.5 to 1	50
Children	
1 to 3	15
4 to 8	25
9 to 13	45
Adults	
Men 14 to 18	75
Men 19+	90
Women 14 to 18	65
Women 19+	75
Pregnant women	85
Nursing women	120

The numbers in the table are for people who don't smoke. Smokers have below-normal levels of Vitamin C—as much as 40 percent lower in pack-a-day smokers. Cigarettes rob your body of Vitamin C by breaking it down and making you excrete it much faster than normal. The Institute of Medicine now recommends an extra 35 mg a day beyond the RDA for smokers. We think this number is way too low. If you smoke, consider taking 1,000 mg daily. This amount could also help protect you against two types of cancer smokers often get: cancer of the larynx and cancer of the esophagus.

Are You Deficient?

If you don't get much Vitamin C on a regular basis, you might have dry hair, your gums might bleed, and you might bruise easily. After several weeks with no Vitamin C in your diet, you'd start to get scurvy. At first you'd just feel a little tired and irritable, but soon you'd have sore and bleeding gums, loose teeth, fatigue, bruising, sore joints, slow wound healing, anemia, and a decreased ability to fend off infection. In the days before canning and refrigeration, Vitamin C deficiency and even mild scurvy was quite common, especially in the winter when fresh fruits and veggies were scarce.

Luckily, Vitamin C is found in so many common fruits and vegetables that almost everyone in our modern society gets enough to prevent scurvy. But according to ongoing studies of American eating habits, most people get only 70 to 80 mg a day from their food. In other words, many of us barely reach the RDA for Vitamin C from our diet, much less get the 250 mg a day many nutritionists consider a more desirable amount. And if you fall into any of these categories, you may need a lot more Vitamin C than you're actually getting:

- **You smoke.** As mentioned earlier, cigarette smoke breaks down your Vitamin C quickly. Also, you need extra Vitamin C to combat the damage smoking does to your cells. Studies show that people exposed to passive smoke—smoke other people create—also need extra Vitamin C.

- **You have diabetes.** Vitamin C doesn't get into your cells very well if you have diabetes (we'll talk about this more later in the chapter).

- **You have allergies or asthma.** Fighting asthma, allergic reactions, and asthma attacks uses up a lot of your Vitamin C (we'll talk about this more later in the chapter).

- **You're sick with an infectious illness such as a cold or flu.** Your immune system needs plenty of Vitamin C, especially when it's in high gear fighting off an illness. (We'll discuss this some more later on.)

Warning!

Admit it—you started smoking as a teenager so you'd look older. Keep smoking and you'll *really* start to look older. We all get facial lines as we age, but cigarette smokers get more of them—lots more—and sooner. Smoking robs your body of the Vitamin C it needs to build collagen. Without strong collagen to support it, the skin on your face sags, bags, and wrinkles.

◆ **You've just had surgery.** Vitamin C helps heal wounds and fight infection.

◆ **You're under a great deal of stress—physical or psychological.** When you're under stress, your body's systems go into overdrive and use up your Vitamin C extra fast.

◆ **You're an older adult.** Older people need more Cs in general, especially if they take drugs that interfere with Vitamin C absorption. If you're elderly and live alone or in a nursing home, you might not be eating well or getting enough fresh foods, which means you might not be getting enough Cs.

◆ **You're pregnant or breastfeeding.** You're passing a lot of your Vitamin C on to your baby.

◆ **You regularly take aspirin, birth-control pills, antibiotics such as tetracy-cline or sulfa drugs, or certain other drugs such as steroids.** These drugs either block Vitamin C from being absorbed into your body or break it down too fast.

◆ **You abuse alcohol.** People who abuse alcohol generally don't eat properly. Also, alcohol may destroy Vitamin C.

Your teeth won't fall out if you have a mild Vitamin C deficiency, but you might have these symptoms: fatigue and tiring easily, appetite loss, muscle weakness, bruising easily, and frequent infections.

Fatigue, appetite loss, and weakness could all be caused by other things, but the clincher is bruising easily. A shortage of Vitamin C weakens the walls of your blood vessels. They break easily, causing bruises and even nosebleeds. If you think low Vitamin C is the problem, try supplementing with 500 mg a day. You should feel a lot better and stop getting bruises within a week.

Low Vitamin C can lead you into a downward spiral of bad health. The deficiency means you're tired all the time—too tired to eat properly. So you eat poorly and get sick more often, which means that you take in even less Vitamin C and use up that lower amount to help fight the infection, meaning you stay deficient and eat less and get sick more often, which means … you get the picture. Break out of the cycle with a better diet and Vitamin C supplements.

Eating Your Cs

You know from all those OJ commercials that oranges and other citrus fruits are a great way to get your Cs. But did you know that there's as much Vitamin C in one kiwi as there is in an orange? Or that a tangerine has less than half the Vitamin C of an orange?

There's some Vitamin C in just about every fruit and green vegetable. Strawberries, melons, and cranberries are high in Vitamin C. Tropical fruits such as guavas, mangos, and papayas are all high in Vitamin C—as high as oranges or higher.

The food that's richest of all in Vitamin C is acerola, a large red berry that's native to the West Indies. One cup of raw acerola berries has a whopping 1,600 mg of Vitamin C, compared to just 80 mg for a medium-sized orange. But don't ask the produce manager at your supermarket where the acerola is. Ripe acerola berries have a pleasantly tart taste, but they're not really grown to be eaten. Instead, juice from the berries is made into a powder that's used as a supplement or added to other foods to raise their Vitamin C level.

Dark-green, leafy vegetables such as spinach and kale are fairly good sources of Vitamin C. Vegetables such as broccoli, Brussels sprouts, potatoes, turnips, and tomatoes are also good dietary sources. Peppers of all sorts—from sweet to ultra hot—are high in Vitamin C. In fact, the average American now eats about 7 pounds of peppers a year. Half a cup of chopped green bell (sweet) peppers has 45 mg. Half a cup of chopped red bell peppers has 95 mg, while an equal amount of chopped yellow bell peppers has a whopping 341 mg. If you're planning to get your Vitamin C from peppers, stick to the sweet ones—we defy anyone to eat half a cup of Scotch bonnets!

There's some, though not a lot, of Vitamin C in meat, poultry, fish, milk, and dairy products. Beans generally have little or no Vitamin C, and there's none in grains such as oats or wheat. Check the fruits and veggies you eat in the following table.

The Vitamin C in Food

Food	Amount	Vitamin C in mg
Acerola	1 cup	1,644
Apple	1 medium	8
Banana	1 medium	10
Blueberries, fresh	1 cup	19
Broccoli, cooked	½ cup	58
Brussels sprouts	½ cup	48
Cabbage, raw	½ cup	17

continues

The Vitamin C in Food   (continued)

Food	Amount	Vitamin C in mg
Cantaloupe	1 cup, pieces	68
Carrot	1 medium	7
Cauliflower, raw	½ cup	36
Collard greens, cooked	1 cup	15
Cranberry juice	6 oz.	67
Grapefruit, pink	½ medium	47
Grapefruit, white	½ medium	39
Guava	1 medium	165
Honeydew melon	1 cup, pieces	42
Kale, cooked	½ cup	27
Kiwi	1 medium	75
Lemon	1 medium	31
Lime	1 medium	20
Mango	1 medium	57
Orange, navel	1 medium	80
Orange juice, concentrate	8 oz.	97
Orange juice, fresh	8 oz.	124
Papaya	1 medium	188
Peach	1 medium	6
Pear	1 medium	7
Pepper, green bell	½ cup	45
Pepper, yellow bell	1 medium	341
Pepper, red bell	½ cup	95
Pineapple	1 cup, pieces	24
Potato, baked	1 medium	26
Spinach, cooked	½ cup	9
Strawberries	1 cup	85
Tangerine	1 medium	26
Tomato	1 medium	24
Turnips, cooked	½ cup	9

Most people, even those who seem to live on junk food, manage to get some Vitamin C. That's mostly because a lot of prepared foods are fortified with extra Cs. Orange Tang, the breakfast drink of the astronauts, has 60 mg of Vitamin C in a 6-ounce serving—all artificially added.

Citrus for Cs

Citrus Fruit	Amount	Vitamin C in mg
Grapefruit, pink	½ medium	47
Grapefruit, white	½ medium	39
Grapefruit, canned	½ cup	42
Grapefruit juice, canned	8 oz.	72
Grapefruit juice, fresh	8 oz.	94
Lemon	1 medium	31
Lemon juice	1 TB.	7
Lime	1 medium	20
Lime juice	1 TB.	5
Orange, mandarin, canned	½ cup	43
Orange, navel	1 medium	80
Orange, Valencia	1 medium	59
Orange juice, concentrate	8 oz.	97
Orange juice, fresh	8 oz.	124
Orange peel	1 TB.	8
Pummelo	1 cup, pieces	116
Sunny Delight	6 oz.	60
Tang powder	6 oz.	60
Tangerine	1 medium	26

If you eat five servings of fresh fruits and vegetables every day, you'll easily reach 250 mg of Vitamin C or even more. When figuring out your Vitamin C intake for a day, be cautious how you count the fruits and vegetables you get from a salad bar. Although the salad bar is a healthier lunch choice than chicken nuggets and fries, you may not be getting as much Vitamin C as you think. Up to half of it is lost when fruits and vegetables are prepared in advance and left out for a few hours.

Freezing preserves most of the Vitamin C in vegetables. In fact, frozen vegetables have almost as much Vitamin C as fresh. Canned vegetables are cooked and then packed in water, which pretty much destroys the Vitamin C. Finally, a good excuse not to eat those mushy green vegetables from the cafeteria steam table!

Frozen fruits have somewhat less Vitamin C than fresh, but canned fruits have almost none. Most canned fruits also have a lot of added sugar, which most of us don't really need, so go for the fresh fruits whenever you can.

Getting the Most from Vitamin C

Because Vitamin C is water-soluble, it's almost impossible to overdose or reach toxic levels, even when you take large doses—the excess passes harmlessly out in your urine. The usual safety range is from 500 to 4,000 mg a day. Large doses sometimes cause stomach upsets, diarrhea, and cramping, however. The problem usually starts at doses of more than 2,000 mg, but children and some adults are more sensitive. If you want to take large amounts of Vitamin C, start with smaller doses and gradually build up until you get diarrhea. Cut back until the problem goes away and then stick with that dose. Nutritionists call this "reaching bowel tolerance."

Take your total Vitamin C dose in several small doses spread throughout the day. Each dose is gone from your body within four hours, so spreading them out helps keep your level steady. We suggest taking your supplements with each meal and before bed.

You'll get the most out of your Vitamin C supplements if you take them along with a good daily supplement that contains all the other vitamins and minerals. You need all of them, but especially calcium and magnesium, to use Vitamin C most effectively. Flavonoids also help Vitamin C work better—we'll discuss that more in Chapter 25.

Alcohol and many common drugs such as aspirin and birth-control pills either block Vitamin C in your body or make it break down too fast. Baking soda (sodium bicarbonate), found in some antacids such as Alka-Seltzer, blocks your absorption of Cs. If you take any of these drugs, take your Vitamin C a few hours later to help avoid interference. Also, if you take aspirin, ibuprofen (Advil), or other nonsteroidal, anti-inflammatory drugs and Vitamin C together, you're more likely to get stomach irritation from the aspirin.

Large doses of Vitamin C can interfere with medical tests for sugar and calcium oxalate in the urine, for blood in the stool, and for hemoglobin levels in the blood. If you're scheduled for a medical checkup, cut back on your C supplements for a few days beforehand to avoid false readings.

Thumbs Up/Thumbs Down

Vitamin C Works Better With ...	Vitamin C Is Blocked By ...
All other vitamins and minerals	Alcohol
B vitamins	Some antibiotics
Calcium	Some antihistamines
Flavonoids	Baking soda (sodium bicarbonate)
Magnesium	Barbiturates such as phenobarbital
	Birth-control pills
	Steroids
	Estrogen

Which Type Should I Take?

The Vitamin C shelves have got to be the most confusing place in any health-food store. Do you want to take your Cs in capsules, tablets, or chewable tablets? Or do you prefer powder, liquid, or maybe chewing gum or syrup? Should you buy your Cs as ascorbic acid or buffered ascorbic acid? How about those pricey "all-natural" tablets made from rose hips? And what exactly is esterized Vitamin C? Read on—it's not as complicated as it seems.

Vitamin C is ascorbic acid and ascorbic acid is Vitamin C, whether it's synthesized in a lab or extracted without solvents from rose hips or acerola. In fact, most of the Vitamin C sold today is made from corn and it's all pretty much the same. Stick to a reliable, inexpensive brand and don't waste your money on the stuff that claims it's better because it's "organic" or "natural."

Vitamin C breaks down when it's exposed to light, heat, water, or air. Buy just a few weeks' worth at a time from a store that turns over its stock quickly. Store your Cs in a cool, dark, dry place.

Pick the form of Vitamin C that's most convenient for you. Here's a rundown of the various versions:

♦ **Ascorbic acid tablets and capsules.** These usually contain 500 mg and are meant to be swallowed whole. For most people, this is the most convenient and economical way to take your Cs.

♦ **Chewable tablets.** These usually contain 250 mg. They have a pleasant, mildly tart taste that kids usually like. A few drawbacks: they're more expensive and they often have sweeteners and flavors added. Also, sodium ascorbate is often added to reduce the acidity (which could damage your tooth enamel). Avoid these if you're on a sodium-restricted diet.

Warning!

If you've been taking large doses of Vitamin C for a long time and suddenly stop, you could temporarily get the symptoms of mild scurvy (rebound scurvy) as your body adjusts to the change. Taper off slowly over two to four weeks instead.

♦ **Ascorbic acid powder.** Kids (and plenty of adults, too) don't like to swallow pills. Luckily, this powder can be stirred into fruit juice or sprinkled on applesauce or fruit. The powder has a slightly acid or sour taste. (Don't add the powder to milk—it will curdle.) A level teaspoon of powder has about 2,000 mg.

♦ **Sodium or calcium ascorbate tablets and powder.** If plain ascorbic acid bothers your stomach, try switching to a buffered version that's made from sodium ascorbate or calcium ascorbate. Don't take large doses (more than 3,000 mg)—you'll get too much sodium or calcium. You could also try time-release tablets of plain ascorbic acid. These don't kick in until they reach your intestines, so you avoid stomach upsets. You may not absorb that much, though.

♦ **Potassium ascorbate crystals.** A spoonful of this stuff mixed with an ounce or two of water makes a bubbly, pleasant-tasting drink that has 4,000 mg of Vitamin C. It also has 700 mg of potassium—an amount that could kill a child or someone with a heart or kidney condition. If you want to take Vitamin C this way, talk to your doctor first. Store the crystals in a cool, dry place out of reach of children.

♦ **With bioflavonoids.** Vitamin C tablets are available with added bioflavonoids. The bioflavonoids may be helpful (see Chapter 25 to learn why), but they won't affect how much Vitamin C you absorb. These tablets are expensive. Buy plain old Vitamin C tablets and spend the money you save on more fresh fruits and vegetables—you'll get plenty of bioflavonoids and other good stuff the tasty way.

◆ **Other forms.** If you want, you can get Vitamin C in liquid, wafer, chewing gum, gummy candies, lozenges, syrup, and other forms. If you have a practical reason for choosing these pricier products, go ahead. Read the labels to figure out how much C you're actually getting.

Quack, Quack

The makers of esterized Vitamin C (or Ester-C ascorbate) say it's absorbed faster, used better, and excreted more slowly. It also costs more than plain ascorbic acid. Save your money. There's no major difference.

Some nutritionists tout ascorbyl palmitate, the fat-soluble form of Vitamin C, saying it stays in your body longer. Researchers disagree. But it will cost a whole lot more for no real benefit.

Frontline Antioxidant

It's this simple: *Vitamin C is the most important antioxidant in your body.* You need Vitamin C as your frontline defense against free radicals (remember those destructive molecules from Chapter 1?). Job one for Vitamin C is to capture free radicals and neutralize them before they can do any damage to your cells.

Dealing with free radicals is the main job of lots of other vitamins and minerals in your body. What makes Vitamin C so important? First, because it's water-soluble, it's everywhere in your body—inside all your cells and in the spaces in between. Because free radicals are also everywhere, Vitamin C is always on the spot to track them down. Second, and just as important, other powerful antioxidants such as Vitamin E and antioxidant enzymes such as superoxide dismutase (SOD) and glutathione need Vitamin C to work properly.

Vitamin C is also needed to make other enzymes that round up and remove toxins such as lead and environmental pollutants in your body. In today's society, environmental pollutants of all sorts are almost impossible to avoid. The faster the toxins are booted out, the less damage they can do. Your best protection is a high level of Vitamin C.

Preventing Cardiovascular Disease

According to some pretty careful studies of data from the National Center for Health Statistics, if every adult in the United States took an extra 500 mg of Vitamin C a day, about 100,000 of them wouldn't die of heart disease every year. Not only would all those people still be alive and kicking, they wouldn't be costing *billions* of dollars in health-care costs every year. Here's where Vitamin C pays dividends in both better health and in real dollars and cents. A year's supply of Vitamin C costs around $20; a coronary bypass operation costs around $50,000 or more.

A European study published in the prestigious British medical journal *Lancet* in 2001 showed that a diet rich in Vitamin C lowered the overall risk of death, especially from heart disease and stroke. The study found that even a small increase in Vitamin C intake from food led to a reduced risk of death. Eating just one extra serving a day of fruits or vegetables was associated with a 20 percent lower risk. Overall, the people with the highest levels of Vitamin C in their blood had half the risk of death compared to those with the lowest levels.

In 2003, researchers from the Harvard School of Public Health looked at results from the Nurses' Health Study and found that women who had a Vitamin C intake of 360 mg or more from food and supplements reduced their risk of heart disease by nearly 30 percent. What is very interesting about the study is that the effect was seen most sharply in women who got their Cs from supplements in addition to their food. High levels of dietary Vitamin C didn't seem to help much. Vitamin C supplements are about the most inexpensive supplement you can buy—here's evidence that they're also about the most inexpensive form of life insurance.

Lowering Cholesterol Levels

Studies show that people with high levels of Vitamin C have lower total cholesterol levels. (We went into the details of cholesterol in Chapter 1—if you skipped it, go back and read it now.) They also have lower LDL cholesterol (that's the bad stuff) and higher HDL cholesterol (that's good). So if your total cholesterol is high, can you lower it by taking Vitamin C? It depends. If your C level is low to begin with, raising it will probably help your total cholesterol level by raising your HDL level a bit. If your C level is already high because you're taking 2,000 mg a day, it's not certain that taking more will help—although it definitely won't hurt.

If your total cholesterol is borderline high (above 200 mg/dL but below 240 mg/dL), Vitamin C supplements, along with a low-fat diet, exercise, and weight loss, could bring it down a little. If your cholesterol is above 240 mg/dL, or if you're already taking a statin drug such as Lipitor, Pravachol, or Zocor to lower your cholesterol, talk to your doctor about taking extra Vitamin C before trying it.

Lowering Blood Pressure

High blood pressure (above 140/90) is a big risk factor for heart disease—and also for stroke and kidney disease. (We'll talk about this in detail in Chapters 18 and 26.) Numerous studies show that people with high levels of Vitamin C have blood-pressure readings that are slightly lower than people with low C levels. The difference is about four points in the diastolic (when your heart is relaxed between beats) reading. That may not sound like much, but lowering your diastolic blood pressure by just two points reduces your chance of heart disease by 8 percent. According to a 2000 study in the famed British journal *Lancet*, taking 500 mg a day of Vitamin C can lower high blood pressure by more than 9 percent. It's all evidence that the main reason people with high Vitamin C levels live longer is that they have fewer heart attacks and strokes.

If you have borderline high blood pressure, Vitamin C, along with exercising, losing weight, and quitting smoking, could do a lot to bring it down. If you have high blood pressure or if you're already taking one or more drugs to lower your blood pressure, talk to your doctor about Vitamin C before you try it.

Preventing Stroke

As with heart disease, so with stroke. Several recent studies have shown that the higher your Vitamin C levels, the lower your risk of having a stroke. The benefits may be even greater if you're overweight, have high blood pressure, or smoke. In a Dutch study that followed more than 5,000 healthy adults for more than 6 years, for instance, the people with the lowest levels of Vitamin C in their diet were 30 percent more likely to have a stroke than the people with the highest levels. How high was high? Just 133 mg, or about the amount of Vitamin C in two oranges.

Enhancing Your Immune System

Your immune system protects you against infection. To do that, it makes several different kinds of white blood cells and a whole lot of complicated chemical messengers that tell the white blood cells where to go and what to do. When you're healthy, you have about a *trillion* white blood cells in your body. When you're sick, you make millions more every hour to fight off the illness. All those cells, and all the chemical messengers they rely on, need plenty of Vitamin C to work right. We still don't know for sure whether Vitamin C can keep you from getting sick in the first place, but we do know that it can help you get better faster. If you're sick or have an infection, taking extra Vitamin C will help your immune system fight back efficiently.

Curing the Common Cold

Does Vitamin C keep you from catching a cold, flu, bronchitis, or pneumonia? No. Does it magically "cure" these illnesses? No. Does it help you get better faster if you do? Yes. If you're basically healthy and take 1,000 to 2,000 mg of extra Vitamin C, your cold symptoms will probably be less severe and you'll get better a little faster. The older you are, the more the extra Vitamin C seems to help.

If you're one of those people who seems to get one soggy cold after another all winter long, or maybe just one bad cold that you can't seem to shake off, low Vitamin C could be causing the problem. Which comes first, the cold or the deficiency? It doesn't really matter—each problem is making the other worse. Low Vitamin C makes you more susceptible to illness, and fighting off an illness uses up a lot of Vitamin C. To break the cycle and give your immune system a much-needed boost, try supplementing with 1,000 mg of Vitamin C a day.

Healing Wounds and Recovering from Surgery

One sign of scurvy is wounds that won't heal or old wounds that reopen. That's because you need Vitamin C to make collagen, which is what makes scar tissue and heals wounds. Extra Vitamin C will help you heal faster if you have a cut, scrape, broken bone, burn, or any other sort of wound.

If you have an operation, your Vitamin C levels will probably be low right after the surgery. We don't know exactly why that happens, but it's just the opposite of what you want. To help you heal and fight off infections, your Vitamin C level needs to be high. We strongly suggest taking 1,000 mg a day for at least 2 weeks before the operation and 4 weeks after it. Not only will you heal faster from the operation, you'll be less likely to get bed sores because the collagen under your skin will be stronger.

Fighting Allergies and Asthma

Does summer mean days in the sun to you? Or does it mean days of sneezing and sniffling from pollen allergies? If you're in the sneezing group, it's because your body thinks the pollen is an invading germ that has to be attacked. To do that, your immune system releases chemicals called histamines into your blood. The major casualty of the battle against the "invaders" is you. Your own histamines make you sneeze, wheeze, sniffle, cough, itch, and be generally miserable. Don't you wish you could explain the difference between pollen and germs to your inner self?

Drugs that counteract your natural histamines are called, not surprisingly, antihistamines. There are a lot of different kinds, including many you can buy over the counter in any drugstore. The long lists of cautions and side effects on these drug labels are more than a little scary. Many antihistamines can make you dangerously drowsy. If you have a health problem such as high blood pressure, heart disease, kidney problems, prostate disease, or lung disease, you shouldn't take them. There's an easier, more natural—and cheaper—way to cope with respiratory allergies: Vitamin C. Try taking 1,000 to 2,000 mg a day for several weeks. Your allergies should calm down noticeably and stay that way as long as you keep taking extra Cs. Why? Because Vitamin C keeps your immune system from making as many histamines to begin with and helps you get them out of your bloodstream faster.

Warning!

Even mild asthma is a serious health problem, because it can suddenly get much worse. If you think you have asthma, see your doctor as soon as possible. If you already take medicine for asthma—even nonprescription drugs—don't stop! Talk to your doctor about taking Vitamin C and other supplements before you try them.

Fighting Asthma Attacks

Some people react to pollen and irritants such as air pollution or chalk dust by having an asthma attack. The airways in their lungs swell up, making them wheeze and have trouble breathing. The airways clog up with extra mucus and the muscles that surround them go into spasms, which makes breathing even harder. If you have asthma, you're not alone. Nearly 20 million Americans have it—and the numbers are on the rise, especially among children. Today more than 6 million kids—about 1 in 20—have asthma. It's the most common chronic childhood disease.

There's plenty of evidence to suggest that low intake of Vitamin C is related to asthma. In general, kids with asthma have lower levels of Vitamin C in their blood than kids without the disease, and kids who eat more fruit, especially citrus fruit, have a lower risk of asthma. Overall, having a high Vitamin C level seems to reduce the risk of asthma in kids by about 10 percent.

Passive smoke is another factor in childhood asthma. Kids who are exposed to secondhand smoke have higher asthma rates and also lower levels of Vitamin C. Overall, kids and teens who are exposed to secondhand cigarette smoke have about 20 percent less Vitamin C in their blood than kids and teens who aren't—even though they get equal amounts from their food. If you have kids and smoke, here's another good reason to quit.

Many nutritionists today believe that taking 1,000 to 2,000 mg a day of extra Vitamin C can help reduce the number of asthma attacks you have and also make them less severe. This works for two reasons. First, as we discussed previously, Vitamin C lowers your histamine production, so your allergies won't trigger an asthma attack as often or as severely. Second, the antioxidant effect of Vitamin C protects your lungs and airways against damage from your own free radicals and from outside air pollution.

Vitamin C is even more helpful for asthma if you also take extra magnesium—we'll talk about that more in Chapter 18.

Diabetes and Vitamin C

People with diabetes, especially those with Type 2 diabetes, often have low Vitamin C levels. People with diabetes also often have gum disease, slow wound healing, frequent infections, and problems with the tiny blood vessels of the circulatory system. Sounds a little like scurvy, doesn't it? In a way, it is—and Vitamin C can help.

The hormone insulin, which is made in your pancreas, carries glucose into your cells, where you use it for energy. Insulin also carries Vitamin C into your cells. People with Type 2 diabetes, however, are resistant to their own insulin. Not enough insulin enters their cells, so not much Vitamin C does either. Diabetics need to take in much more than the RDA to be sure enough reaches their cells. If you have diabetes, your doctor will probably recommend that you take 500 or 1,000 mg a day of extra Vitamin C. Some diabetics say that their circulatory problems and other complications get a lot better when they take larger doses, as high as 3,000 mg a day or even more. They also say that they can control their blood sugar better when they take large doses. It's also possible that extra Vitamin C could help prevent diabetic cataracts.

Warning!

If you have diabetes and want to try taking large doses of Vitamin C, talk to your doctor first. If you decide to go ahead, add Vitamin C slowly and check your blood sugar levels often.

Talk to your doctor before you start taking large doses of Vitamin C for diabetes. One possible drawback is that you will have a lot of Vitamin C in your urine, which could give a false negative reading on a test for glucose in the urine. Vitamin C doesn't have any effect on the results of the A1c blood test, which measures your blood sugar over a 3-month period, or on a finger prick test for your blood sugar level.

What about preventing Type 2 diabetes with Vitamin C? A large population-based study in England, published in 2000, showed that the people with the lowest (healthiest) long-term blood sugar levels had the highest levels of Vitamin C—and vice versa. The lower the blood level of Vitamin C, the more likely the individual was to have high blood sugar or diabetes. So will taking Vitamin C supplements prevent Type 2 diabetes? Of course not, especially if you're at risk from other factors, such as being overweight and getting very little exercise. But if you're at risk for diabetes or already have it, taking supplements and improving your diet to get more Vitamin C could help keep the problem under control.

Kidney Stones, Gallstones, and Vitamin C

If you've ever had a kidney stone, your doctor may advise against taking Vitamin C supplements. Recent research shows, however, that there's no real basis for this. In fact, in an ongoing study of male physicians that started in 1986, the ones with the *highest* levels of Vitamin C had the *lowest* risk of kidney stones. And a 1999 study confirmed that people with high levels of Vitamin C in their blood don't have an increased risk of kidney stones.

Vitamin C may also help prevent gallstones, at least in women. A study of more than 13,000 women found that the ones who had the highest blood levels of Vitamin C were 39 percent less likely to have gallstones. For some reason, men don't get the same protective effect. Given that surgery to remove the gallbladder because of gallstones is now one of the most common operations in America, here's another good reason to get those extra Cs.

Cancer and Vitamin C

Before we go any further into Vitamin C and cancer, let's clear up a few things. Yes, Vitamin C can definitely help prevent cancer. No, Vitamin C does not cure cancer. Maybe, Vitamin C helps treat cancer. Let's take these one at a time.

Preventing Cancer

Study after study after study proves that Vitamin C can help protect you against cancer. People with high levels of Vitamin C and other antioxidants are markedly less likely to get cancer of the lung, cervix, colon, pancreas, esophagus, mouth, and stomach. Why? We're still not sure, but it's very likely that the antioxidants gobble up free radicals and damaging toxins before they can damage your cells and trigger cancer. In the case of stomach cancer, Vitamin C blocks the formation of cancer-causing nitrosamines from the nitrates and nitrites found in bacon, hot dogs, and other cured meats.

Curing Cancer

A study by Dr. Linus Pauling in 1976 showed that some terminally ill cancer patients lived as much as a year longer if they took megadoses (more than 10,000 mg) of Vitamin C. A few later studies have backed this up. In all the studies, though, all the patients eventually died—none were cured. No study has ever shown that megadoses of Vitamin C (or any other vitamin, for that matter) cure cancer.

Treating Cancer

If you're being treated for cancer, there's no question that Vitamin C can really help you get through this difficult time. As mentioned previously, Vitamin C could help you bounce back from surgery more quickly. Many people getting radiation treatment or chemotherapy have low Vitamin C levels. Part of the reason is that the treatment can make you tired, nauseated, and cause appetite loss and taste changes—all factors that reduce your interest in eating well. The other part is that the treatment is making you produce huge amounts of free radicals, so any Vitamin C you get from your food is going to mop them up. Unless you take supplements, you won't have any left over for other things, such as keeping your immune system active. Cancer treatment lowers your immunity, making you more likely to get sick or pick up an infection.

Discuss nutrition and supplements, especially Vitamin C, with your doctor *before* you start your cancer treatment. In many cases they could make a big difference in how well you do and even improve how well the drugs you take work. On the other hand, there is some evidence to suggest that some tumors actually grow faster if you take high doses of antioxidants.

Making Babies with Vitamin C

Okay guys, stop snickering and pay attention. If you and your partner want a baby and nothing's happening, the problem could be the quality of your sperm. Don't panic—there's a good chance that Vitamin C can make you a father.

Your seminal fluid contains lots of Vitamin C—much more even than your blood. It's there to protect the delicate genetic material in your sperm from free-radical damage. If your Vitamin C level in general is low (because you smoke, for example), your sperm count is probably low as well. Studies show that taking 1,000 mg of Vitamin C daily can raise your sperm count by quite a bit.

Food for Thought

If your sperm count is low, taking just 1,000 mg of Vitamin C a day for a few weeks could raise it by 100 percent or more

Another common cause of male infertility is antibodies that cling to your sperm, making them clump together instead of swimming freely to their destination. You probably have the antibodies because you have a chronic infection such as prostatitis. Even after you take antibiotics to clear up the infection, you'll still be making the antibodies. Here's where Vitamin C can help. Taking 1,000 mg daily for 2 to 3 months is quite likely to stop those antibodies from hitching rides. In one study, every participant had a pregnant wife at the end of 60 days.

Saving Babies with Vitamin C

About one in ten pregnant women develop a very serious condition known as pre-eclampsia. The symptoms include dangerously high blood pressure, swelling of the face and ankles, and protein in the urine. The babies of mothers with pre-eclampsia are likely to be born prematurely and to have developmental problems. Several studies, starting in the 1990s, showed that daily doses of Vitamin C and Vitamin E during pregnancy seemed to help prevent pre-eclampsia. But in 2006, two important studies showed that the vitamins didn't necessarily help and might even be harmful.

The first study gave Vitamin C and Vitamin E to one group of healthy pregnant women and compared them to another group that took placebos. There was virtually no difference in how many ended up with pre-eclampsia—it happened to about 6 percent of the mothers in both groups. In the second study, one group of women at high risk of pre-eclampsia took Vitamin C and Vitamin E; another group took placebos. The women in the vitamin group had a slightly higher risk of having a low birthweight baby; they were also at greater risk of developing high blood pressure. In the end, there was virtually no difference between the groups in the rate of pre-eclampsia: 15 percent of the vitamin group got it, compared to 16 percent of the placebo group.

The amounts of Vitamin C and Vitamin E in prenatal supplements aren't enough to have any impact on pre-eclampsia, so there doesn't seem to be any reason not to take them. If you're pregnant, discuss all supplements with your doctor before you try them.

A common reason for a baby to be born weeks or even months early is that the membrane that holds the amniotic fluid breaks too soon. Some strong recent studies show that this is a lot more likely to happen to women whose C levels are low. Could taking Vitamin C supplements help prevent the problem? Quite probably, but if you're pregnant, talk to your doctor before taking extra Vitamin C supplements.

C-ing Is Believing

Vitamin C can help prevent cataracts—clouding of the lens in your eye that can lead to blindness—as you grow older. Cataracts are very common among older adults; 45 percent of people older than age 75 have them. A 1997 study by researchers at Tufts University and Harvard University School of Medicine found that taking Vitamin C supplements over a long period—10 years or more—lowered the risk of cataracts among older women by an amazing 77 percent. Even women who had other risk factors for cataracts, such as smoking, were protected if they took Vitamin C supplements. The researchers believe the antioxidant powers of Vitamin C are the key here. The extra Cs mop up free radicals in your eyes before they can damage the delicate lens. How much Vitamin C do you need for eye protection? The study suggests 250 mg a day does the trick.

Early onset cataracts, which develop before age 60, might also be preventable with Vitamin C. In a long-term study of women younger than age 60 and without diabetes (diabetes independently raises your risk of cataracts), the ones who got the most Vitamin C had the lowest risk of early onset cataracts. The women who got 362 mg a day from their food had a 57 percent lower risk than those who ate less than 140 mg a day. Women who took Vitamin C supplements every day over 10 years reduced their risk by 60 percent over women who didn't take supplements.

Other Health Problems Helped by Vitamin C

We could go on—and on and on—about the wonders of Vitamin C, but let's just hit a few highlights instead:

- ◆ **Protecting against mental decline.** Vitamin C can help protect you against mental decline, dementia, and Alzheimer's disease as you age. One recent study showed that taking Vitamin C in combination with Vitamin E could significantly reduce your risk of Alzheimer's and dementia. We'll discuss this in more detail in Chapter 15.

◆ **Treating lead poisoning.** Vitamin C helps you excrete lead faster. High lead levels have recently been linked to high blood pressure in adults, another reason Vitamin C may help blood pressure.

◆ **Preventing gum disease (gingivitis).** You may be more at risk for getting gum disease if you have even a slight Vitamin C deficiency. Remember, bleeding gums are an early sign of scurvy.

◆ **Preventing osteoporosis.** According to recent studies, older women with high dietary intakes of Vitamin C have stronger bones than those with low intakes. The women with the strongest bones have high dietary intakes of both Vitamin C and calcium—and they don't smoke.

◆ **Slowing Parkinson's disease.** High doses of antioxidant vitamins such as Vitamin C and Vitamin E could slow down the progress of Parkinson's disease in the early stages. If you have Parkinson's, discuss taking antioxidants and other supplements with your doctor before you try them.

◆ **Relieving symptoms of Peripheral Artery Disease (PAD).** In PAD, clogged arteries in the feet and legs impair bloodflow, leading to difficulty walking and an increased risk of heart attack and stroke. People with PAD have low Vitamin C levels, so it's possible that taking supplements may help relieve the symptoms of pain and cramping.

Other health problems that may be helped by Vitamin C supplements include herpes, eczema, hepatitis, chronic fatigue syndrome, rheumatoid arthritis, and many others. There aren't many studies of Vitamin C for these problems, so we can't say for sure that it helps. It doesn't hurt, though, and many patients do feel better when they take extra Cs.

The Least You Need to Know

◆ Vitamin C is your body's main antioxidant vitamin.

◆ You need Vitamin C to build connective tissue, heal wounds, and keep your immune system running properly.

◆ Although the adult RDA for Vitamin C is 75 mg a day for an adult woman and 90 mg a day for an adult man, most doctors and nutritionists believe that that amount is far too low and recommend 250 to 500 mg of Vitamin C a day.

◆ Foods high in Vitamin C include citrus fruits; strawberries; melons; cranberries; tomatoes; peppers; dark-green, leafy vegetables; potatoes; turnips; and broccoli.

◆ Vitamin C can help diabetes, high blood pressure, and high cholesterol, as well as help prevent heart disease and stroke.

◆ Vitamin C can also help prevent vision loss, asthma, and gallstones.

Vitamin D: Look on the Sunny Side

In This Chapter

- Why you need Vitamin D
- How your body makes Vitamin D from sunshine
- What foods are high in Vitamin D
- How Vitamin D builds strong bones
- How Vitamin D helps prevent cancer

Go out in the sun without sunscreen? Are you kidding? Risk sunburn, wrinkles, or even skin cancer? Go on, live dangerously—but just for 10 minutes a day. On a nice afternoon in July, that's all the sunshine you need to get your daily dose (and then some) of Vitamin D. Your body makes this important vitamin from sunlight on your skin.

Vitamin D is essential for keeping your bones and your immune system healthy—and it could also keep you from getting colon cancer and some other types of cancer as well. So the next time you sneak out early from the office to go to the beach, don't feel guilty, feel healthy! But remember to put on your sunscreen as soon as you've gotten enough rays for your Vitamin D.

Why You Need Vitamin D

It's the calcium in milk that helps make your bones strong, right? Right—but without the Vitamin D, or *calciferol*, that's also added to milk, the calcium won't work. Vitamin D's most important role is to regulate how much calcium you absorb from your food. Most of that calcium goes to build strong bones and teeth. You also need calcium to send messages along your nerves and to help your muscles contract (such as when your heart beats). Vitamin D regulates the amount of calcium in your blood and makes sure you always have enough. We're just starting to realize that Vitamin D also plays a role in a lot of other body functions. Your immune system needs Vitamin D, and it may help prevent cancer, especially colon cancer. The future for this vitamin looks very sunny!

def•i•ni•tion

Vitamin D in general is sometimes called **calciferol**. The form of Vitamin D you make in your body from sunshine is called Vitamin D_3, or **cholecalciferol**.

The Sunshine Vitamin

Vitamin D is the eccentric uncle of the vitamin family—it does things its own way. To get all the other vitamins, you have to eat them. To get Vitamin D, all you have to do is go outside. That's because you actually make Vitamin D when the sun shines on your skin. How? Basically, the ultraviolet light in the sunshine makes a type of cholesterol that's found just under your skin turn into something called Vitamin D_3, or *cholecalciferol*. The Vitamin D_3 gets carried to your liver, where it gets changed into a more active form; from there, it goes to your kidneys where it becomes even more active. Some of the Vitamin D_3 stays in your liver and kidneys, where it helps you reabsorb calcium from your blood. Some goes to your bones to help them hold on to their calcium. The rest goes to your intestines to help you absorb calcium from your food.

Even eccentric uncles act normal sometimes, though—and so does Vitamin D. It's found naturally in a few foods, but in a slightly different form called Vitamin D_2, or *ergocalciferol*. Vitamin D supplements contain either cholecalciferol or ergocalciferol—both work, but cholecalciferol is more active. Look for supplements that contain this form.

Food for Thought _____

The form of Vitamin D you get from foods and in some supplements is called Vitamin D₂, or *ergocalciferol* (it's also sometimes called calcifidiol or calcitrol). The *ergo-* part comes from ergot, a fungus that grows on rye plants. Substances in ergot cause hallucinations—in fact, LSD was first made from ergot. It also contains ergosterol, which is converted by ultraviolet light into Vitamin D₂. Don't worry—Vitamin D was first discovered in ergot, but your daily supplement is made from yeast or fish liver and can't cause hallucinations.

The AI for Vitamin D

For years, many researchers said the RDA was too low for older people. You just naturally make less Vitamin D in your skin as you get older—which is one of the reasons older people tend to have fragile bones. In 1997, the recommended amounts for Vitamin D were changed to account for age changes. The Institute of Medicine decided not to set an RDA, though. Instead, the Vitamin D amounts are now called *Adequate Intakes* (*AIs*) and are based on the amounts needed "to sustain a defined nutritional status." In other words, the AI is the amount you need to maintain a basic level of good health.

Although the AI is given in micrograms, the Vitamin D in food and supplements is generally measured in *International Units* (*IU*). One mcg equals 40 IU. We use both measurements in the AI chart for Vitamin D.

Adequate Intakes for Vitamin D

Age in Years/Sex	Vitamin D in mcg	Vitamin D in IU
Infants, Children, and Adolescents		
0 to 18	5	200
Adults		
19 to 50	5	200
51 to 70	10	400
70+	15	600
Pregnant women	5	200
Nursing women	5	200

Many nutritionists and doctors feel that you need even more Vitamin D as you get older to keep your bones strong and avoid osteoporosis (bones that are thin, brittle, and break easily). An important study published in *The New England Journal of Medicine* in 1997 backs them up. The study showed that men and women older than age 65 can cut their risk of a bone fracture in half if they take 700 IU of Vitamin D and 500 mg of calcium every day. (We'll talk more about osteoporosis in Chapter 17.) Additional studies have shown that even when older adults get the AI for Vitamin D, nearly 40 percent are still deficient. Today many researchers believe that the AI needs to be increased even more, to 1,000 IU daily. The best way to get more Vitamin D? Get outside in the sunlight more—without sunscreen.

Are You D-ficient?

You might be—a surprisingly large number of Americans are. In fact, a study in 1998 showed that on average nearly half of us are deficient in Vitamin D. Among healthy young people, the rate of deficiency is about 42 percent! Among hospitalized elderly people, the rate is even higher—about 57 percent. And among African American women aged 15 to 49, 10 to 30 percent are deficient, even though they get the RDA every day.

Food for Thought

If you don't get outside much, sitting by a sunny window won't help—the ultraviolet light you need to make Vitamin D is blocked by window glass. Sunscreen with a sun protection factor (SPF) higher than 8 will block ultraviolet from your skin so well that you won't make any Vitamin D.

A major reason for a deficiency is being D-prived of sunlight. As a rule of thumb, 5 to 10 minutes of daily sun exposure in the summer is enough. As the shockingly high number of people low on Ds shows, not too many of us are getting outdoors enough. That might not be the only reason, however. Among people who take a daily multivitamin with 400 IU of Vitamin D, 46 percent still have low levels. The recent studies suggest that 400 IU just isn't enough for good health and strong bones.

Vitamin D is fat-soluble, so when you make a lot (by spending a day at the beach, for example), some of it gets stored in your fatty tissues and your liver. When you've made enough to last for a while, your body automatically stops making more. If you're outside a lot in the nice weather, you probably store enough Ds to carry you well into the winter.

On the other hand, it's hard to tell whether you're getting the AI every day, because you can't really know how much Vitamin D you're making from sunshine. If you live in a sunny climate such as Florida or Arizona, you probably get plenty year-round just from your normal outdoor activities. If you live in a very rainy, foggy, or overcast climate, or in an area that has a lot of air pollution, you might not, because the ultraviolet light from the sun is blocked. You also might not be getting enough Vitamin D if your skin is very dark.

Food for Thought

How much sun is enough for optimum Vitamin D production? Not a lot. Five to ten minutes of sun exposure between 10 A.M. and 2 P.M. daily in the summer is enough to carry you through the whole year. If you have darker skin, stay in the sun a bit longer. When you're outside in the sun, put your sunscreen on only after the first 5 or 10 minutes.

You might be deficient in Vitamin D if …

◆ **You're an older adult.** You're now making only about half as much Vitamin D in your skin as when you were younger.

◆ **You don't get any sunlight.** People who are housebound or live in nursing homes are especially at risk, but if you work long hours indoors, you might be at risk, too.

◆ **You have kidney or liver disease.** You can't convert Vitamin D_3 into its more active forms. Talk to your doctor about supplements.

◆ **You take drugs such as cholestyramine (Questran) or colestipol (Colestid) to lower your cholesterol.** These drugs block your absorption of Vitamin D and other fat-soluble vitamins. Talk to your doctor about supplements.

◆ **You take corticosteroid drugs such as cortisone, prednisone, or dexamethasone for allergies, asthma, arthritis, or some other health problem.** These drugs can deplete your Vitamin D_3 level. Talk to your doctor about supplements.

◆ **You take anticonvulsant drugs such as phenytoin (Dilantin) or phenobarbital.** These drugs interfere with how you use your Vitamin D. Talk to your doctor about supplements.

◆ **You're a strict vegetarian or vegan.** There's very little Vitamin D in plant foods. If you don't drink milk and also don't get outside much, you—and your vegan kids—might not be getting enough Vitamin D.

◆ **You abuse alcohol.** Alcohol blocks your ability to absorb Vitamin D in your intestines and store it in your liver.

Kids who don't get enough Vitamin D develop rickets—their bones don't grow and harden properly. Fortunately, most kids get plenty of Vitamin D and rickets is rare. Infants who are breastfed exclusively, however, can get rickets, because breast milk is low in Vitamin D and babies don't get exposed to much sunlight. The American Academy of Pediatrics recommends giving breastfed infants a daily multivitamin containing 200 IU of Vitamin D. Over-the-counter drops work well.

Today, older adults, especially people who don't get much sun because they're in nursing homes or can't get out much, are the ones most likely to be short on Vitamin D. The deficiency shows up as osteomalacia—soft, weak, and painful bones. Osteoporosis is caused mostly by a shortage of calcium, but Vitamin D plays a crucial role as well. In fact, about a third of all elderly patients with hip fractures turn out to be low on Vitamin D. We'll talk a lot more about the crucial balance of Vitamin D, Vitamin K, and calcium when we get to calcium in Chapter 17.

Eating Your Ds

Long before anyone knew what caused rickets (Vitamin D wasn't discovered until the 1930s), they knew that choking down a daily spoonful of awful-tasting cod-liver oil prevented it. Fish oil contains a lot of Vitamin D, so you get some from eating fish liver, mackerel, herring, sardines, salmon, tuna, and other oily fish.

There aren't that many other foods that naturally have Vitamin D. Beef liver, egg yolks, butter, and margarine all have some, though not a lot. Plant foods have almost none, but Vitamin D is added to a lot of breakfast cereals. Take a look at the following chart to find the foods that are naturally high in Vitamin D.

def•i•ni•tion

Fortified milk, milk that has Vitamin D and (sometimes) Vitamin A added to it, has been around since the 1930s. As part of a public-health drive to eliminate rickets, milk producers began adding 400 IU of Vitamin D to every quart of milk. The program worked—rickets soon became rare. It's still rare today, mostly because 90 percent of all milk producers in the United States fortify their milk.

Today almost all the Vitamin D people get from their diets comes from *fortified milk*. There isn't naturally much Vitamin D in milk, but milk producers have been adding 400 IU of it to every quart of milk—whole, skim, low-fat, and nonfat—for decades. It's the reason rickets has practically disappeared. There's no Vitamin D in most milk products, though. Cheese, yogurt, cottage cheese, and other dairy foods aren't made with fortified milk, so they don't have much or any Vitamin D. Also, raw milk, most organic milk, and goat's milk don't have added Vitamin D. Margarine, however, is fortified with Vitamin D. How much of your Vitamin D requirement do you get from food?

The Vitamin D in Foods

Food	Amount	Vitamin D in IU
Butter	1 pat	2
Cheddar cheese	1 oz.	2.8
Cod-liver oil	1 tsp.	460
Egg	1 large	25
Herring, fresh	3 oz.	270
Liver, beef	3 oz.	26
Mackerel, fresh	3 oz.	943
Margarine	1 TB.	21
Milk	8 oz.	100
Salmon, fresh	3 oz.	350
Sardines, canned	3 oz.	1,000
Shrimp	3 oz.	129

Getting the Most from Vitamin D

If you spend a lot of time in the sun, your body automatically stops making Vitamin D after you've stored up enough. In other words, you can't overdose on yourself.

The same definitely isn't true of Vitamin D supplements. Of all the vitamins, this is the one you need to be most careful with. Large doses can make calcium build up in your blood, which could have serious consequences—although this is very unlikely in doses less than 1,000 IU. Too much Vitamin D might also increase your risk of a heart attack or kidney stones.

If you fall into one of the risk categories we talked about earlier, you probably need Vitamin D supplements. How about if you don't? Most people get only about 50 to 70 IU in their diets, so if you're not outside much, supplements might be a good idea—especially in the winter.

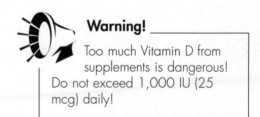

Warning!

Too much Vitamin D from supplements is dangerous! Do not exceed 1,000 IU (25 mcg) daily!

Now You're Cooking

You'll absorb your Ds a lot better if you take them with some dietary fat. Take D supplements with a meal.

Most multivitamin supplements now have 400 IU, which meets the AI for people younger than 50 even if you never get any sun or drink any milk. If you decide to take additional supplements, be on the safe side and keep your total daily dose to no more than 1,000 IU. Talk to your pediatrician before giving Vitamin D supplements to babies and children.

Vitamin D and Cancer

We've known for a long time that colon cancer and breast cancer are more common among people in northern climates—places where it's too cold for part of the year to get much sun. Is there a Vitamin D connection?

Yes, when it comes to colon cancer—and maybe also breast, ovarian, and prostate cancer, and maybe other cancers as well. Some researchers believe that Vitamin D deficiency contributes to 100,000 additional cases of cancer and 30,000 annual cancer deaths.

D-feating Colon Cancer

According to recent studies, people who get a lot of Vitamin D from their food and supplements are much less likely to get colon cancer. In one study, men who got at least 645 IU of Vitamin D from their food had a 40 percent reduction in their risk of colon polyps—the amount of sun they got didn't seem to matter. In another study, people who already had colon polyps and who took a combination of Vitamin D and calcium supplements had a reduced risk of recurrence. The higher the Vitamin D dose, the lower the risk.

D-fending Against Breast and Ovarian Cancer

In the United States, breast cancer rates are lower in the sunny Southwest and higher in the cloudy Northeast. Does the difference in sunshine exposure explain why? Quite possibly. In 2006 scientists looked at 13 different studies on Vitamin D and breast cancer and seven studies on Vitamin D and ovarian cancer. In both cases they concluded that a daily dose of 1,000 IU of Vitamin D could lower the risk of developing these cancers by about a third. The link between low Vitamin D and these cancers is similar to the link between cigarette smoke and lung cancer.

D-stroying Prostate Cancer

Recent research shows that your risk of prostate cancer is related to your sun exposure. Researchers compared a group of men in San Francisco with advanced prostate cancer with a similar group of healthy men. Among the men who averaged 20 hours of sun exposure each week—and therefore had high Vitamin D levels—the risk of prostate cancer was halved. Similar results have come from the Physicians' Health Study. Among the 15,000 men in this study, those with the highest levels of Vitamin D in their blood were half as likely to develop aggressive prostate cancer as those with the lowest levels.

Not only does Vitamin D help prevent prostate cancer, it may help treat it. Vitamin D in supplement form can inhibit the spread of prostate cancer cells in the body. Also, combining Vitamin D with the chemotherapy drug docetaxel (Taxotere) for advanced prostate cancer may be twice as effective as docetaxel alone.

Other Health Problems Helped by Vitamin D

Vitamin D can help strengthen your immune system in general. In particular, you need it to make monocytes, special white blood cells that fight off infections. About 5 percent of your white blood cells are monocytes, so a shortage of Vitamin D could leave you wide open to infection.

Helping Psoriasis

Psoriasis is a chronic skin disease that makes your skin get itchy, red, flaky patches. Sunshine seems to help clear up the patches for some people. Likewise, a prescription skin cream that has a form of Vitamin D in it seems to help in mild cases. Just taking a lot of Vitamin D in supplements doesn't, though—and it could be dangerous. If you have psoriasis, talk to your doctor about using calcipotriene (Dovonex) cream.

Helping Your Hearing

The smallest bones in your body are in your ears. In each ear, three tiny bones transmit sounds from your eardrum to another tiny bone called the cochlea. The snail-shaped cochlea sends the sounds to your brain. If any of the tiny bones is damaged, the sound doesn't get sent very well.

Many adults lose some of their hearing as they grow older. In fact, more than one out of every four adults older than age 65 has some hearing loss. In some cases, a shortage of Vitamin D may have damaged the delicate ear bones—and it's possible that taking Vitamin D supplements can help restore some hearing. This doesn't work in every case, of course, so talk to your doctor before you try it.

Preventing Falls

Falls in the elderly are a major cause of injury and even death. Taking Vitamin D supplements alone can reduce the risk of falling among older people by 22 percent. When Vitamin D supplements are combined with calcium, the risk of falling among older women drops even more, by 46 percent. Among less active women, the effect is even greater, dropping their risk by 65 percent. What about older men? For unknown reasons, adding calcium doesn't seem to help them. Overall, the supplements seem to help by increasing muscle strength.

A study in Scotland of 548 older adults who fell and broke a hip found that nearly all of them were deficient in Vitamin D. Other studies show, however, that taking Vitamin D supplements alone isn't enough to keep elderly people with osteoporosis from getting a bone fracture (see Chapter 17 on calcium to learn more about this). Keeping your bones strong as you age involves a number of factors—and getting enough Vitamin D from sunshine and supplements if needed is just one part of the puzzle.

D for Autoimmune Diseases

The crippling autoimmune disease multiple sclerosis is very rare among people living near the equator and becomes progressively more common the further you go to the poles. Researchers have long suspected a link between MS and a lack of Vitamin D from low sun exposure. Recent studies have shown that women who get at least 400 IU of Vitamin D daily have only a 60 percent less risk of getting MS compared to women who get lower amounts each day. Similarly, Vitamin D may help prevent rheumatoid arthritis (RA), another crippling autoimmune disease. Women with the highest levels of Vitamin D are about a third less likely to develop the disease.

The Least You Need to Know

- Vitamin D is a fat-soluble vitamin.
- Vitamin D is essential for strong bones.
- Vitamin D may also help prevent cancer.
- The Adequate Intake (AI) for Vitamin D is 5 mcg or 200 IU for people younger than age 50. You need more Vitamin D as you get older.
- Your body makes Vitamin D from sunshine on your skin. You also get some from your food.
- Most foods don't have much Vitamin D. The best source is fortified milk.

Vitamin E: E for Excellent

In This Chapter

- ◆ Learning why you need Vitamin E
- ◆ Learning whether Vitamin E can help prevent heart disease
- ◆ Boosting your immunity with Vitamin E
- ◆ Helping prevent cancer with Vitamin E
- ◆ Needing extra Vitamin E as you get older

On the vitamin report card, E stands for excellent. Vitamin E is an honor student in cancer prevention. And it's an A+ student in immune system improvement. All that, and it plays well with others, too. Vitamin E teams up with Vitamin A and Vitamin C to give you maximum antioxidant protection.

When it comes to heart disease and cancer, Vitamin E was once thought to be at the head of the class. Recent research has lowered Vitamin E's class standing, but this supplement hasn't flunked out yet. We'll explain why later in this chapter.

Why You Need Vitamin E

You need Vitamin E for one big reason: free radicals. We know, we know—we're always talking about these dangerous little vandals. What makes Vitamin E so special? Vitamin E is special because it's especially good at protecting your cell membranes against free radicals—and damage to your cell membranes is often the first step down a slippery slope that can lead to cancer, heart disease, and other health problems.

Vitamin E works so well as an antioxidant because it's a fat-soluble vitamin—and your cell membranes are made up mostly of fat. Vitamin E gets into the membrane and lassoes any free radicals that try to get through.

Vitamin E also teams up with Vitamin A, beta carotene, and Vitamin C, the other major antioxidant vitamins, to give you extra protection.

The Alpha, Beta, and Gamma of E

Vitamin E is a family of different compounds, all working together to protect you against roaming free radicals. The family is divided into two branches: the *tocopherols* and their cousins the tocotrienols.

def•i•ni•tion

In 1922, researchers found that lab rats on a diet of highly processed foods with no fats couldn't have babies. When the rats were given wheat-germ oil—high in Vitamin E—they became fertile again. Vitamin E was originally called **tocopherol**, from the Greek words *tokos*, "offspring," and *pheros*, "to bear."

The tocopherol clan has four members: alpha, beta, gamma, and delta tocopherol (aren't scientists imaginative?). For a long time, we thought that only alpha-tocopherol was really important and that the others were just along for the ride. That's because alpha-tocopherol is the most common and the most active form, the one that works the hardest to fend off free radicals. It turns out, though, that the other forms of tocopherol also help fend off free radicals pretty well. Gamma tocopherol, for example, seems best in protecting you against free radicals from nitrogen oxides. (That's the stuff that makes acid rain—imagine what it can do to your cell membranes!)

But just as your mother always compares you unfavorably to your well-behaved older brother, nutritionists compare all the other Vitamin E family members to alpha-tocopherol. Gamma tocopherol, for example, is only about 20 percent as active as alpha-tocopherol.

The four tocotrienol cousins (also called alpha, beta, gamma, and delta) are members of the E family found in some plant foods such as rice and barley. They're not as active as the tocopherols, but on their own they have antioxidant powers. In fact, they may be even better than the tocopherols at protecting you against some types of free radicals, especially the pesky peroxyl radical, which is formed when high-energy radiation such as ultraviolet light bombards your body. Tocotrienols may also help in cancer prevention and in keeping down your cholesterol.

The RDA for Vitamin E

The RDA for Vitamin E was adjusted in 2000 by the Institute of Medicine, but by only a tiny amount—the recommended amount for adult women was raised to 15 mg. Many nutritionally oriented health-care providers think this is still way too low. The RDA is based on natural alpha-tocopherol, because that's the most active form of Vitamin E. Nutritionists often count the Vitamin E in food in milligrams, because foods contain mixed tocopherols. Scientific types like to count the Vitamin E in terms of International Units (IUs) of alpha-tocopherol, because that's the most common and active form. One mg of natural Vitamin E is equal to 1.49 IU; 1 mg of synthetic Vitamin E is equal to 1.1 IU. We're going to assume that you'll take natural Vitamin E, for reasons we'll discuss later in this chapter, so the RDA is shown both ways in the chart.

The RDA for Vitamin E

Age in Years/Sex	Vitamin E in mg	Vitamin E in IU
Children		
1 to 3	6	9
4 to 8	7	10
9 to 13	11	16
Adults		
14+	15	22
Pregnant women	15	22
Nursing women	19	28

As with the other RDAs, the amount of Vitamin E is very small. It's the bare minimum you need to avoid deficiency. Much larger doses of 400 IU (18 times the RDA) or even more are very safe—in fact, many of the studies judging the value of Vitamin E for preventing heart disease, cancer, and other health problems use doses that high or even higher.

Are You Deficient?

Vitamin E deficiency doesn't have any dramatic effects—your teeth don't fall out, and you don't go blind. If you don't get the RDA for a long time—several months or even years—you eventually get nerve damage, especially to the nerves in the spinal cord, and sometimes damage to the retina of your eye. The damage is hard to spot, though, and it takes a long time to show up. Damage from a serious Vitamin E deficiency is very rare because almost everyone gets somewhere between 7 and 11 mg of Vitamin E just from the foods they eat. But what about a mild Vitamin E shortage? Unfortunately, that seems to be fairly common. According to a 1999 study, almost 30 percent of U.S. adults turn out to be low on Vitamin E. The problem is particularly serious among African Americans—about 41 percent turn out to be low on Es. For everyone, the reason seems to be low dietary intake. As we'll discuss in a moment, there's not that much Vitamin E in foods.

> **Food for Thought**
>
> If you take a blood-thinning drug such as warfarin (Coumadin), heparin, or aspirin, your doctor may recommend against also taking Vitamin E because the combination could thin your blood too much. In fact, studies have shown that Vitamin E does have an additive effect with aspirin, but not with warfarin or heparin. Even so, discuss taking Vitamin E supplements with your doctor before you try them.

Diet aside, there are a few medical conditions that can make you deficient in Vitamin E:

◆ **You have cystic fibrosis.** You can't digest fats well, so you don't absorb enough Vitamin E. Talk to your doctor about supplements.

◆ **You have Crohn's disease or ulcerative colitis.** You can't absorb Vitamin E well through your intestines. Talk to your doctor about supplements.

◆ **You have liver disease.** You can't use Vitamin E properly. Talk to your doctor about supplements.

◆ **You're on a very low-fat, low-calorie diet.** You might not be getting enough Vitamin E from your food. Also, you need a little fat in your food to absorb Vitamin E.

◆ **You take drugs such as cholestyramine (Questran) or colestipol (Colestid) to lower your cholesterol.** These drugs block your absorption of Vitamin E and other fat-soluble vitamins. Talk to your doctor about supplements.

Eating Your Es

There just aren't that many foods with Vitamin E in them. The best dietary sources are vegetable oils, seeds, wheat germ, and nuts. There's a little Vitamin E in plant foods such as avocados, asparagus, mangos, and sweet potatoes, but it's hardly worth mentioning. Animal foods such as meat and milk have practically no Vitamin E. Here's the breakdown:

Foods High in Vitamin E

Food	Amount	Vitamin E in mg
Almond oil	1 TB.	5.30
Almonds, dry-roasted	1 oz.	6.72
Apple	1 medium	0.81
Asparagus, cooked	4 spears	0.81
Avocado	½ medium	2.32
Corn oil	1 TB.	1.90
Hazelnuts	1 oz.	6.70
Mango	1 medium	2.32
Olive oil	1 TB.	1.67
Peanut butter	2 TB.	3.00
Peanut oil	1 TB.	1.60
Peanuts	1 oz.	2.56
Safflower oil	1 TB.	4.60
Sunflower oil	1 TB.	6.30
Sunflower seeds	1 oz.	14.18
Sweet potato	1 medium	5.93
Wheat germ	¼ cup	4.08
Wheat-germ oil	1 TB.	20.30

Vegetable oils in general have Vitamin E, but there's a lot of variation. About 90 percent of the Vitamin E in safflower oil is alpha-tocopherol, but it's only about 10 percent in corn oil. The Vitamin E in soybean oil, which is used in a lot of prepared salad dressings, is mostly gamma tocopherol.

Getting the Most from Vitamin E

The possible health benefits of extra Vitamin E really kick in only at daily amounts of more than 100 IU. There's no way you can eat that much Vitamin E—in fact, it's hard to eat even 25 IU. To get 100 IU from food, you'd have to eat about 15 ounces of almonds (which would have more than 2,500 calories) or swallow 5 tablespoons of wheat-germ oil (600 calories) or 22 tablespoons of safflower oil (more than 2,600 calories). Supplements are the way to go. But which kind?

Natural or Synthetic?

Natural Vitamin E is made from vegetable oil, usually from soybeans or safflower seeds; synthetic Vitamin E is made chemically. Natural Vitamin E is about twice as expensive, but it's also more active. You absorb it better and it stays in your system longer. Natural E is definitely the best choice.

When you look at the label on the vitamin jar, you can easily tell the difference. Natural Vitamin E is called d-alpha-tocopherol and the synthetic version is called dl-alpha-tocopherol. Look for supplements that have just the *d-* prefix.

I'm All Mixed Up

Vitamin E isn't just Vitamin E—it's the whole family. To make sure you're getting everything the family has to offer, choose a mixed supplement that has all the tocopherols, from alpha to delta; you can also get supplements that have tocotrienols. Most of the Es in a mixed supplement still come from alpha-tocopherol, because it's the most active form.

Wet or Dry?

Vitamin E supplements are available in dry and wet forms. In the dry form, the alpha-tocopherol is chemically bound to succinate; in the wet form, it's bound to acetate. Acetate and succinate are weak acids found naturally in your body—they're added to keep the Vitamin E from reacting with oxygen in the air and don't affect you in any way.

Dry Vitamin E is made into tablets or capsules. Wet Vitamin E is more like an oil, so it's usually sold as softgel capsules or as a liquid. If you have trouble digesting fats or oils, pick the dry succinate form. Otherwise, choose the wet form—you'll absorb the Es better.

Thumbs Up/Thumbs Down

Vitamin E Works Better With ...	Vitamin E Is Harmed By ...
Small amounts of dietary fat	Antacids
Selenium	Some cholesterol-lowering drugs
Vitamin A	
Beta carotene	
Vitamin C	

What About Selenium?

The trace mineral selenium helps Vitamin E work better and longer in your body. (We'll talk more about selenium in Chapter 21.) You need only very tiny amounts of it—the amount in your daily multivitamin/mineral supplement is usually plenty. If you think you're not getting enough selenium, though, try one of the natural Vitamin E supplements that has added selenium.

Vitamin E and Heart Disease: Excellent or Ex?

In the 1990s, four really important studies published in major medical journals seemed to show that people who took Vitamin E supplements had less heart disease. Two of the studies were based on results from the long-running Nurses' Health Study and the Physicians' Health Study, which followed large groups of women and men over several decades. Both showed that the participants who took at least 100 IU of supplemental Vitamin E for at least 2 years had a lower risk of heart disease. Among the women nurses, the drop was substantial—the Vitamin E takers reduced their risk by about two thirds. Another study, the Cambridge Heart Antioxidant Study (CHAOS), looked at 40,000 men who already had heart disease and found that Vitamin E kept their heart disease from getting worse. In fact, the men who took at least 400 IU of Vitamin E cut their chances of a nonfatal heart attack by an amazing 77 percent. Finally, a long-term study of more than 34,000 postmenopausal women showed that those who ate the most foods high in Vitamin E but didn't take E supplements had strikingly less heart disease.

The studies were very exciting, because they seemed to point the way to a safe, inexpensive way of lowering your risk of heart disease. Even so, the basic idea needed to be tested more rigorously in controlled experiments comparing Vitamin E to other approaches. That's exactly what researchers did starting in the late 1990s. The results were a big disappointment: study after study, all carefully designed and published in prestigious medical journals, showed that Vitamin E had little or no benefit. Or did it? As we'll see, the studies mostly looked at older people with existing heart disease, so the studies don't necessarily tell us much about how Vitamin E can help healthy people of *any* age protect their hearts.

Let's look a little more closely at some of the major studies to see what they said. In 2004, results from the Primary Prevention Project, an ongoing study in Italy, showed that Vitamin E supplements didn't reduce the risk of heart attack, stroke, or death among nearly 5,000 people who were at high risk because they had health problems such as diabetes or high blood pressure. Similar results came in 2005 from the ongoing Women's Health Study, which followed nearly 40,000 healthy women at least 45 years old from 1992 to 2004. The women who took 600 IU of Vitamin E every other day didn't have any fewer heart attacks or strokes than those who took a placebo. Overall, however, the women in the Vitamin E group had a 24 percent reduction in their risk of death from heart disease. Two large studies, the Heart Outcomes Prevention Evaluation (HOPE) trial and the HOPE-TOO trial, looked at more than 9,000 men and women who were older than age 55 and were at high risk of a heart attack or stroke because they had cardiovascular disease or diabetes plus another risk factor, such as high blood pressure. In a 10-year period, half took 400 IU of Vitamin E and half took a placebo. The results, published in 2006, showed that both groups had almost identical numbers of heart attacks and strokes. Vitamin E supplements had no apparent effect on cardiovascular outcomes.

The evidence seems clear: Vitamin E isn't quite the magic bullet researchers had hoped to find for fighting heart disease and cancer (we'll talk about that later in this chapter). Does that mean Vitamin E is useless? No. It's important to remember that studies looked at older people who were already at high risk for heart disease because of conditions such as diabetes. The people in the studies were taking prescription medications to treat their health problems. The drugs could keep the Vitamin E from helping or cover up any help the Es did provide. Finally, the studies were all short-term, lasting only 5 years or less, and none showed any harm from taking extra Es.

What these studies don't tell us is what happens when healthy people at normal risk for heart disease take Vitamin E supplements for a long time. Will they have lower rates of heart disease and stroke as they get older? The earlier studies suggest they will, but we can't say for sure. Research continues, and when the next edition of this book comes out, things could be very different yet again. In the meantime, we think taking extra Vitamin E is still a good idea.

It's also important to remember that vitamins from food and supplements are just one aspect of good health. Giving up smoking, drinking less alcohol, losing weight, getting exercise, and eating better all do a lot more to help prevent heart disease than taking supplements can. Lifestyle counts.

Food for Thought

In 2004, a meta-analysis of many studies of Vitamin E claimed that taking supplements could very, very slightly increase your overall risk of death. The studies the analysis was based on were all elderly patients who were already ill. Most researchers agree that the study is seriously flawed and that the supplements don't raise your risk of death.

E-luding Cancer

The evidence that Vitamin E helps prevent cancer isn't as dramatic as for heart disease, and it, too, has been put to the test in recent years. For every study that seems to show that Vitamin E helps prevent a type of cancer, another study seems to show it doesn't. For most cancers, the evidence is just too inconclusive. All we can do right now is take a look at some of the more promising areas.

Remember the ABC study (Alpha-Tocopherol, Beta-Carotene Cancer Prevention Study) from Chapter 3? That's where we talked about the beta carotene part of the study—and the news wasn't so great. Here's where we get to talk about the alpha-tocopherol (Vitamin E) part—and the news here is a lot better. The ABC study looked at more than 29,000 middle-aged male smokers in Finland in a 10-year period. One group of participants took 50 mg a day of supplemental Vitamin E for a period of 5 to 8 years. The result? Their risk of getting prostate cancer was reduced by a third—and among those who did get prostate cancer, the death rate was reduced by 41 percent. In addition, the men who had the highest blood levels of Vitamin E, whether from diet or supplements, lowered their risk of lung cancer by about 20 percent. Among the men who were light smokers and had been smoking for the shortest time, the reduction was even more dramatic—anywhere from 40 to 50 percent.

Warning!

Very large doses of Vitamin E (thousands of IU) can block your use of Vitamin A.

Because there's already some evidence that Vitamin E and selenium can help ward off prostate cancer, the National Cancer Institute is sponsoring a major long-term study to look more closely at this cancer-killing combo. The Selenium and Vitamin E Cancer Prevention Trial (SELECT) got under way in 2004 with 32,400 men participating. The men are randomly assigned to take various combinations of selenium, Vitamin E, and placebos every day for 7 to 12 years; they're checked for prostate cancer every 6 months. The first results should be available around 2013. Until then, there's no way to say for sure if taking extra Vitamin E can help prevent prostate cancer in healthy men. Look for the update in a future edition of this book!

In 2004, the results of a 5-year study showed that high dietary intake of Vitamin E in the form of alpha-tocopherol, significantly reduced the risk of bladder cancer. High Vitamin E from dietary sources alone reduced risk by 42 percent; getting a lot of Es from supplements and diet reduced the risk a touch more, by 44 percent.

Excellent for the Elderly

As you get older, your immune system naturally slows down. That makes you more likely to get sick with a serious infection that you can't fight off, such as pneumonia.

There's recently been some excellent news for older adults about Vitamin E and immunity—and it comes from the prestigious *Journal of the American Medical Association*. In a 1997 article, researchers showed that taking Vitamin E can give your immune system a real boost. Healthy volunteers, all older than age 65, took Vitamin E supplements for 33 weeks. Tests at the end of that time showed that their immune systems were much more active. The best results came from taking 200 mg a day; taking more didn't seem to help more.

Another example of how Vitamin E can boost immunity also comes from the pages of the *Journal of the American Medical Association*, this time from a 2004 study. Half of more than 600 elderly residents of a nursing home were given a daily Vitamin E supplement containing 200 IU; the other half got a placebo. During the course of a year, the Vitamin E group had significantly fewer colds compared to the placebo group. That might not seem like a particularly important result, but upper respiratory infections in the elderly can lead to complications such as pneumonia and death. Anything that reduces risk so safely is good.

If you're older than 60, it's probably time to start taking those extra Es—but talk to your doctor first, especially if you have any chronic health problems.

Thanks for the Memories

There's some pretty good evidence that Vitamin E can help prevent Alzheimer's disease (AD) in older adults. For instance, a study in 2004 looked at nearly 5,000 people aged 65 or older and found that those who took supplements of both Vitamin C and Vitamin E were 78 percent less likely to show signs of Alzheimer's disease than those who didn't take supplements. No benefit was found from taking either vitamin by itself or from taking just a daily multivitamin.

Researchers had hoped from earlier studies that Vitamin E might also help slow down AD after it happened. Some studies in the 1990s suggested that Vitamin E in large doses (as high as 2,000 IU daily) seemed to slow down—but not stop or prevent—Alzheimer's. But a 2005 study looked at a large group of patients with mild cognitive impairment. Half the group took the drug Aricept (donepezil), which is used to treat early AD, and half took Vitamin E supplements. After 3 years, Vitamin E showed no effect on the risk of progression to full AD. In both groups, about the same number of people got worse.

Vitamin E could help reduce poor memory problems in elderly people without Alzheimer's. Researchers have noted a strong connection in the elderly between low Vitamin E levels and memory poor enough to cause problems with the activities of daily living, such as managing money and preparing meals. High Vitamin E intake from food appears to help protect against cognitive decline. There aren't any studies yet to show that adding Vitamin E to your diet will help improve poor memory, but it seems pretty clear that making sure you get plenty of Vitamin E from a good diet will help keep your memory sharp as you age.

Other Health Problems Helped by Vitamin E

Vitamin E can be helpful for a lot of health problems, although it's not a cure for any of them. Here's a rundown of some current medical thinking:

- ◆ **Male infertility.** Some men are infertile because of free radicals. Why? You probably haven't ever given this much thought, but the cell membranes of sperm are very fatty, so they're especially vulnerable to attack by free radicals. Taking Vitamin E supplements can help mop up enough free radicals to prevent the damage. In one study, 5 out of 15 infertile men became fathers after just one month of 200 IU a day.

- **Benign breast disease.** If you want to make your doctor squirm, ask him or her why this perfectly natural condition is called a disease. Benign breast disease makes your breasts feel "lumpy." They might also swell and become tender when you're getting your period. It's uncomfortable and annoying, but usually benign breast disease isn't dangerous or a sign of breast cancer. We don't know exactly why this works, but taking anywhere from 200 to 600 IU of Vitamin E a day seems to relieve the symptoms for a lot of women.

- **Diabetes.** Vitamin E supplements have been suggested for treating or preventing just about every complication this disease can have. It's possible that Vitamin E can help people with Type 2 diabetes better control their blood sugar, prevent and treat diabetic neuropathy, reduce the risk of heart attack and stroke, and avoid kidney disease and eye problems. If you have diabetes and want to try Vitamin E supplements, talk to your doctor first.

- **Eye health.** The delicate blood vessels in your eyes are easily damaged by free radicals. A good supply of Vitamin E helps prevent the damage by sopping up the free radicals before they can do any harm. Likewise, Vitamin E helps protect the lens of your eye from free radical damage. People with low levels of Vitamin E are more likely to develop cataracts (clouding of the lens) as they get older. Studies show that long-term use of Vitamin E supplements can cut cataract risk.

- **Intermittent claudication and leg cramps.** Intermittent *what?* This is an annoying circulation problem that's caused by hardening of arteries in the legs. It makes your calf muscles ache and cramp up when you walk even a short distance. Vitamin E seems to help some people. If you want to try it, start with 200 IU daily for a week. If that doesn't help, try slowly increasing the dose, but don't go higher than 600 IU. Vitamin E also helps another annoying problem—nighttime leg cramps. Small doses of just 200 IU often do the trick. Take it with your evening meal.

- **Parkinson's disease.** A diet rich in Vitamin E may help prevent Parkinson's disease. A promising long-term study that looked at using Vitamin E, along with the drug selegiline (Deprenyl), to slow down the progression of this devastating brain disease showed that Vitamin E had no effect. If you have Parkinson's, talk to your doctor about Vitamin E and other supplements before you try them.

- **Lou Gehrig's disease, also known as amytrophic lateral sclerosis (ALS).** A 2005 study showed that people who regularly take Vitamin E supplements sharply reduce their risk of this lethal but relatively rare disease.

Some athletes claim Vitamin E improves their performance, although there's no real evidence for this. Other people claim Vitamin E miraculously cures everything from acne to gallstones. Although just about everybody can benefit from getting some extra Vitamin E, use your common sense. Talk to your doctor before you try big doses of Vitamin E for any reason.

The Least You Need to Know

- ◆ The adult RDA for Vitamin E is 15 mg or 22 IU.

- ◆ Many doctors today recommend taking 100 IU to 400 IU of Vitamin E every day.

- ◆ To get more than the RDA for Vitamin E, you'll need to take supplements.

- ◆ Vitamin E is safe in large doses.

- ◆ Vitamin E supplements may help prevent cancer and can boost the immunity of older adults.

Chapter 16

Vitamin K: The Band-Aid in Your Blood

In This Chapter

- ◆ Why you need Vitamin K
- ◆ Which foods are high in Vitamin K
- ◆ How Vitamin K helps your blood clot
- ◆ How Vitamin K helps keep your bones strong

When you cut your finger slicing onions in the kitchen, what happens? First, you swear under your breath. Next, you grab a paper towel and press it against the cut. A few minutes later, the bleeding stops. You slap on a Band-Aid and go back to fixing dinner. But what made the bleeding stop? Without going into all the gory (get it?) details, it's Vitamin K—the same stuff that stops all your other bleeding, too, such as when you cut yourself shaving, barked your shins on someone's bike in the driveway, and gave yourself a paper cut at the office.

Life is full of minor injuries, of course, which is why your blood needs to be full of Vitamin K. For most people, that's not a problem—a real shortage of Vitamin K is pretty rare.

Why You Need Vitamin K

Vitamin K is essential for making the blood clots that quickly stop the bleeding whenever you injure yourself. This fat-soluble vitamin actually comes in three different forms.

First, there's Vitamin K_1, or *phylloquinone*. This is the form of Vitamin K found in plant foods. Next, there's Vitamin K_2 (you were expecting some other number?), also called *menaquinone*. This is the form friendly bacteria in your intestines make for you. If you guessed that the last form would be called Vitamin K_3, you're absolutely right. This is the artificial form, also called *menadione*. All your Vitamin K ends up in your liver, where it's used to make some of the substances that make your blood clot.

Vitamin K is mostly needed to help you stop bleeding, but it has some other jobs as well. The most important is the crucial role Vitamin K_1 plays in building your bones. Vitamin K is needed to help you hold on to the calcium in your bones and make sure it's getting to the right place. There's also some interesting research on Vitamin K and cancer.

Food for Thought

In the late 1920s and early 1930s, Danish researchers discovered a substance that was essential for forming blood clots. They called it Vitamin K, for the Danish word *koagulation*, which is similar to the English word "coagulation" and refers to blood clotting.

def•i•ni•tion

Vitamin K_1, or **phylloquinone** (also sometimes called *phytonadione*), is the form found in plant foods. Vitamin K_2, or **menaquinone,** is the form made in your intestines by friendly bacteria. Vitamin K_3, or **menadione** (also sometimes called *menadiol*), is the synthetic form. It's more active than the natural forms.

The AI for Vitamin K

There's been an AI for Vitamin K only since 1989. Up until then, researchers thought that all the Vitamin K you needed was made for you by friendly bacteria in your intestines. In fact, though, the bacteria make only half or less of what you need. You get the rest mostly from—you guessed it—green, leafy vegetables. In 2000, the Institute of Medicine increased the AI slightly for adults. Check out the following table to make sure you're getting enough Vitamin K.

The AI for Vitamin K

Age in Years/Sex	Vitamin K in mcg
Infants	
0 to 0.5	2.0
0.5 to 1	2.5
Children	
1 to 3	30
4 to 8	55
9 to 13	60
Young Adults and Adults	
Men 14 to 18	75
Men 19+	120
Women 14 to 18	75
Women 19+	90
Pregnant women	90
Nursing women	90

Are You Deficient?

As a rule, Vitamin K deficiency is extremely rare—almost everyone gets more than enough from their own bacteria and from their food. Sometimes newborn babies don't have enough Vitamin K because they don't yet have any bacteria to make it in their intestines. To make up for that and prevent a serious bleeding problem called *hemorraghic disease of the newborn*, most newborns are given an injection of a tiny amount of Vitamin K soon after birth.

When adults get Vitamin K deficiency, it's generally because they eat very few green vegetables or because they have been taking oral antibiotics for a long time. Antibiotics kill off the intestinal bacteria that make Vitamin K. Sometimes Vitamin K deficiency is caused by liver disease or a problem digesting fat. You might be deficient if …

   ◆ **You have serious liver disease.** You can't use Vitamin K properly. Your doctor will probably recommend Vitamin K shots.

◆ **You have Crohn's disease, ulcerative colitis, or some other serious intestinal problem.** You can't absorb fats well, so you don't absorb much Vitamin K from your food. Talk to your doctor about supplements.

◆ **You've been taking antibiotic pills for a long time (at least several weeks).** Tetracycline, neomycin, and cephalosporin kill the bad bacteria—but they also kill the friendly bacteria that make Vitamin K in your intestines. Eating more Vitamin K foods should help, but talk to your doctor first.

◆ **You take drugs such as cholestyramine (Questran) or colestipol (Colestid) to lower your cholesterol.** These drugs block your absorption of Vitamin K and other fat-soluble vitamins. Talk to your doctor about supplements.

The major symptom of Vitamin K deficiency is that your blood clots very slowly, so you bleed for a long time even from minor injuries. Vitamin K deficiency causes big black-and-blue marks from very slight bruises or even for no reason, nosebleeds, blood in your urine, and intestinal bleeding.

If you have Vitamin K–deficiency symptoms, see your doctor at once. You'll need blood tests to check your clotting time and your prothrombin level (we'll explain about prothrombin a little later in this chapter). If the results show a deficiency, you may need more tests to figure out why. In the meantime, your doctor will probably give you Vitamin K shots. These can take a while to kick in, though, so you may also have to take Vitamin K supplements.

Eating Your Ks

A lot of foods haven't ever been analyzed to find out how much Vitamin K they have. And in the ones that have been studied, the K amounts are variable—some sources give amounts that are a lot different than others. In general, though, all the dark-green, leafy vegetables, such as kale, broccoli, lettuce, and cabbage, are good choices. Strawberries are also good. Some animal foods, including egg yolks and liver, have small amounts of Vitamin K.

Making sure you eat foods rich in Vitamin K has a big payoff, at least for women. A recent study of more than 120,000 female nurses showed that among middle-aged and older women, the ones with the most Vitamin K in their diet had the lowest risk of a

> **Now You're Cooking**
>
> There are 199 mcg of Vitamin K in an ounce of green tea leaves—but not in any other kind of tea. That sounds like a lot, until you realize that it takes a dozen tea bags to make an ounce. In other words, a cup of green tea has only about 16 mcg of Vitamin K.

hip fracture. (We'll talk more about this study and the role of Vitamin K in building healthy bones in the following section.)

Foods High in Vitamin K

Food	Amount	Vitamin K in mcg
Beef liver	3 oz.	89
Broccoli, raw	½ cup	58
Cabbage, raw	½ cup	52
Cauliflower, raw	½ cup	96
Egg	1 large	25
Milk, skim	1 cup	10
Potato, baked	1 medium	6
Soybean oil	1 TB.	76
Spinach, raw	½ cup	74
Strawberries	1 cup	21
Tomato, raw	1 medium	28
Turnip greens, raw	½ cup	182
Wheat germ	1 oz.	10

Getting the Most from Vitamin K

Most people get more RDA for Vitamin K from their food than needed and don't ever need a supplement. Not too many multivitamins have even small amounts of Vitamin K in them, although you can buy K supplements in 100 mcg capsules. In fact, because supplements should be used only if your doctor has diagnosed a real Vitamin K deficiency, you should probably skip these. If you want to make sure you're getting enough Vitamin K, the best approach is to eat your vegetables.

If you're low on Vitamin K because of an intestinal problem that makes it hard for you to digest fats, you may need supplements to treat or prevent clotting problems. Discuss this with your doctor—don't supplement on your own.

If your doctor advises Vitamin K supplements, you will probably have to take only 100 mcg a day. Any more than that could be toxic and might cause liver damage. Vitamin K supplements are made with phytonadione, a water-soluble version of Vitamin K_1.

Vitamin K and Clotting

Your blood normally has a number of different clotting factors—substances that help it form clots to stop bleeding from cuts, bruises, and other injuries. You need Vitamin K to help your liver make prothrombin (factor II), the most important of the clotting factors. Some of the other factors, including factors VII, IX, and X, are also made in your liver and also depend on Vitamin K. Without clotting factors, your blood clots very slowly or not at all, so even a small cut can bleed for a long time and a minor bang can cause a big bruise.

Vitamin K and Osteoporosis

You need Vitamin K to help your bones grab onto calcium, put it in the right place, and hold onto it after it's there. If you don't have enough Ks, you won't be able to form new bone very well. In the long run, a shortage of Vitamin K can lead to osteoporosis, or bones that are brittle and break easily. (We'll talk a lot more about osteoporosis when we talk about calcium in Chapter 17.) There's some evidence that Vitamin K supplements can help reduce bone loss and increase bone density. In a 2006 meta-analysis that looked at 13 trials, researchers found that taking Vitamin K supplements reduces bone loss and cuts the risk of fractures.

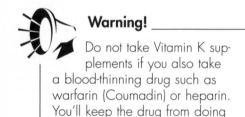

Warning!

Do not take Vitamin K supplements if you also take a blood-thinning drug such as warfarin (Coumadin) or heparin. You'll keep the drug from doing its job.

How much Vitamin K do you have to eat to protect your bones? At least the AI of 90 mcg a day for women and 120 mcg for men. In a study of female nurses, the nurses with the strongest bones averaged just more than 100 mcg daily, so women might want to aim for a bit more.

The anticlotting drugs warfarin (Coumadin) and heparin are often prescribed for elderly people with heart trouble or who are at risk of stroke or other health dangers caused by blood clots. There's a big problem with these drugs, however: they work by blocking your use of Vitamin K, which in turn can weaken your bones. Long-term use of these drugs has been shown to increase your risk of fracturing a vertebra or rib. If your doctor prescribes these drugs, be sure to discuss the increased risk of osteoporosis with him or her.

K Kills Cancer Cells

But so far, only in the test tube. Vitamin K seems to slow down or kill tumor cells in the lab just as well as powerful drugs. Some studies are looking at combining Vitamin K with standard anticancer drugs to help them work better. We don't know how well this works yet.

The Least You Need to Know

- ◆ You need Vitamin K to help your blood clot properly.

- ◆ The adult AI for Vitamin K is 90 mcg for women and 120 mcg for men.

- ◆ Green, leafy vegetables are the best food source of Vitamin K. Friendly bacteria in your intestines also make some of your Vitamin K.

- ◆ Vitamin K deficiency is very rare, so supplements aren't needed.

- ◆ Vitamin K plays an important role in building strong bones and preventing osteoporosis.

Part 3

Minerals: The Elements of Good Health

Ever feel a little rocky? It's not surprising—you have enough different minerals in your body to keep a geologist busy for days!

You need the essential minerals every bit as much as you need vitamins. In fact, without the minerals, your vitamins can't do their jobs, and vice versa. And like vitamins, some minerals have important roles in helping you prevent and treat health problems. All the minerals in your body add up to a market value of just a few dollars. But when it comes to your good health, they're worth more than their weight in gold.

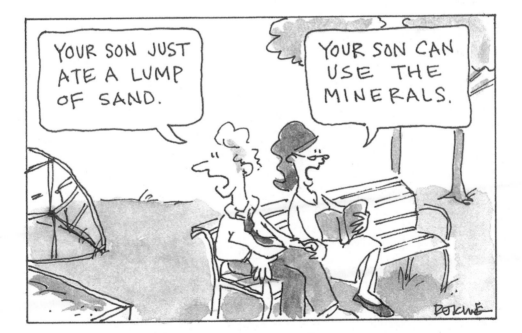

Chapter 17

Calcium: Drink Your Milk!

In This Chapter

- ◆ Why everyone needs calcium—and why women need extra
- ◆ How calcium keeps your bones strong all your life
- ◆ What foods are high in calcium
- ◆ How to choose the right calcium supplement
- ◆ How calcium may help your blood pressure and your heart
- ◆ How calcium may help PMS

Close your eyes and think back to your childhood. You can probably still hear your mother saying, "Drink your milk! It's good for you." You might even find yourself saying the same thing to your own kids today. Well, your mom was right—and so are you. Milk is the best food source of calcium, and kids need plenty of calcium to build strong bones.

Close your eyes and think back again, this time to your teen years. You can probably still hear yourself saying to your mother, "Aw, Mom, milk's a kid's drink." Your mom was right—and you were wrong. Milk—or more precisely, the calcium in milk—isn't just for kids. You need calcium all through your life to keep your bones strong.

Why You Need Calcium

Calcium is by far the most abundant mineral in your body. It makes up about 2 percent of your total body weight, or between 2 and 3 pounds if you're an average adult. Most of your calcium—98 percent of it—is in your bones. Another 1 percent is in your teeth, and the last 1 percent circulates in your blood. Small as the amount of calcium in your blood is, it's very important—so important that your body will pull calcium from your bones to make sure there's enough in your blood. Among other things, calcium helps regulate your heartbeat, control your blood pressure, clot your blood, contract your muscles, and send messages along your nerves. Calcium is needed to make many different hormones and enzymes, especially the ones that control your digestion and how you make energy and use fats. It also helps build your connective tissue and may help prevent high blood pressure and colon cancer.

Boning Up on Calcium

How many bones are in your skeleton? Give up? You have 206. Every single one of them is made up mostly of calcium phosphate, a very hard, dense mixture made when calcium and phosphorus combine. (We'll talk about phosphorus a little later in this chapter.)

Your bones may be hard, but they're also living tissue. You're constantly breaking down old bone and building new bone. From the time you're born until you get to be about 30 to 35 years old, you build up bone faster than you lose it, so your bones get bigger and denser, and you reach what's called peak bone mass. You could think of it as building up a bone savings account. After about age 35, you start to slowly break down bone faster than you can rebuild it—you start to draw on your saved-up bone. Some slow bone loss is a normal part of getting older, but if you don't get enough calcium, the process can start to happen too fast, especially in older women who've reached menopause. As adults—both men and women—age, they naturally draw down their bone savings account and lose some bone density. This thinning is called *osteopenia*. If you lose too much bone, though, you empty out your bone savings account. At that point, your bones are thin, brittle, and break very easily. You've got *osteoporosis*.

def•i•ni•tion

Osteopenia means bones that have become thin but not dangerously so. **Osteoporosis** means bones that break easily because they are thin, porous, and brittle. Osteoporosis has several related causes, but too little calcium in the diet plays a big part in causing it.

Here's where calcium comes in. If your bones are strong to begin with, and if you keep giving them plenty of calcium as you get older, you'll help keep your bones strong throughout your life. And even if osteopenia or osteoporosis has already set in, calcium may help slow it down.

We'll be talking a lot about the role of calcium in preventing and treating osteoporosis all through this chapter. That's because osteoporosis is a very serious health problem. It affects some 10 million Americans—four out of five of them older women. More than half of all Americans aged 50 or older are at risk. You need calcium now to avoid the crippling broken bones osteoporosis can cause.

Food for Thought

Osteoporosis is a silent disease—bone loss doesn't have any symptoms. That's why doctors recommend that all women older than age 65, and younger women who have extra risk factors, have a bone mineral density (BMD) test. Talk to your doctor about having this quick, painless x-ray procedure. For more information, check the website of the National Osteoporosis Foundation at www.nof.org.

The RDA for Calcium

In 1994, the National Institutes of Health (NIH) had a major conference on osteoporosis. A panel of experts looked at all the latest information on the importance of calcium and recommended much higher daily intakes of calcium for everyone. Here's the chart with their recommendations:

NIH Consensus Panel on Optimal Calcium Intake

Age in Years/Sex	Calcium in mg
Infants	
0 to 0.5	400
0.5 to 1	600
Children	
1 to 10	800 to 1,200
11 to 24	1,200 to 1,500

continues

NIH Consensus Panel on Optimal Calcium Intake   (continued)

Age in Years/Sex	Calcium in mg
Adults	
Men 25 to 65	1,000
Men and women older than 65	1,500
Women 25 to 49	1,000
Women 50 to 65, taking estrogen	1,000
Women 50 to 65, not taking estrogen	1,500
Pregnant women	1,200 to 1,500
Nursing women	1,200 to 1,500

In 1997, the Food and Nutrition Board of the Institute of Medicine caught up to the NIH. The old RDA for calcium, set by the Food and Nutrition Board back in 1989, was scrapped in favor of a higher standard. Here's the new and improved RDA for calcium:

The RDA for Calcium

Age in Years/Sex	Calcium in mg
Infants	
0 to 0.5	210
0.5 to 1	270
Children	
1 to 3	500
4 to 8	800
9 to 18	1,300
Adults	
19 to 30	1,000
31 to 50	1,000
51+	1,200

Age in Years/Sex	Calcium in mg
Pregnant Women	
14 to 18	1,300
19 to 30	1,000
31 to 50	1,000
Nursing Women	
14 to 18	1,300
19 to 30	1,000
31 to 50	1,000

When you compare the charts, you see that the biggest difference between them is the amounts for older adults and pregnant and nursing women. The NIH suggests somewhat higher amounts for these groups and also suggests different amounts based on your sex and whether you take estrogen after menopause. (We'll explain more about estrogen and older women a little later in this chapter.) The overall message is clear from both charts: you need plenty of calcium, especially as you get older.

Are You Deficient?

More than half of all young people today don't meet the RDA for calcium. That means they're not getting the calcium they need during the crucial childhood, teen, and young-adult years to build up their bone mass. If you don't get enough calcium during these critical years, you don't build up your bone savings account, which could lead to big trouble when you're older.

It's not just kids who don't get enough calcium. Most women in the United States eat less than 600 mg of calcium a day. In fact, calcium is the one nutrient most likely to be missing in the typical American diet. According to U.S. Department of Agriculture surveys, 78 percent of adult women aren't getting the RDA for calcium. Among girls ages 12 to 19, 87 percent aren't getting enough—at a time when they need calcium more than ever to build their peak bone mass. Men do better, but even so, only 55 percent of adult men are getting enough calcium. It's no wonder that today we have a virtual epidemic of osteoporosis—and that we'll have even more cases in the future as the population gets older. By one estimate, the number of hip fractures in the United States may triple by the year 2040.

Poor diet is bad enough, but a number of common drugs can rob your body of calcium. This is such an important topic that we have to deal with it separately.

Calcium-Robbing Drugs

Some common prescription and over-the-counter drugs can rob your body of calcium and lead to osteoporosis. If you regularly take any of these drugs, talk to your doctor about calcium supplements.

Cortisone and Other Steroid Drugs

A lot of people take drugs called glucocorticoids, which are synthetic versions of the steroid hormones your body naturally produces. This large class of drugs includes cortisone, hydrocortisone, prednisone, and dexamethasone. These drugs are lifesavers for some 30 million Americans who have severe asthma, lupus, rheumatoid arthritis, inflammatory bowel disease, and other medical problems. But—and this is a big but—they can also cause bone loss by breaking down bone faster than you can rebuild it. For a long time, doctors thought you had to worry only if you were taking high doses. Recent studies show, however, that taking even small doses—fewer than 10 mg a day—for a long time can cause osteoporosis. (The small doses in inhaled asthma medications containing steroids don't seem to affect bone density.) So if you're taking any sort of steroid drug, talk to your doctor about having a bone density test and taking calcium and Vitamin D supplements. You should also follow all the lifestyle suggestions we'll talk about a little further on to avoid osteoporosis.

Thyroid Drugs

Many people, especially middle-aged women, don't produce enough hormones from their thyroid gland and need to take supplements (Synthroid or another drug), usually for the rest of their lives. There's no question that they need the supplements, but large doses over a long period can lead to bone loss. If you take thyroid drugs, check your dose with your doctor once a year—your need may change and you may be able to take less. Also talk to your doctor about calcium supplements.

Drugs for High Cholesterol

Cholestyramine (Questran), a drug used to treat high cholesterol, can block your absorption of calcium and fat-soluble vitamins such as Vitamin D. Talk to your doctor about calcium supplements.

Aluminum Antacids

If you often take nonprescription antacids that contain aluminum (Maalox, Rolaids, Gelusil, and others), your body may start storing aluminum in your bones instead of calcium. You could end up with weakened bones—especially if you also have kidney problems. If you take these antacids only now and then, you don't have to worry. But if you often take antacids for heartburn, talk to your doctor about other ways to control it.

Alcohol and Tobacco

Heavy drinkers and people who smoke have a higher risk for osteoporosis. If you do both, you're at even greater risk. Smokers have lower bone density than nonsmokers (we don't really know why). In fact, a recent study showed that smoking doubles your risk of a hip fracture, even if you don't have osteoporosis. Alcohol interferes with your absorption of calcium. Also, heavy drinkers often don't eat very well and don't get enough calcium in their food. People under the influence tend to fall—and combined with osteoporosis this leads to broken bones.

Other Prescription Drugs and Calcium

Valuable as calcium supplements are, they can sometimes interfere with prescription drugs you might have to take. Doctors usually recommend taking your calcium supplements 2 hours apart from any other drugs to prevent problems. There are some cases, though, where you might even need to skip the supplements. If you take any of these drugs, be very careful about your extra calcium:

- ◆ **Digitalis.** If you take calcium supplements with this heart medicine, you might get dangerous irregular heartbeats. Try to get enough calcium from your foods and avoid supplements.

- ◆ **Phenytoin (Dilantin).** Calcium and phenytoin (a drug used to treat epilepsy and other problems) react to each other. The calcium can keep the phenytoin from working right, while the phenytoin can keep you from absorbing the calcium. Talk

> ### Now You're Cooking
>
> All milk—regular, skim, low-fat, 1 percent, 2 percent, and nonfat—has the same amount of calcium: about 300 mg in 8 ounces. It's the same for all other dairy foods: low-fat and regular have the same amount of calcium.

to your doctor about calcium supplements before you try them. If you decide to take calcium supplements, take them three hours after you take your phenytoin.

◆ **Antibiotics such as tetracycline and fluroquinolones, including ciprofloxacin (Cipro).** Calcium from milk, dairy products, and supplements keep these antibiotics from working well to fight infection. Take them on an empty stomach. Wait at least an hour before drinking milk or eating any dairy products. You usually have to take antibiotics for only a week or 10 days, so it's probably best to just skip your calcium supplements for that time. If you take a multi-supplement that has calcium, take it a couple of hours apart from your medicine.

◆ **Calcibind (cellulose sodium phosphate).** This drug is used to prevent kidney stones. If you take it, don't take calcium supplements. In fact, you need to avoid calcium completely, even calcium from food. Your doctor will explain how to take Calcibind and what foods to avoid.

◆ **Thiazide diuretics.** These drugs are used to treat high blood pressure and some other conditions. They can interact with calcium supplements and raise the amount of calcium in your system too high. If you take this type of drug, talk to your doctor about calcium supplements.

◆ **Iron supplements.** Calcium supplements can interfere with your absorption of iron from supplements. If you take iron supplements, take your calcium supplements a few hours apart—unless you take calcium citrate. That type of calcium supplement is okay to take with iron.

Can calcium help make a drug work better? In the case of metformin (Glucophage), a drug used to treat Type 2 diabetes, the answer is yes. Metformin can reduce your ability to absorb the B vitamin cobalamin. Calcium supplements can help you absorb the cobalamin better. If you take metformin, discuss all dietary supplements with your doctor before you try them.

Eating Your Calcium

The NIH panel says that the preferred way to get enough calcium is through your food. Fortunately, lots of favorite foods are rich in calcium—and a lot of common foods, including orange juice, are now available with added calcium.

Milk and dairy products are by far the best sources of calcium. There's about 300 mg of calcium in one 8-ounce glass of milk. (Milk also has Vitamin D, which you need to absorb calcium better and also to build your bones.) Yogurt usually has even more calcium than milk, and many yogurt makers are now adding extra calcium. The amounts vary from brand to brand, though, so read the labels carefully. An ounce of cheddar cheese has 200 mg, while an ounce of mozzarella has 147 mg and a cup of low-fat cottage cheese has 138 mg.

Here's the best news of all: ice cream is a good source of calcium. There's 85 mg in half a cup of plain vanilla ice cream. So next time you order a double-scoop cone, forget the calories and think of the calcium!

Other good dietary sources of calcium are dark-green, leafy vegetables, including broccoli, kale, and spinach. Beans; nuts; tofu (bean curd); and fish with soft, tiny bones (canned sardines and salmon are good choices) also give you plenty of calcium. English muffins turn out to be a good source of calcium—there's about 90 mg in each one. Use the following chart to pick the calcium-rich foods you need.

Food for Thought

Can't drink milk because it gives you gas, cramps, or even diarrhea? You're lactose intolerant—you don't make lactase naturally, an enzyme that helps you digest milk. Lactose intolerance is quite common, but that's no excuse to skip your milk. A lot of people who can't drink regular milk do fine with lactose-reduced or lactose-free milk. You can also add lactase drops to your regular milk or chew some lactase tablets before drinking it. Look for lactase products at your drugstore or health-food store.

Foods High in Calcium

Food	Amount	Calcium in mg
Almonds, dry-roasted	1 oz.	80
American cheese	1 oz.	124
Black beans	1 cup	47
Brie cheese	1 oz.	52
Broccoli, cooked	½ cup	36
Cabbage, cooked	½ cup	25
Cheddar cheese	1 oz.	204
Chickpeas	1 cup	78
Colby cheese	1 oz.	194

Foods High in Calcium   (continued)

Food	Amount	Calcium in mg
Collard greens, cooked	½ cup	15
Cottage cheese, low-fat	1 cup	138
Egg	1 large	25
English muffin	1 regular	90
Ice cream, vanilla	½ cup	85
Kale, cooked	½ cup	47
Kidney beans	1 cup	50
Milk	8 oz.	300
Mozzarella cheese	1 oz.	147
Navy beans	1 cup	128
Okra	½ cup	50
Peanuts	1 oz.	15
Potato, baked	1 medium	20
Pudding, instant, chocolate	½ cup	149
Ricotta cheese, part-skim	½ cup	337
Salmon, with bones	3 oz.	203
Sardines, with bones	3 oz.	92
Spinach, cooked	½ cup	122
Sunflower seeds	1 oz.	34
Sweet potato, baked	1 medium	32
Swiss chard, cooked	½ cup	51
Swiss cheese, processed	1 oz.	272
Tofu, uncooked	½ cup	130
Turnip greens, cooked	½ cup	99
Yogurt, plain, low-fat	8 oz.	415

Cooking green veggies and beans breaks down the tough cell walls and releases the calcium so that you can absorb it better. Because calcium is a mineral, cooking doesn't affect it. Cook the greens lightly, though, to protect the other vitamins in them.

Picking the Right Calcium Supplement

Let's face it: the only way a lot of us are going to get enough calcium each day is to take supplements. But just look at how many different supplements are on the shelf at the store. How can you pick the right one for you from all those choices?

It's not as complicated as it looks.

For starters, you need to know that you can't buy pure calcium—for complicated chemistry reasons, it's always combined with another harmless element. Your body breaks down this combination and absorbs the calcium. What this means is that a 500 mg tablet doesn't have 500 mg of calcium—it has a mixture of calcium and something else. The amount of actual calcium in the tablet is the *elemental calcium.* Today many manufacturers list just the elemental amount on the label, so you can figure out how much calcium you're really getting much more easily. Keeping that in mind, let's look at the different calcium combinations (check out the chart that appeared earlier in this chapter for the quick version):

♦ **Calcium carbonate.** The cheapest supplement, calcium carbonate is also the highest in elemental calcium: 40 percent. This is the form of calcium found in Tums and many generic versions. It has one big drawback: it dissolves slowly in your stomach, so you may not get the full benefit of all the calcium.

♦ **Calcium phosphate (also called tribasic calcium phosphate).** This form is 39 percent elemental calcium. You don't need the extra phosphorus that comes with these tablets—skip them.

def•i•ni•tion

The actual amount of usable calcium in a supplement is called the **elemental calcium.** It's given on the label as a percentage of the total in the supplement. For example, a 1,000 mg tablet of calcium carbonate is 40 percent elemental calcium—so you get only 400 mg of calcium from it. So that you don't have to do all that mental arithmetic, many manufacturers now list on the label only the amount of elemental calcium.

Food for Thought

If you don't like to drink milk but still want to get the calcium, try soy milk or almond milk. These nondairy products are packed with about as much calcium as an equal amount of milk, but have no lactose, no cholesterol, less fat, and fewer calories. They're great as a drink or in a shake.

- **Calcium citrate.** This is the form many doctors and nutritionists recommend. Calcium citrate is only 21 percent elemental calcium, and it's relatively expensive. On the big plus side, it dissolves easily even if you don't have much stomach acid, so you're more likely to absorb all the calcium before the pill passes out of your stomach. Many people naturally produce less acid as they age, so calcium citrate is a good choice for older adults. It's also good for people taking acid-blocking drugs such as ranitidine (Axid, Pepcid, Tagamet, and Zantac) or omeprazole (Prilosec). If you get kidney stones, calcium citrate is the best choice.

- **Calcium lactate.** This form is found in many generic calcium supplements. It has only 13 percent elemental calcium and is relatively expensive. On the other hand, it dissolves easily even if you're low on stomach acid; so, like calcium citrate, it's a good choice for older adults and people who take acid-blocking drugs.

- **Calcium gluconate.** This form is also found in many generics, but it has only 9 percent elemental calcium. It's not a very good choice.

- **Calcium glubionate.** This is a concentrated syrup form that contains 6.5 percent elemental calcium. You'd need to take 12 teaspoons a day to get 1,000 mg of calcium. Calcium glubionate is on the expensive side. It's useful for children and people who have trouble swallowing pills, because it can be mixed into juice or water.

Calcium Supplements to Avoid

Adding to all the calcium confusion are three forms you should not take, no matter how large the word "natural" is on the label.

- **Bone meal.** A powder made from the ground bones of cattle, bone meal has more than 1,500 mg of calcium in a 5 g serving, along with other minerals such as phosphorus and zinc. The FDA warns that bone meal may contain dangerously high amounts of lead.

- **Dolomite.** This is a mineral also known as calcium magnesium carbonate. It contains calcium—and also magnesium, which you may not want or shouldn't take. The FDA warns that dolomite may contain dangerously high amounts of lead.

Quack, Quack

Can coral calcium cure cancer? Of course not. Those infomercials for calcium supplements made from marine coral claim that the ratio of calcium to magnesium and the other trace minerals found in this product will magically cure all sorts of things. The Federal Trade Commission and the FDA disagree—these ads were yanked for making false and unsubstantiated claims.

◆ **Oyster-shell calcium.** Actually, this is calcium carbonate, but it's made from ground-up oyster shells. These supplements may also contain too much lead and sometimes other contaminants such as mercury and cadmium. Don't use them if you're allergic to shellfish.

Getting the Most from Calcium

Your body uses calcium around the clock, so try to space out your calcium over the day. If you can, have calcium-rich foods with every meal. If you take supplements, spread them out through the day, and don't take more than 600 mg at a time.

Should you take calcium supplements with meals or on an empty stomach? It's hard to say. On the one hand, you need stomach acid to make the supplement dissolve, and you make acid when you eat. On the other hand, the food you eat along with the supplement could block your absorption of the calcium—especially if you eat foods that are high in fiber—while at the same time calcium could block your absorption of other minerals from your food.

We've run out of hands, so do what most doctors recommend: take your calcium supplements between meals, but with a small protein snack—a few spoonfuls of yogurt, a piece of cheese, or maybe a leftover chicken leg—to make your stomach produce acid.

 Food for Thought

Some chewable antacids contain calcium in the form of calcium carbonate. This isn't a very good way to get your calcium. Ordinarily your stomach acid separates the calcium from the carbonate. Antacid tablets, however, are designed to neutralize your stomach acid—so most of the calcium won't be released and will just pass through your body instead. You'll also get other ingredients you may not want, such as aluminum and sugar.

If you have trouble choking down those big 500 mg calcium tablets, your last excuse not to take extra calcium is gone. A number of manufacturers now make tasty chewable and liquid calcium supplements. The only hard part is choosing your favorite flavor.

If milk is good and calcium supplements are good, isn't it even better to take them together? No—take them an hour or two apart so your body can absorb the most calcium from both.

Warning! _____

Don't take calcium supplements if you have kidney disease!

Calcium citrate dissolves faster than calcium carbonate, but it has less elemental calcium. To get the benefits of both forms, you could try a combination formula. Two popular brands are Os-Cal and Caltrate.

Most people don't have any side effects from taking calcium supplements even in high doses. To be on the safe side, though, don't take more than 2,000 mg of calcium in a day—that's your total intake, including food and supplements.

Sometimes people who take calcium supplements get constipation. If this happens to you, space out your supplements more across the day and be sure to drink plenty of water.

In very rare cases, too much calcium (more than 2,000 mg a day for a long time) can cause hypercalcemia, or an overload of calcium in the blood. The symptoms include appetite loss, drowsiness, constipation, dry mouth, headache, and weakness. Stop taking the supplements and call your doctor.

The Dynamic Duo: Calcium and Vitamin D

Vitamin D and calcium work together to keep your blood level of calcium normal. You also need Vitamin D to help your bones hold on to their calcium. For the best protection against osteoporosis, try to get about 200 IU of Vitamin D daily. (See Chapter 14 for more information.)

Some calcium supplements also contain Vitamin D and sometimes also Vitamin K. As you know from our earlier chapters on these vitamins, they're important for the complex process of bone remodeling, so you might want to choose a calcium supplement that has them both. To avoid getting too much Vitamin D, though, don't take any other supplements that contain it.

The dynamic duo has a sidekick: magnesium. This mineral is crucial for bone health because it helps you absorb calcium and use Vitamin D properly. The rule of thumb is half as much magnesium as calcium. So if you're getting 1,000 mg of calcium a day from food and supplements, you need 500 mg of magnesium. You can get calcium supplements that also have magnesium in them, but that may not be a good idea (see Chapter 18 for why).

Thumbs Up/Thumbs Down

Calcium Is Helped By ...	Calcium Is Blocked By ...
Vitamin D	Alcohol
Vitamin K	Tobacco
Magnesium	High-fiber foods
	Foods high in oxalic acid
	Cortisone-like drugs
	Tetracycline
	Thyroid drugs
	Thiazide diuretics
	Aluminum antacids
	Some drugs for high cholesterol

The Function of Phosphorus

Phosphorus is needed to build the structure of your bones and teeth, and it also plays important roles in almost every body process. For all its importance, phosphorus is so widespread in every food you eat that it's almost impossible to be deficient in it. (We'll explain all about phosphorus in Chapter 21 on trace minerals.) There's about 30 mg of phosphorus in a 12-ounce can of diet soda. Some researchers have suggested that the phosphorus in diet soda can play a role in causing osteoporosis. The theory is that the phosphoric acid in the soda has to be neutralized by calcium carbonate in the body, which keeps the calcium from being used to build bone instead. It's more likely, however, that the detrimental effects of drinking a lot of diet soda isn't because of the phosphorus but because the soda replaces milk in the diet.

Avoiding Osteoporosis

Are you at risk for osteoporosis? Answer the questions in this chart and add up your "Yes" answers. The more "Yes" answers you have, the greater your risk.

Are You at Risk for Osteoporosis?

	Yes	No
1. Do you have a small, thin frame?	❑	❑
2. Are you white or Asian?	❑	❑
3. Are you over age 50?	❑	❑
4. Have you passed menopause?	❑	❑
5. Did your mother have osteoporosis?	❑	❑
6. Did you reach menopause early or have a hysterectomy?	❑	❑
7. Do you take thyroid medicine?	❑	❑
8. Do you take cortisone-like drugs?	❑	❑
9. Is your diet low in calcium-rich foods?	❑	❑
10. Are you physically inactive?	❑	❑
11. Do you smoke?	❑	❑
12. Do you drink a lot of alcohol?	❑	❑

If you're at risk, what should you do? Getting more calcium is just one of the steps you need to take at once. Here are the others:

◆ Get regular exercise. Regular weight-bearing exercise—walking, jogging, dancing, skating, climbing stairs—helps keep your bones strong. (Swimming, yoga, and bike-riding are good exercise, but they won't strengthen your bones.) Walking for half an hour just three times a week could make a big difference.

◆ If you smoke, stop.

◆ Limit your alcohol to two drinks a day.

◆ If you're a woman past menopause, talk to your doctor about low-dose hormone replacement therapy (HRT) in combination with calcium and Vitamin D supplements to help restore lost bone.

◆ If you already show signs of bone loss, talk to your doctor about prescription drugs to slow bone loss and build new bone. Some of the newest drugs are easy to take and very helpful.

◆ Do everything you can to avoid falls that could break bones. For example: remove scatter rugs and electrical cords you could trip over; put night lights by stairs; install a grab bar and nonskid tape in the shower or tub; wear flat, rubber-soled shoes.

Food for Thought _____

When a woman reaches menopause, she makes a lot less of the hormone estrogen. But estrogen helps control how quickly you lose calcium from your bones, so when you make less of it, you start losing bone faster—a lot faster if you also have other risk factors. For the first 6 to 10 years after menopause, you could lose bone quickly, as fast as about 3 percent of your total every year. Over 10 years, then, you could lose more than 30 percent of your total bone density. By that point, your bones could be so thin that even a hard hug from a grandkid could make a rib break.

Not for Women Only

Osteoporosis is a problem for all older adults—not just women. The odds are lower if you're a man, but even so, some two million men already have osteoporosis and about three million are at risk. In fact, a third of all hip fractures from osteoporosis happen to men. And when they do, it's serious—a third of all the men who get these fractures die within a year.

Just as bone loss gets worse in older women when they start producing less estrogen, it gets worse in older men when they naturally start making less of the male hormone testosterone.

Even so, hormones don't seem to really be the main reason for osteoporosis in men. Not enough calcium in the diet and not enough exercise are important factors, but medications, smoking cigarettes, and drinking heavily also play big roles.

Warning! _____

According to the National Osteoporosis Foundation, osteoporosis affects more than 20 million American women. Every year osteoporosis causes about 1.5 million bone fractures in older adults. As a woman, your risk of getting a bone fracture from osteoporosis is equal to your total risk of getting breast, uterine, and ovarian cancer.

Because osteoporosis is seen as such a problem for women, doctors sometimes overlook it in older men. If you fall into any of the risk categories, talk to your doctor.

Warning! _____

You don't have to wait for a fracture to tell whether your bones are thinning. One early warning sign is trouble with your teeth. If your dentures stop fitting right, it might be because of bone loss in your jaw. If you're at risk for osteoporosis, talk to your doctor about having a bone-density test. New x-ray techniques make this quick, safe, and easy.

Calcium and High Blood Pressure

Calcium may help prevent or treat high blood pressure in some people. If you don't eat much calcium, you're more likely to get high blood pressure than someone who gets the RDA or more. In general, the higher the level of calcium in your blood, the lower your blood pressure. According to one study, taking 1,000 mg a day of extra calcium also lowers your diastolic blood pressure (that's the pressure when your heart is relaxed between beats), but it doesn't seem to do anything for your systolic pressure (when your heart is contracting and the pressure is highest).

Other studies show that taking calcium supplements (anywhere from 400 to 1,000 mg) can lower blood pressure for some people, especially African Americans and people who are sensitive to salt.

The results of the Dietary Approaches to Stop Hypertension (DASH) study, first published in 1997, showed that a diet high in fresh fruits and vegetables and low-fat dairy products was the most effective for lowering blood pressure, especially when compared to the typical American diet. The DASH diet is high in calcium—it has more than 1,200 mg, compared to just 450 in the typical American diet. A follow-up study called DASH-Sodium showed that the DASH diet without limiting salt worked as well to lower blood pressure as did a diet that strictly limited salt intake.

If your blood pressure is on the high side but you don't yet need medicine to lower it, take a look at your calcium level. Try to raise your intake to at least 1,000 mg a day, preferably by adding foods rich in calcium to your diet. After a few months, you may notice a drop in your blood pressure.

Warning!

If you take medicine for high blood pressure, keep taking it. Talk to your doctor about calcium supplements before you try them.

Pregnant women sometimes have trouble with high blood pressure. Calcium supplements seem to help. Because pregnant women need extra calcium anyway, this is another good reason to be sure you're getting 1,000 mg a day—enough for you and your growing baby.

Calcium and Colon Cancer

The research here is promising. In general, the lower your calcium intake, the more likely you are to get colon cancer, possibly because calcium blocks the growth of cancer cells. Also, people who have had colorectal polyps (benign tumors that can develop into cancer) are at less risk of having them come back if they take calcium supplements—and that translates into a lower risk of colon cancer. Colon cancer is one of the top three causes of cancer death, but it's very treatable if caught in time. If you're at risk of colon cancer (if one of your parents had it, for example), getting 1,500 to 2,000 mg of calcium a day could be a sensible precaution.

Calcium and Other Cancers

The evidence for calcium and other cancers is mixed, and much of it is still preliminary. Here's where we stand:

◆ **Prostate cancer.** Some studies suggest that a high intake of calcium or a high intake of dairy foods is associated with an increased risk of prostate cancer. But other studies don't show a connection or even show a protective effect. Bottom line? Men should probably avoid going over the RDA for calcium.

◆ **Ovarian cancer.** Women who get a lot of dietary calcium from dairy foods may lower their risk of this deadly cancer. But is it the calcium that helps or something else in the dairy products? No answer on this one yet.

◆ **Breast cancer.** Early research suggested that Vitamin D and calcium supplements could protect women against breast cancer. In 2006, results from the long-running Women's Health Initiative study showed that the supplements had no effect. There were problems with the design of the study, however, and it's almost impossible to separate out the effects of Vitamin D and calcium from the diet. Bottom line here? We still don't know.

Calcium and Kidney Stones

For years, doctors warned patients who had kidney stones to avoid calcium. The idea was that the calcium combined with oxalate—a natural substance found in green, leafy vegetables such as spinach—to form the painful stones.

In fact, the opposite may be true. Recent studies show that high calcium intake actually decreases the risk of kidney stones. If you've ever had a kidney stone, there's no longer really much reason to give up the bone-protecting benefits of calcium. To be on the safe side, though, try to get most of your calcium from food, not supplements. If you do take supplements, take them with meals to block your uptake of oxalates. And be sure to drink plenty of water every day.

Calcium and Heart Disease

Two important studies in 1997 pointed out a link between atherosclerosis (arteries clogged with fatty deposits called plaque) and osteoporosis. In the first study, researchers found that women who had the most bone loss from osteoporosis were also the most likely to have calcium-containing plaque blocking their carotid arteries. Because the carotid arteries carry blood to the brain, these women were at higher risk of having a stroke. The second study showed that men and women with low Vitamin D levels also had higher rates of calcium-containing plaque in the arteries leading to their hearts, making them more vulnerable to heart attacks.

These studies were followed in 1999 by two more. One showed older women who had high calcium intakes had a 30 to 35 percent reduction in their risk of ischemic (bloodflow–blocking) heart disease. The other showed that adding 400 mg of calcium a day to the diets of middle-aged women cut their risk of strokes. Overall, what the studies suggest is that a good level of calcium intake—enough to help prevent osteoporosis—may also help prevent heart attacks and strokes. We expect to see a lot more studies like these in the future, but why wait? Start getting more calcium now.

Calcium and PMS

If your calcium level drops too low, you get irritable and depressed. Sound familiar? That's the way a lot of women feel in the days before their period. Could PMS really just be your body's way of telling you to eat more calcium? According to a 1998 study, yes. In this study of women who had severe PMS, half took a 300 mg calcium supplement four times a day; the other half took a sugar pill. Of course, the participants didn't know which they were taking. After 3 months, the women taking the calcium had sharply reduced PMS symptoms—their depression, mood swings, food cravings, water retention, and pain were much better. The women on sugar pills didn't show much improvement. Another study in 2005 looked at the diets of a large group of women and found that the ones who got the most calcium from their food had the fewest PMS symptoms.

If you want to try calcium for PMS, start by trying to get more calcium from your diet. If you want to try supplements, bear in mind that you have to take them every day, that the effect takes a few cycles to really kick in, and that while calcium could cut your PMS symptoms in half, you might still need to take other steps.

Calcium and Weight Loss

We saved the best for last. Calcium could be your secret weapon for dieting. In 2000, researchers reported a surprising finding: mice placed on a high-calcium, low-calorie diet lost weight at double the rate of mice on the same low-calorie diet but with less calcium. Was it possible that the magic pill for weight loss had finally been found?

Not so fast. Some studies, mostly of the observational kind that look at the diets of large groups of people, suggest that dairy foods, which are high in calcium, may help with weight loss for people watching their calories and may also slow weight gain among middle-aged people. Other observational studies haven't proven the calcium/weight-loss connection. Clinical studies, where the amount of calories and calcium in the diet are carefully controlled, have been small and have had mixed results.

If you're dieting or watching your weight, low-fat dairy products are a good idea anyway—and if they help you with your weight management, so much the better.

The Least You Need to Know

- You need calcium, the most abundant mineral in your body, along with Vitamin D to build strong bones and keep them that way throughout your life.
- The adult DRI for calcium is between 1,000 and 1,200 mg.
- Milk and other dairy foods are the best source of calcium. Dark-green, leafy vegetables such as kale also have calcium.
- Many different kinds of calcium supplements are available. Calcium citrate supplements are best for most people.
- Calcium can help prevent osteoporosis as well as high blood pressure, colon cancer, and heart disease.
- Calcium can help reduce the symptoms of PMS.

Magnesium: Magnificent for Your Heart

In This Chapter

- ◆ Learning why you need magnesium
- ◆ Finding foods high in magnesium
- ◆ Helping your heart with magnesium
- ◆ Helping your blood pressure with magnesium
- ◆ Helping relieve asthma with magnesium
- ◆ Helping diabetes with magnesium

If sometimes you feel like a nut, go for it! Nuts are high in magnesium, and this magnificent mineral helps maintain your maximum health. Magnesium makes your muscles relax—and that plays a big role in keeping your heartbeat healthy and holding down your blood pressure.

Today many doctors have realized that magnesium makes a big difference for some patients. Magnesium is becoming a mainstream medication for people with migraines, asthma, and diabetes. Getting enough magnesium helps these people control their medical problems. Magnesium has one other major mission: it helps keep your bones strong by working with calcium throughout your life.

Why You Need Magnesium

Every single cell in your body needs magnesium to produce energy. You also need magnesium to make more than 300 different enzymes, to send messages along your nerves, to make your muscles relax, to maintain strong bones and teeth, to help your heart beat, and to keep your blood pressure at normal levels. Magnesium seems to help some health problems, such as asthma and diabetes, and can be very valuable for treating heart-rhythm problems.

You also need magnesium to use other vitamins and minerals properly. Vitamin C and calcium both work better, for example, when there's plenty of magnesium around.

To do all that, you need a fair amount of magnesium. In fact, your body contains about 25 g of magnesium—it's the fourth most abundant mineral in your body. Most of it's in your bones and teeth, but you also have a lot in your muscles and blood. The amount in your blood is very important for keeping your body's functions in balance. In fact, magnesium is involved in more than 300 biochemical reactions in your body. Just as you need calcium to make your muscles contract—when your heart beats, for example—you need magnesium to make them relax again. That's why the levels of calcium and magnesium in your blood have to be steady and why you need to be sure you're getting enough of both. If you don't have enough of them, your body will pull these minerals from your bones and put them into your blood, which can lead to weakened bones.

The RDA for Magnesium

In 1989, the RDA for magnesium was lowered somewhat, especially for children and pregnant women. As usual, the reasoning was that most people were getting less than even the lowered amount, but they seemed healthy enough anyway. In 1997, the recommended amounts for magnesium were raised a little. Here's a chart with the new guidelines:

The RDA for Magnesium

Age in Years/Sex	Magnesium in mg
Infants	
0 to 0.5	30
0.5 to 1	75
Children	
1 to 3	80
4 to 8	130
9 to 13	240
Boys 14 to 18	410
Girls 14 to 18	360
Adults	
Men 19 to 30	400
Men 31+	420
Women 19 to 30	310
Women 31+	320
Pregnant Women	
18 and younger	400
19 to 30	350
31 to 50	360
Nursing Women	
18 and younger	360
19 to 30	310
31 to 50	320

Many researchers believe the RDA is still too low to prevent some health problems.

The research into the value of larger doses is now pretty solid. Many nutritionists and doctors now suggest 500 mg a day for adults. This amount could do a lot to help keep your blood pressure normal and prevent heart disease.

Are You Deficient?

A lot of people don't get enough magnesium from their food to meet even the lowered RDA. By some estimates, in fact, nearly three quarters of all Americans don't. Even so, very few healthy people are really deficient—you'd have to have very low amounts of magnesium for a long time to have any symptoms. If you're not basically healthy, though, you could become deficient, especially if you have any of these health problems:

◆ **You abuse alcohol.** Most alcohol abusers have poor diets that are too low in magnesium and other nutrients. Low blood levels of magnesium are found in 30 to 60 percent of alcoholics.

◆ **You have diabetes.** You may be excreting a lot of your magnesium in your urine—we'll talk about that some more later in this chapter.

◆ **You have Crohn's disease, celiac disease, or another chronic illness that affects your intestines.** You may not be absorbing enough magnesium from your food. Discuss supplements with your doctor.

◆ **You have kidney disease.** Your kidneys may not be handling magnesium very well. Your doctor can prescribe medications that prevent magnesium deficiency. Don't take supplements!

◆ **You've been vomiting a lot or having severe diarrhea.** You lose a lot of magnesium when this happens.

◆ **You use *diuretic drugs*.** Diuretics make you pass more urine, which lowers your level. This can become a real problem if you often use nonprescription diuretics ("water pills") without telling your doctor. It can also be a problem with prescription diuretics such as thiazide diuretics and furosemide (Lasix). Discuss supplements with your doctor.

Warning!

Nonprescription diuretics ("water pills") or herbal diuretics such as buchu or uva ursi ("dieter's tea") can make you pass too much urine and make your levels of magnesium and other important minerals such as potassium drop too low.

def•i•ni•tion

Diuretic drugs make your kidneys produce more urine, which removes water—and also some minerals and vitamins—from your body. These drugs can lower your magnesium level and may also affect your potassium level (see Chapter 20 for more information on potassium).

◆ **You are receiving the anticancer drug cisplatin.** This drug causes you to lose a lot of magnesium in your urine. Discuss supplements with your doctor.

◆ **You're an older adult.** Older adults tend to have low magnesium levels because they absorb less of it and excrete more. Also, older adults are more likely to be taking drugs that interact with magnesium. Discuss supplements with your doctor.

A lot of people get some of their magnesium from the water they drink. In many areas, the water is "hard"—it has a lot of minerals such as calcium and magnesium in it. (A lot of bottled mineral waters also have magnesium, usually more than 6 mg per quart.) People who live in areas where the water is "soft" and where the water contains few minerals, or people who drink only distilled water, might be low on magnesium.

If you don't get enough magnesium, all your tissues are affected, but you'll feel it most in your heart, nerves, and kidneys. Generally, deficiency symptoms include nausea, loss of appetite, muscle weakness or tremors, and irritability. You might also have a rapid heartbeat. Severe magnesium deficiency can cause your heart to beat irregularly. Many nutritionists and doctors feel that breathing problems such as asthma are caused in part by magnesium deficiency. Extra magnesium can sometimes be very helpful for people with asthma. (We'll talk more about magnesium for heart problems and asthma later in this chapter.)

Eating Your Magnesium

Magnesium is found in lots of foods. Good sources include nuts; beans; dark-green, leafy vegetables (of course); whole grains; and seafood. Most people get a lot of their daily magnesium from milk, which has about 34 mg per cup. Soy foods such as miso and tofu (bean curd) are high in magnesium; soy milk actually has more magnesium than cow's milk. There isn't much magnesium in meat or foods that have been refined or processed a lot—just compare the 23 mg in a slice of whole-wheat bread to the measly 5 mg in a slice of white bread.

Looking at the chart, you can see some delicious ways to get magnesium from your food. A peanut butter sandwich on whole-wheat bread, for example, easily gives you nearly 100 mg.

The Magnesium in Food

Food	Amount	Magnesium in mg
Almonds, dry-roasted	1 oz.	84
Banana	1 medium	33
Black beans	1 cup	121
Bread, white	1 slice	5
Bread, whole-wheat	1 slice	23
Broccoli, cooked	½ cup	19
Cashews, dry-roasted	1 oz.	72
Chickpeas	1 cup	78
Flounder	3 oz.	50
Kidney beans	1 cup	80
Lentils	1 cup	71
Lima beans	1 cup	82
Milk, low-fat	8 oz.	34
Miso	½ cup	58
Oatmeal, cooked	1 cup	56
Okra	½ cup	46
Peanut butter	2 TB.	51
Peanuts	1 oz.	52
Peas	½ cup	31
Pinto beans, canned	1 cup	64
Potato, baked with skin	1 medium	55
Shrimp	3 oz.	29
Soy milk	1 cup	45
Spinach, cooked	½ cup	79
Swiss chard	½ cup	76
Tofu	½ cup	118
Walnuts	1 oz.	48
Wheat germ	½ cup	69
White beans	1 cup	113
Yogurt	8 oz.	40

Getting the Most from Magnesium

It's not that easy to get the RDA for magnesium just from your food—and it's even harder to get 500 mg a day that way. Even so, that's the best way to get your magnesium, along with all the other valuable vitamins and minerals found in magnesium-rich foods. If you want to take a supplement, remember that your daily multi-supplement probably has 10 to 50 mg of magnesium. Between your food and your multi, you won't need a large dose of supplemental magnesium to make up the difference. That's good because large doses of magnesium—more than 600 mg—can give you diarrhea. And bear in mind that many over-the-counter antacids and laxatives contain magnesium. Frequent use of these products could raise your magnesium level too high, especially if you also take supplements.

The magnesium in supplements is always combined with some other harmless substance to make it stable. At the vitamin counter you'll find a lot of different choices, with names such as magnesium citrate and magnesium gluconate. We suggest taking magnesium chloride or magnesium lactate because you absorb these best. Avoid magnesium oxide—most people find it hard to tolerate. For the most benefit, take between 200 and 500 mg a day; don't consume more than 500 mg. Spread out your magnesium over the day and take the supplements with meals. If you get diarrhea from the supplements, cut back on your dose.

Your kidneys are very good at removing excess magnesium, so you're unlikely to have problems other than diarrhea from taking too much. The excess will just pass out harmlessly in your urine, unless you have kidney problems.

> ### Now You're Cooking
>
> You now have an extra good reason for eating that double-fudge brownie: chocolate is high in magnesium! Here's how much: ¼ cup of chocolate chips—35 mg; 1 ounce of unsweetened baking chocolate—88 mg; 1 tablespoon of unsweetened cocoa powder—25 mg.

Food for Thought

Magnesium is the main ingredient in many antacids such as Maalox and Mylanta. Antacids aren't the same as magnesium supplements. If you use antacids a lot, you'll probably get diarrhea. That leads us to the other use of magnesium: in larger amounts, it's a laxative in products such as milk of magnesia (magnesium hydroxide) and Epsom salts. Use these laxatives only if your doctor recommends them, and not as a source of supplemental magnesium.

Thumbs Up/Thumbs Down

Magnesium Works Better With ...	Magnesium Is Blocked By ...
Calcium	Alcohol
Potassium	Excess amounts of calcium
Thiamin	Fat-soluble vitamins
Vitamin C	(Vitamins A, E, and K)
Vitamin D	

Magnesium and Your Heart

Low levels of magnesium seem to be related to some types of heart problems. In 2003 a study of more than 7,000 men who took part in the long-term Honolulu Heart Program showed that the rate of heart disease was significantly lower in those with the highest daily magnesium intake (more than 340 mg) compared to those with the lowest (fewer than 186 mg).

Because magnesium helps your muscles relax, a shortage may cause a spasm in one of your coronary arteries. The spasm blocks the bloodflow and can cause a heart attack. Some doctors think that a shortage of magnesium is behind many sudden heart attacks, especially in people who don't have a history of heart disease. In fact, intravenous magnesium is sometimes used in emergency rooms as a treatment for heart attacks.

def•i•ni•tion

Cardiac arrhythmias cause your heart to beat irregularly. Sometimes the arrhythmia makes you have an extra heartbeat or skip one; it could also make your heart beat too fast. Cardiac arrhythmias can be serious. See your doctor at once if you're having symptoms.

Magnesium may also protect against heart attacks caused by blood clots. Magnesium helps keep the clots from forming by making your platelets (tiny blood cells that form clots) less "sticky." This makes them less likely to lump together into an artery-clogging clot.

Too little magnesium can also cause *cardiac arrhythmias*. When that happens, your heart beats irregularly. You might skip a beat or have an extra one, or your heart could beat too fast. If the problem is serious enough, your heartbeat won't quickly return to normal and you could die suddenly. Studies suggest that people with low levels of magnesium are more likely to die suddenly from heart-rhythm problems.

For people who already have heart problems, magnesium can help improve their ability to exercise and relieve angina, or chest pain caused by exertion.

Warning! ⎯⎯⎯⎯⎯

Don't take magnesium supplements or antacids containing magnesium if you have congestive heart failure!

Magnesium Manages Blood Pressure

Magnesium helps your muscles relax. If you don't have enough magnesium, the walls of your blood vessels could tighten up, which raises your blood pressure. As it turns out, many people with high blood pressure don't eat enough magnesium. When they get more in their diet—up to 600 mg a day—their blood pressure drops. This doesn't work for everybody, though, so we can't say for sure that magnesium will make your high blood pressure go down. Even so, many doctors suggest that you try eating more magnesium-rich foods if you have high blood pressure. This recommendation has been borne out by the latest results from the Dietary Approaches to Stop Hypertension (DASH) study, which showed that a diet with plenty of magnesium is a positive lifestyle modification for people with high blood pressure and for people who have prehypertension—blood pressure that is getting close to being too high.

Pregnant women sometimes get dangerously high blood pressure, especially in the last few months of pregnancy. Magnesium may help prevent this problem. If you're pregnant, your doctor will probably prescribe a multi-supplement that has magnesium in it. Don't take additional magnesium supplements unless your doctor recommends them.

Warning! ⎯⎯⎯⎯⎯

Even mild asthma is a serious health problem because it can suddenly get much worse. If you already take medicine for asthma—even non-prescription drugs—don't stop! Talk to your doctor about taking magnesium and other supplements before you try them.

Help for Asthma

When you have an asthma attack, the muscles lining the airways in your lungs contract. This makes the airways get too narrow, so you have trouble breathing. Magnesium helps the muscles relax, so the airways open up and you can breathe more easily. In emergency rooms, intravenous magnesium is used to treat severe asthma attacks. Don't try to treat an attack on your own by swallowing magnesium supplements, though—it doesn't work and could be dangerous. Take your medicine instead.

If you have asthma, it might be because your diet is low in magnesium. Getting more through supplements and magnesium-rich foods—up to 1,000 mg a day—could help prevent attacks and make your attacks less severe. For the best results, spread out your dose over the day.

Magnesium and Diabetes

High blood pressure is often a problem for people with diabetes—and people with diabetes often have low magnesium levels. Is there a connection? Some doctors think there is and recommend magnesium supplements for diabetic patients. Because magnesium plays an important role in carbohydrate metabolism, this mineral may also help diabetics control their blood sugar better and help prevent complications later, such as eye problems, kidney disease, and heart disease.

There's also some evidence that older people who are at risk for diabetes because they already have high blood sugar or simply because they are getting older can prevent it by getting more magnesium. Several long-running studies, such as the Nurse's Health Study, the Health Professionals' Follow-up Study, and the Iowa Women's Health Study have all shown that older adults with low magnesium intake from food are more likely to develop Type 2 diabetes.

If you have diabetes or are at risk for it, try to get as much magnesium as you can from your diet by eating more whole grains; nuts; and green, leafy veggies. You might also want to consider taking between 200 and 300 mg a day in supplements. Talk to your doctor about taking supplements before you try them, especially if you have kidney problems because of your diabetes.

Magnesium and Colon Cancer

In 2006, an important study in Sweden showed that women who got the most magnesium from their diet had the lowest risk of colon cancer. The risk was directly related to the daily intake: the women who had the highest intake (255 mg or more) were only 60 percent as likely to develop colorectal cancer as the women with the lowest intake (fewer than 209 mg). Here's yet another good reason to eat more beans; nuts; whole grains; and green, leafy vegetables such as kale.

Magnesium for Healthy Bones

We talked a lot about the importance of calcium for strong bones in the previous chapter. But calcium isn't the only mineral you need to keep your bones healthy—you also need enough magnesium. The magnesium helps keep your calcium levels in balance and makes sure you produce enough Vitamin D.

The general rule of thumb is that you need twice as much calcium as magnesium to prevent osteoporosis (bones that are thin, brittle, and break easily). Because women need more calcium as they get older, they also need more magnesium. According to the RDA, women aged 25 to 50 need 1,000 mg of calcium a day, so they also need to get 500 mg of magnesium. If you're a woman older than age 50 and you're not taking estrogen, you probably need 1,500 mg of calcium and 750 mg of magnesium every day. This amount is hard to get through your diet alone—consider taking magnesium and calcium supplements.

Warning!

Don't take magnesium supplements, antacids, or laxatives containing magnesium if you also take the antibiotic drugs ciprofloxacin (Cipro) or tetracycline! The magnesium will block the drugs from entering your bloodstream! If you take prescription diuretics, insulin, or digitalis, you may need more magnesium. Discuss magnesium supplements with your doctor before you try them!

If you've been diagnosed with osteoporosis, magnesium supplements may be as important—or even more important—as calcium supplements for slowing and reversing bone loss. Discuss your treatment options with your doctor before you start taking magnesium supplements.

Magnesium and Migraines

People who get migraine headaches often have low magnesium levels. Does that mean that low magnesium causes migraines? Could be, although we're still not sure why. If you get migraines, try to get 500 mg of magnesium a day through your diet and by taking a magnesium supplement. This daily amount could reduce the number of attacks you get. It seems to work particularly well as a preventive measure for women who get migraines as part of their menstrual cycle.

One very interesting recent study showed that in about half the cases, intravenous magnesium stopped migraine headaches in their tracks. Unfortunately, when you have a migraine, just swallowing magnesium supplements doesn't have the same effect.

Other Problems Helped by Magnesium

There's a lot of controversy over whether magnesium helps some other health problems. We're not too sure about some of these—magnesium doesn't seem to do anything for prostate trouble, gallstones, body odor (we'll never understand how that one got started), or depression, for example, although some people claim it does. Let's look at two cases where the evidence shows that magnesium helps:

♦ **Premenstrual syndrome (PMS).** Some women swear that magnesium supplements relieve uncomfortable PMS symptoms, especially breast tenderness, headaches, and irritability. If you get severe PMS, try taking 300 to 500 mg a day for the 2 weeks leading up to your period. If you get severe cramps from your period, keep taking the magnesium during that time—it may help reduce cramping. Magnesium may help even more if you combine it with pyridoxine (refer to Chapter 8 for more information about this).

Warning!

Don't take magnesium supplements, antacids, or laxatives containing magnesium if you have kidney disease!

♦ **Preventing kidney stones.** Magnesium supplements seem to help keep calcium kidney stones from coming back. All you need is 100 to 300 mg a day. The magnesium seems to help more if you also take 10 mg a day of pyridoxine. If you get kidney stones, talk to your doctor about magnesium supplements before you try them.

The Least You Need to Know

♦ Magnesium is a mineral needed for more than 300 different roles in your body.

♦ The adult RDA for magnesium is between 280 and 350 mg a day. Many researchers feel this is too low and suggest 500 mg a day.

♦ Foods high in magnesium include nuts; beans; dark-green, leafy vegetables; and milk.

♦ Magnesium may help prevent heart-rhythm problems and high blood pressure.

♦ Magnesium may be helpful for people with asthma and diabetes. It may also help prevent migraine headaches.

♦ Magnesium is very important for building strong bones and preventing osteoporosis.

♦ A diet high in magnesium-rich foods may help prevent colon cancer.

Zinc: Immune System Booster

In This Chapter

- ◆ Why you need zinc
- ◆ Which foods are high in zinc
- ◆ How zinc helps colds
- ◆ How zinc helps prostate problems
- ◆ Why you need zinc for healthy skin, hair, and nails

Look up zinc in the encyclopedia and you'll learn all about this important industrial metal. You'll learn about how it's used to make pipes and galvanized metals that resist corrosion. You'll learn that 6.8 million metric tons of zinc are used every year. You might even learn that there are 338 zinc mines in the world. What you won't learn is that the same stuff that galvanizes metal is also incredibly important for your health.

Zinc is very important for your immune system. In fact, if you have a bad cold, taking extra zinc could get you back on your feet several days sooner. Zinc also helps you heal quickly from wounds, keeps your skin healthy, helps preserve your eyesight, helps you absorb iron from your diet, and might even improve your memory. It's no surprise that today many doctors and nutritionists tell their patients to "think zinc!"

Why You Need Zinc

More than 100 different enzymes in your body depend on zinc to work properly. Here's just one example: you need zinc to make the enzyme alcohol dehydrogenase, which breaks down alcohol. If you're deficient in zinc, your body can't process alcohol and you get very drunk on just a small amount.

You also need zinc to make many hormones, including the ones that tell your immune system what to do when you're under attack from germs. Zinc is essential for making the hormones that control growth and for the important male hormone testosterone. You have some zinc in every one of your body's cells, but most of it's in your skin, hair, nails, and eyes—and in your prostate gland if you're male. All told, your body contains more than 2.2 g of zinc.

The RDA for Zinc

Even though you use zinc in many important body processes, you don't need to eat much of it. Technically speaking, zinc is a trace element—a mineral you need in only very small amounts (we'll talk more about trace elements in Chapter 21). The adult RDA for zinc is 12 mg a day or less—an amount that most everybody easily gets from food. Check out the chart to see what your zinc need is.

The RDA for Zinc

Age/Sex	Zinc in mg
Infants	
0 to 6 months	2
6 months to 1 year	3
Children	
1 to 3 years	3
4 to 8 years	5
9 to 13 years	8

Age/Sex	Zinc in mg
Adults	
Males 14+ years	11
Females 14+ years	8
Pregnant women	11
Nursing women	12

Are You Deficient?

The first hint that zinc is an important nutrient came almost a century ago in Egypt, when doctors noticed that young, poor boys who ate almost nothing but unleavened bread were very short and underdeveloped. It turned out that their diet had enough zinc, but they couldn't absorb it because their diet was high in phytates, a substance found in high-fiber grain foods that blocks the uptake of zinc. After they got more variety in their diet, they started growing normally again.

In our modern society, such a serious zinc deficiency is very rare. A slight deficiency in zinc, however, isn't that uncommon. Surveys show that many women get only about half the RDA. You might be on the low side for zinc if …

◆ **You're a strict vegetarian or vegan.** Animal foods such as fish and meat are the best dietary sources of zinc. Fruits have virtually none. Children who don't eat animal foods are more at risk for zinc deficiency. Vegetarians should aim to get 50 percent more than the RDA from their food to make up for the decreased absorption of zinc from only plant foods.

◆ **You eat a very high-fiber diet.** The fiber, especially fiber from whole grains, contains phytates that bind up the zinc in your diet and keeps you from absorbing it. A diet that contains mostly tortillas made from corn, for example, is very high in phytates and may cause deficiency. Aim to get 50 percent more than the RDA from your food to make up for the decreased absorption of zinc caused by the phytates.

◆ **You have Crohn's disease, celiac disease, or another disease that affects how you absorb nutrients.** You may not be absorbing enough zinc from your food.

◆ **You're pregnant or breastfeeding.** You're passing a lot of your zinc on to your baby. If your diet is on the low side for zinc to begin with, you might be deficient. Talk to your doctor about supplements.

◆ **You're older than age 50.** Your ability to absorb zinc from your food drops as you get older.

◆ **You abuse alcohol.** Alcohol abusers don't eat very well in general. Even moderate amounts of alcohol flush out the zinc stored in your liver and make you excrete it.

Zinc deficiency has a number of symptoms: slowed growth in children, slow wound healing, frequent infections, skin irritations, hair loss, and loss of your sense of taste.

Generally speaking, you don't have to worry much about being deficient in this mineral. Anyone in the Westernized world who eats a reasonably well-balanced diet will get plenty of zinc. Worldwide, however, an estimated one in five people is deficient because of poor diet.

Eating Your Zinc

The best food source of zinc by far is oysters. There are about 12 mg in a single raw oyster. Other foods that are good sources of zinc are shellfish, lean meat, poultry, and organ meats. You absorb only about 20 to 40 percent of the zinc you get from animal foods, and you absorb even less from the zinc in plant foods.

> **Now You're Cooking**
>
> Did you know pure maple syrup is a good source of zinc? There's 0.8 mg in 1 tablespoon.

There's a fair amount of zinc in beans, nuts, seeds, and whole grains, but your body can't use it very well. That's because these foods also have a lot of fiber, and the phytates in the fiber combine with zinc and keep a lot of it from being absorbed. Fruits are low in zinc. For the best food sources of zinc, check the chart.

The Zinc in Food

Food	Amount	Zinc in mg
Almonds, dry-roasted	1 oz.	1.4
Beef, ground	3 oz.	4.6
Beef liver	3 oz.	5.2
Black beans	1 cup	1.9
Bread, whole-wheat	1 slice	0.4
Cashews, dry-roasted	1 oz.	1.6

Food	Amount	Zinc in mg
Cheddar cheese	1 oz.	0.9
Chicken, without skin	3 oz.	2.10
Chickpeas	1 cup	2.5
Egg	1 large	0.5
Flounder	3 oz.	0.5
Kidney beans	1 cup	1.9
Lentils	1 cup	2.5
Lima beans	1 cup	1.8
Milk, 1 percent	8 oz.	1.0
Oatmeal	1 cup	1.1
Oysters, canned	3 oz.	77.3
Oysters, raw	6 medium	76.4
Oysters, smoked	3 oz.	103.0
Peas, split	½ cup	0.9
Peanut butter	2 TB.	0.9
Peanuts	1 oz.	0.9
Pecans	1 oz.	1.6
Sunflower seeds	1 oz.	1.4
Swiss cheese	1 oz.	1.1
Turkey	3 oz.	1.7
Walnuts	1 oz.	0.8
Wheat germ	¼ cup	3.6
White beans	1 cup	2.5
Yogurt	8 oz.	2.0

Warning!

Don't take zinc supplements if you're taking the antibiotic drugs tetracycline or ciprofloxacin (Cipro). The zinc will keep the drug from being absorbed into your bloodstream.

Getting the Most from Zinc

You have a lot of choices at the vitamin counter when you're looking for a zinc supplement. What you want is a form that you can easily absorb, so we suggest zinc gluconate as your first choice and zinc acetate as your second. Zinc citrate and zinc monomethionate are also good options. Zinc picolinate is sometimes promoted as being more absorbable than other forms, but there's not much evidence for this. Zinc sulfate is the cheapest form of zinc supplement and it's widely used, but it's more likely to upset your stomach. Avoid zinc oxide—that form is really useful only in skin creams meant to block sunlight.

Most good multi-supplements have the RDA for zinc. If you want to get more, try zinc supplements; they usually come in 10-, 30-, or 50-mg capsules. Zinc supplements in large amounts can block your absorption of calcium, copper, and iron. It's especially important to keep your copper and zinc levels in balance. If you regularly take extra zinc, be sure you're also getting some extra copper, and take the supplement a few hours apart from each other.

Take zinc supplements with meals to avoid stomach upsets. For the best absorption, don't take zinc with a high-fiber meal. The fiber will reduce the amount you absorb.

Taking zinc in large doses (more than 60 mg per day) for a long period of time could lead to problems absorbing copper, lowered immunity, and lowered HDL cholesterol levels. Large doses of zinc could be toxic; however, it would be almost impossible to take enough zinc supplements to poison yourself—you'd throw it all up long before that.

Fighting Off Colds

The next time you catch a cold, some pretty good studies suggest that zinc can help you get over it a couple days quicker. Your immune system needs zinc to work at top efficiency. In fact, your infection-fighting white blood cells contain a lot of the zinc in your body. Giving them a zinc boost when you have a cold seems to help them fight off the virus faster. It also seems to reduce cold symptoms such as a runny nose, coughing, and hoarseness.

For treating a cold with zinc, the best approach seems to be lozenges containing at least 13 mg of zinc gluconate combined with glycine. (Lozenges made with zinc acetate don't seem to help.) The glycine is a sweetener that helps cover up the terrible taste. Dextrose, sucrose, and maltose are also sometimes used. Any other sweetener and many flavorings can interfere with the antiviral action of the zinc.

Put the lozenge in your mouth and let it dissolve slowly. Don't chew it or swallow it. Repeat every 2 hours or so for no more than a week. Adults shouldn't take more than eight lozenges a day. Limit children to no more than six a day. You can buy zinc lozenges in any health-food store; many pharmacies now carry them as well. Most lozenges contain anywhere from 10 to 25 mg. Just swallowing zinc supplements won't help your cold symptoms at all.

There are some drawbacks to zinc lozenges. Even though they're flavored to disguise their awful taste, they can leave a metallic aftertaste in your mouth. If you take a lot of them, they can affect your sense of taste and smell—your sense of taste and smell should return to normal a few days after you stop taking the extra zinc.

Warning!

Nasal sprays and gels containing zinc are marketed as cold treatments. There's no evidence these work, but there have been some reports of people losing their sense of smell after using them.

Zinc may be a very useful immune-system booster in general. It seems to give a real boost to your *thymus gland*, especially if you're older than age 40. By then, your thymus may have naturally shrunk quite a bit, so it's not producing the hormones it used to—and those hormones stimulate your body to produce infection-fighting blood cells. Getting a little extra zinc—just 15 to 30 mg—every day may get your thymus moving again. That means your immune system will work better and fight off illness faster.

def•i•ni•tion

Your **thymus gland** is a small but very important organ found in your neck just above your breastbone. It plays a very important role in your health by making some of the hormones that tell your immune system what to do. When you're born, your thymus is quite large. By the time you're a teenager, it's shrunk a lot, and by the time you're 40, it's shrunk even more. For a long time researchers thought that was normal, but recent studies show that zinc can revitalize your thymus and get it working again.

Zinc Club for Men

Are the guys just kidding around when they tell you to eat oysters for a better sex life? Believe it or not, they're right. Oysters are by far the food highest in zinc—and you need plenty of zinc to make testosterone and other male hormones. You also need zinc to make healthy sperm and semen, so getting more zinc in your diet could help solve male infertility. In one study, men with low sperm counts took zinc supplements for 6 weeks. Their testosterone levels and sperm counts went up, and nearly half of them had pregnant wives before the study was over.

Zinc can also be very helpful for treating and possibly even preventing prostate problems. Your *prostate gland* is a small organ that wraps around the *urethra* at the neck of the bladder. As you get older, your prostate often naturally gets bigger, a condition called *benign prostatic hypertrophy* (*BPH*). The enlarged gland squeezes the urethra and causes a need to go frequently (and also other urination problems). Sometimes the problems get so bad that medication or even surgery is needed.

A healthy prostate gland naturally has a lot of zinc in it, but men with BPH often have low zinc levels. Taking an extra 50 mg a day in zinc supplements seems to help some men with mild BPH by shrinking the prostate. It doesn't press as much against the urethra, and you can urinate more easily. It takes a while for the zinc to kick in—stay with the supplements for 3 to 6 months before you decide they're not working.

def•i•ni•tion

A small male organ called the **prostate gland** wraps around the **urethra,** the tube that carries urine from your kidneys to your bladder. The prostate makes some of the fluids found in semen. As males get older (especially older than age 50), the prostate may enlarge and start pressing on the urethra, a condition called **benign prostatic hypertrophy** (BPH). The main symptom is the need to urinate frequently.

What about zinc to help prevent prostate cancer? No firm answers here yet, but some good ongoing research suggests it can be valuable. But don't overdo it—a 2003 study from the National Cancer Institute suggests that men who take more than 100 mg a day of supplemental zinc have an increased risk of advanced prostate cancer. Stick to the amount in your daily multi-supplement.

Finally, guys, despite rumors to the contrary, zinc doesn't stop balding or restore lost hair.

Healthy Skin, Nails, and Hair

Zinc is really important for healthy skin. A shortage of zinc is often behind minor skin rashes and irritations that don't seem to have any real cause. These often clear up when patients start eating a diet higher in zinc or take zinc supplements. Zinc also sometimes helps people with psoriasis.

Sometimes a zinc shortage causes white spots on the fingernails or nails that break easily. Adding zinc to your diet could clear up the problem.

A form of zinc is used in some dandruff shampoos to control flaking. It's possible that you also absorb some of the zinc into your body through your scalp if you use one of these shampoos, but don't count on it. On the other hand, just eating more high-zinc foods or taking zinc supplements won't solve your dandruff problem.

Zinc for Healing

Zinc is essential for healing wounds. Several studies have shown that patients recovering from surgery heal faster if they get enough zinc. The effect is dramatic if the patient was low on zinc to begin with; it didn't work as well on patients who had good zinc levels. If you're scheduled for an operation, talk to your doctor about taking zinc supplements for a few weeks before and after. It could make a difference in how quickly you recover.

Think Zinc

Can zinc help make your kids smarter? Quite possibly. Several intriguing studies over the past few years have shown that kids who got a little extra zinc—20 mg every day instead of the RDA of 8 to 11 mg—did better on memory tests. They also seemed to be able to pay attention longer. That ties in with studies suggesting that zinc supplements may help kids with attention deficit hyperactivity disorder (ADHD). If your child is taking medication for ADHD, discuss zinc supplements with the doctor.

Zinc for Other Problems

Some zinc zanies recommend it for all sorts of health problems. Here are some ways zinc may make a difference:

◆ **Diabetes.** Some people with Type 2 diabetes may be too low on zinc because they don't absorb it well and also excrete it quickly. Zinc supplements could help. Zinc might also help with two other problems diabetics often have: slow wound healing and frequent infections. Don't overdo it, however: one study showed that more than 50 mg daily increased blood sugar levels in people with Type 2 diabetes.

◆ **Age-related macular degeneration.** This serious eye problem is the leading cause of blindness in older adults. Your eyes naturally contain a lot of zinc—and a lot of it is concentrated in your retina, the part of your eye affected by macular degeneration. Zinc supplements could help prevent or slow down vision loss from macular degeneration.

◆ **Memory.** Can't remember where you left the car keys? Maybe you're not getting enough zinc. People who get the RDA do better on memory tests than those who don't.

Does zinc help Alzheimer's disease, rheumatoid arthritis, anorexia nervosa, or liver disease? Probably not, but we don't know for sure—the information in all cases is contradictory.

The Least You Need to Know

◆ You need zinc to make more than 100 different enzymes and many hormones, including testosterone.

◆ The adult RDA for zinc is 11 mg for men and 8 mg for women.

◆ Oysters are very high in zinc. Lean meats, beans, nuts, and seeds are also good food sources of zinc.

◆ Zinc can help relieve cold symptoms and boost your immune system.

◆ Zinc can help male infertility and can relieve symptoms of benign prostatic hypertrophy.

◆ Zinc is important for healthy skin, hair, and nails and helps wounds heal faster.

Chapter 20

Electrolytes: Keeping Your Body in Balance

In This Chapter

- ◆ Why potassium, sodium, and chloride are vital to your health
- ◆ Why you need to keep your electrolytes in balance
- ◆ How sodium raises your blood pressure and how potassium lowers it
- ◆ How potassium can prevent strokes

Here's a chapter that should get you all charged up about an easy way to improve your health. We're talking about your *electrolytes*—the potassium, sodium, and chloride in your body. These minerals are electrically charged, so they can carry nutrients into and out of your cells. They also carry messages along your nerves and help control your heartbeat. Most important of all, your electrolytes have a lot to do with controlling your blood pressure.

Eat too much sodium and not enough potassium, and your blood pressure could shoot up to unhealthy levels. Cut back on the sodium and increase your potassium, though, and you'll be helping your blood pressure stay normal. The most electrifying thing of all is that you can do that easily, starting today, just by making some easy changes in your diet. And if you keep your blood pressure where it should be, other health problems, such as heart disease and kidney trouble, may never get started.

What's an Electrolyte?

Electrolytes are minerals that dissolve in water and carry electrical charges. In your body, potassium, sodium, and chloride are the electrolyte minerals. And because you're made mostly of water, these minerals are found everywhere in your body: inside your cells, in the spaces between cells, in your blood, in your lymph, and everywhere else. Each tiny particle of sodium and potassium in your body has a positive charge; each tiny particle of chloride has a negative one. Because electrolytes have electrical charges, they can move easily back and forth through your cell membranes. Why is that so important? Because as they move into a cell, they carry other nutrients with them; and as they move out, they carry out waste products and excess water.

Potassium, sodium, and chloride are very closely linked—so closely that we really can't talk about them separately. Here's why: to keep your body in balance, your cells need to have a lot of potassium inside them and a lot of sodium in the fluids outside them. To keep the balance, sodium and potassium constantly move back and forth through your cell membranes.

You can see the link between sodium and potassium. Where does the chloride come in? Sodium combines easily with other elements. Here's a good example: remember that familiar formula NaCl from science class? Na is the chemical symbol for sodium, and Cl means chloride. Put them together and you have sodium chloride, better known as ordinary table salt. You mostly need the sodium found in salt (table salt is about 40 percent sodium), but your body also needs the chloride. Among other things, you use it to make hydrochloric acid, the powerful digestive juice in your stomach.

Why You Need Electrolytes

All three electrolytes—potassium, sodium, and chloride—keep the amount of water in your body in balance, carry impulses along your nerves, help make your muscles contract and relax, and keep your body from becoming too acidic or alkaline. You need electrolytes to carry glucose (blood sugar) and other nutrients into your cells and to carry waste products and extra water out again. Electrolytes also regulate your blood pressure and your heartbeat. In fact, sodium and potassium are so important for controlling your blood pressure that we'll talk about that more later in this chapter.

The RDAs for Electrolytes

Now that you know how important electrolytes are for keeping you alive, here's a surprise: there are no RDAs for them. Why? Every single living cell on Earth—plant or animal—needs potassium, sodium, and chloride, which means that there's plenty of them in your food. Because the electrolytes are so easy to eat, nobody ever really gets deficient. By the logic of the RDAs, then, there's no reason to bother setting a minimum amount, because everybody gets whatever it is anyway. In 2004, however, the Institute of Medicine issued Adequate Intakes (AIs) for sodium, chloride, and potassium. When you look at the chart, you'll see that the amounts are really pretty small.

Adequate Intakes for Potassium, Sodium, and Chloride

Age in Years	Potassium in mg	Sodium in mg	Chloride in mg
Infants			
0 to 0.5	400	120	180
0.5 to 1	0.7	370	570
Children and Adults			
1 to 3	3,000	1,000	1,500
4 to 8	3,800	1,200	1,900
9 to 13	4,500	1,500	2,300
14 to 50	4,700	1,500	2,300
51 to 70	4,700	1,300	2,000
70+	4,700	1,200	1,800

For the sake of comparison, figure there are about 2,300 mg of sodium in a teaspoon of salt. To stay healthy, you need to get only a bit more than half a teaspoon of salt every day.

Are You Deficient?

Ordinarily, you can't be deficient in electrolytes. You don't really need that much to begin with, and everyone gets plenty from their food.

The one exception is if you get sick with something that makes you vomit a lot or have severe diarrhea. In that case, you might quickly lose so many electrolytes (especially potassium) with the fluid that you run short. Unless you replace the fluids and electrolytes quickly, this can be serious—especially in small children.

If you're low on potassium, you might get muscle cramps in your legs (this sometimes happens to athletes who sweat a lot in really hot weather). If you're low on potassium, you'll feel nauseated and very weak and listless. You'll start to feel better as soon as you get some more potassium into your system. In really severe cases, your heart could fail, but that's very unlikely for most people.

Food for Thought

If you have severe vomiting or diarrhea, you need to replace the electrolytes and water you lose. Sports drinks are one way to go, or you can try this home remedy: in a large glass, combine 8 ounces of apple, orange, or any other fruit juice with half a teaspoon of honey and a pinch of ordinary table salt. In another glass, combine 8 ounces of plain water and a pinch of baking soda (sodium bicarbonate). Take a few sips from one glass, then a few sips from the other until you've drunk them both. The fruit juice contains the potassium you need, while the salt and baking soda provide sodium. The sugar from the juice and honey helps you absorb the electrolytes.

Sodium and chloride deficiencies are uncommon, because you get both elements from salt. Even when you sweat buckets, you still have plenty of salt in your body. It's much more important to replace the lost water.

Drink Up!

You've probably heard that for optimal health, you need to drink water 8 × 8: Eight 8-ounce servings, or 64 ounces, every day. Even though this advice is repeated all over the place, in 2004 the Institute of Medicine shot it down. According to the IOM, a woman needs to get about 91 ounces of fluid every day, and a man needs about 125. Most people seem to get these amounts just from the normal fluids they drink, such as coffee, soft drinks, juice, and water, and from the water in foods such as fruits and vegetables. You'll probably get enough fluid every day if you eat a normal diet and are guided by your thirst when it comes to drinking.

Potassium Pitfalls

Sodium, chloride, and potassium work together to keep the amount of water in your cells and around them (as in your blood) just what it ought to be. Sometimes the water balance gets a little out of whack. Extra hormones might make women hold on to too much water and get a little bloated. This often happens to women before and during their menstrual periods. To relieve the discomfort, some women use nonprescription diuretic drugs ("water pills") and herbs such as buchu and uva ursi ("dieter's tea"). Diuretics reduce the amount of water in your body by making you produce more urine, but that can also make you excrete more electrolytes than you take in. You could accidentally make yourself sick, especially if you take too much or use them too often. Avoid using nonprescription diuretics—they may do more harm than good.

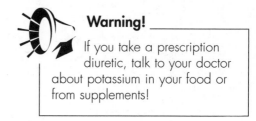

Warning!

If you take a prescription diuretic, talk to your doctor about potassium in your food or from supplements!

If you have a heart condition, you might retain too much water because your heart isn't pumping very well. That can put a serious strain on it, so your doctor may prescribe a diuretic drug to help your body eliminate the retained fluid. Diuretics are also often prescribed to treat high blood pressure.

If your doctor prescribes a diuretic, it may be a "potassium-sparing" one such as triamterene (Dyazide, Maxzide) that doesn't affect your potassium levels. Other diuretics such as furosemide (Lasix) *do* affect your potassium levels. If you need to take a diuretic that affects your potassium, your doctor may also tell you to eat potassium-rich foods or prescribe a potassium supplement.

Other Prescription Drugs

Digoxin (Lanoxin) is a digitalis-type drug that is often prescribed for people with heart failure and heart-rhythm problems. If you also take a diuretic that lowers your potassium level, the combination of low potassium and digoxin could make your heart stop suddenly. On the other hand, if your potassium level gets too high, it could

Warning!

If you take digoxin or any other digitalis-type heart medicine, talk to your doctor about potassium in your food or from supplements!

combine with the digoxin and make your heart rhythm get out of control. So if you take any sort of digitalis-type drug for your heart, follow your doctor's instructions and be very careful about your potassium. Don't use salt substitutes, because they simply substitute potassium for sodium.

Warning!

If you take an ACE-inhibitor drug for high blood pressure or your heart, talk to your doctor about potassium in your food or from supplements!

Another type of drug called an ACE inhibitor (Capoten, Capozide) is sometimes prescribed to treat heart problems and high blood pressure. These drugs can make your potassium level go up. If you also take a potassium supplement or use a salt substitute, you could make your potassium level skyrocket—and that could make your heart beat irregularly or even stop. If you take an ACE inhibitor, follow your doctor's instructions and be very careful about your potassium. Don't use salt substitutes.

Eating Your Electrolytes

Potassium is found in almost all foods, including fruits, vegetables, beans, meat, milk, and grains. Beans, fruits, and vegetables (especially potatoes) are the best natural sources. Some sodium and chloride are found in almost all foods.

We get plenty of both in the form of sodium chloride—the chemical name for plain old table salt. In fact, salt is so common in foods that we're not going to list any here. We'll stick to foods that are good sources of potassium.

The Potassium in Food

Food	Amount	Potassium in mg
Avocado	½ medium	550
Banana	1 medium	451
Beef, ground	3 oz.	205
Black beans	1 cup	801
Broccoli, cooked	½ cup	228
Cantaloupe	1 cup	494
Carrot, raw	1 medium	233
Cauliflower, cooked	½ cup	200

Food	Amount	Potassium in mg
Chicken	3 oz.	195
Chickpeas	1 cup	477
Corn	½ cup	204
Flounder	3 oz.	292
Kidney beans	1 cup	713
Kiwi	1 medium	252
Lentils	1 cup	731
Milk	8 oz.	381
Okra	½ cup	257
Orange	1 medium	250
Orange juice	8 oz.	474
Potato, baked with skin	1 medium	844
Prune juice	8 oz.	706
Spinach, cooked	½ cup	419
Strawberries	1 cup	247
Sweet potato	1 medium	397
Tomato	1 medium	273
Tomato juice	6 oz.	658
Watermelon	1 cup	186
Wheat germ	¼ cup	259

Getting the Most from Electrolytes

We don't recommend taking potassium supplements unless your doctor prescribes them for you. If you think you need extra potassium, the best way is to eat it. The nonprescription potassium supplements sold in health-food stores contain only 99 mg (the FDA won't let them be bigger). That's about the amount of potassium in two big bites of a banana or a couple big swallows of orange juice—without the stomach upset potassium pills can cause. You easily excrete any excess potassium in your urine.

Warning!

People with kidney disease must avoid sodium and potassium! Follow your doctor's instructions!

There's almost never any need for extra sodium or chloride. Most of us get plenty of salt from our food (or even too much) and don't need extra, even in very hot weather or when we're sweating a lot. An exception might be someone running an ultra marathon in very hot weather and losing a lot of electrolytes from excess sweating.

Quack, Quack
If you sweat a lot from an athletic activity or hard work in hot weather, do you need those expensive sports drinks? No way! Drink a lot of plain water instead. It's important to replace the lost fluid. If you want to replace the lost potassium, have a piece of fruit or some OJ—there's nearly 500 mg in 8 ounces.

Shaking Up Salt

The American Heart Association recommends limiting sodium to just one teaspoon daily, but most Americans get twice that amount or more each day. Almost all the excess salt comes from prepared and packaged foods and from restaurant food. Salt is hard to avoid. We sprinkle salt on our food as a seasoning, and it is added to almost every processed food. Condiments such as ketchup and soy sauce are loaded with salt. Baked goods made with sodium bicarbonate are full of sodium. And you can tell from their names that many food additives, such as monosodium glutamate (MSG) and sodium nitrite, have a lot of sodium. Too much sodium and not enough potassium are the culprits behind many cases of high blood pressure (we'll talk more about that soon). For now, let's just say that almost all doctors and researchers agree: we eat too much salt. Cutting back on salt could reduce your chances of high blood pressure, stroke, kidney problems, and heart disease. It's an easy way to improve your health.

Step one is to just put the salt shaker away. We add salt to food to season it, not because we need it—our foods naturally have all the salt we need. If you stop adding salt, your food may taste a little bland at first, but after a few days you won't notice the difference.

The next step is to cut back on processed foods that are high in salt—lunch meats and snack foods would be good places to start. Other easy steps are choosing no-salt or low-salt foods. Try switching to unsalted butter, for example.

About half the extra salt we get comes from processed foods, but picking a low-sodium version can be a little confusing. Plenty of processed foods today claim to be low in sodium, but the labels all seem to say different things. Here's how the FDA says to sort out the claims:

- ◆ **Sodium-free or salt-free.** Less than 5 mg per serving.

- ◆ **Very low sodium.** 35 mg or less per serving.

- ◆ **Low sodium.** 140 mg or less per serving.

- ◆ **Light in sodium.** At least 50 percent less sodium per serving than the food ordinarily has.

- ◆ **Lightly salted.** At least 50 percent less sodium per serving than the food ordinarily has.

- ◆ **Reduced or less sodium.** At least 25 percent less sodium per serving than the food ordinarily has.

- ◆ **Unsalted, no salt added, without added salt.** No salt has been added during processing, even though salt is ordinarily added to that food.

> ### Now You're Cooking
>
> Salt substitutes swap sodium chloride for potassium chloride. Give them a try, but only to season your food at the table. Using potassium chloride for cooking gives food a bitter taste. If you need to restrict your potassium, don't use salt substitutes—most have more than 600 mg in just a quarter teaspoon. And watch out for "lite salt" products—these still contain a lot of sodium.

There's one more requirement. If the label mentions only lowered salt or sodium, a line in the Nutrition Facts panel must say "Not a sodium-free food" or "Not for control of sodium in the diet." Still confused? We don't blame you. Here's a good way to choose: look for the words "free" or "low" to get the least sodium.

Electrifying News on High Blood Pressure

We know from many studies that people who eat a low-potassium, high-sodium diet are more likely to have high blood pressure. We know that if you already have high blood pressure, eating less sodium helps bring it down. We know that uncontrolled high blood pressure can lead to heart disease, kidney disease, and strokes. What we still don't know is exactly why sodium has such an impact on your blood pressure.

The balance between your potassium and sodium levels is important for keeping your blood pressure down. Many researchers believe that a good balance is roughly five parts potassium, or even more, to one part sodium. Unfortunately, our high-salt diets give many of us balances that are more similar to one part potassium to two parts sodium, or twice as much sodium as potassium. It's not surprising that about 30 percent of American adults—some 50 million people—have high blood pressure. Among adults older than age 65, more than half have high blood pressure.

About half of all people who have high blood pressure are salt-sensitive—sodium in their diet makes their blood pressure zoom up. These people should try very hard to reduce their sodium intake. Older people and African Americans are most likely to be salt-sensitive, but it makes sense for everyone to cut back. Studies show that overall, the average person who consumes less salt has lower blood pressure. In fact, a 1997 study in the prestigious British medical journal *The Lancet* suggests that older people who lower their salt intake also sharply lower their risk of stroke, even if they don't have high blood pressure.

Just cutting back on sodium isn't the whole solution. Many people with high blood pressure also benefit from *increasing* their potassium. When they do, they get a more natural balance in their electrolytes, and their blood pressure goes down. You don't need pills or supplements to get the benefits: just eating fewer salty foods and more foods rich in potassium will help. In many cases, lowering your sodium intake to fewer than 2,000 mg a day and raising your potassium intake to more than 3,500 mg a day has a very beneficial effect, especially for older people.

Proof that this works came in 1997—and was confirmed in 2000 by follow-up research—as part of the important Dietary Approaches to Stop Hypertension (DASH) study. Some people in the study ate a typical American diet; others ate a diet that was much lower in fat and much higher in fruits and vegetables—which are high in potassium. All the people in the study got about 3,000 mg a day of sodium. But the people who ate the typical American diet got only 1,700 mg of potassium, whereas the people who ate lots more fruits and vegetables got about 4,700 mg of potassium. Guess whose blood pressures dropped? You're right. The typical Americans didn't improve at all, but the fruit and vegetable eaters saw their blood pressures drop substantially. And the higher their blood pressures were to begin with, the more they dropped.

What if you already take medicine for high blood pressure? Keep taking it as you cut back on sodium in your diet and try to get more dietary potassium. Reducing your sodium almost always makes the drug work better. Cut back enough and make some lifestyle changes, and you might be able to take a smaller dose or maybe even stop taking medicine altogether. *Never* stop taking any medicine, but especially high–blood-pressure drugs, on your own. Always talk to your doctor first.

Preventing Strokes with Potassium

Even if you don't have high blood pressure, potassium could help protect you against having a stroke. If your potassium intake is low, your odds of a stroke go up, no matter what other risk factors you may have, such as cigarette smoking or being overweight.

According to several long-term studies of older adults, just one daily serving of a potassium-rich food could substantially cut your risk of a stroke by an amazing 40 percent. That's just one banana, glass of orange juice, or baked potato. And if you eat more than one serving a day, your odds against a stroke might improve even more. The benefit is strongest for people who already have high blood pressure.

The Least You Need to Know

◆ Sodium, chloride, and potassium are electrolytes, minerals that have electrical charges and carry nutrients into and out of your cells.

◆ Electrolytes help regulate your blood pressure and heartbeat.

◆ Most people get plenty of potassium from their food and too much sodium from salt (sodium chloride).

◆ Good food sources of potassium include beans, fruits, and vegetables.

◆ Too much sodium in your diet may raise your blood pressure to unhealthy levels, but potassium in your diet could help lower it.

◆ Potassium could help protect you against having a stroke.

Chapter 21

The Trace Minerals: A Little Goes a Long Way

In This Chapter

◆ Finding out what trace minerals are and why you need them

◆ Knowing the roles of iron, iodine, chromium, and selenium

◆ Learning the roles of boron, copper, manganese, molybdenum, and other less-important trace minerals

◆ Avoiding certain trace minerals

True or false: your body needs arsenic. Amazingly, the answer is true! Trace minerals—minerals you need in only tiny amounts—are full of surprises like that. Most of the trace minerals in your body do many important things, from carrying oxygen to building your bones to making the hormones and enzymes that tell your body what to do. You also have some trace minerals that don't seem to do anything useful at all.

The world of trace minerals is still being explored. We weren't even sure you needed boron, for example, until well into the 1980s. More roles for these tiny powerhouses are sure to be discovered as research continues.

What's a Trace Mineral?

If you have less than a teaspoon of a mineral in your body, it's a *trace mineral*—one that you need, but only in very small amounts. In the human body, 15 substances are considered necessary trace minerals (check out the chart for the whole list).

Although you need all the trace minerals, some are more important than others. Zinc, for example, is so important that we gave it its own chapter (see Chapter 19). Some of the other trace minerals, such as nickel, are so minor and so easy to get from your food that there just isn't a lot to say about them. We'll concentrate on the trace minerals that could make a real difference to your health. Not every trace mineral has an RDA or even an Adequate Intake (AI) amount. We just don't know about some of them, such as nickel and boron.

The Trace Minerals

Mineral	Function	Adult RDA or AI
Boron	Builds healthy bones	None
Chromium	Controls blood sugar	20 to 35 mcg
Cobalt	Needed for cobalamin (Vitamin B_{12})	None
Copper	Needed for antioxidant enzymes, red blood cells, and other enzymes	700 to 900 mcg
Fluoride	Protects against tooth decay; builds healthy bones	3.0 to 4.0 mg
Iodine	Needed for thyroid hormones	150 mcg
Iron	Needed for hemoglobin in red blood cells	8.0 to 18.0 mg
Manganese	Needed for protein digestion and tissue formation	1.8 to 2.3 mg
Molybdenum	Needed for normal growth and development	45 mcg
Nickel	Needed to make some enzymes and hormones	None
Selenium	Needed for the antioxidant enzyme glutathione	55 mcg
Silicon	Builds healthy bones	None
Tin	Unknown	None

Mineral	Function	Adult RDA or AI
Vanadium	Unknown	None
Zinc	Builds a healthy immune system	8.0 to 11.0 mg

Why You Need Trace Minerals

You might not need much of a trace mineral, but some are especially important when it comes to making the many different enzymes, hormones, and other chemical messengers your body uses every minute of every day. You need iodine to make thyroid hormones, which in turn control some very important parts of your metabolism, including your body weight. You need the trace mineral iron to carry oxygen in your blood and also to make other enzymes. Some trace minerals, such as selenium, are used to make the powerful natural antioxidants that protect you against free radicals. And some trace minerals work closely with vitamins to make them more active and long-lasting.

We still don't completely understand the roles of some other trace minerals, such as manganese. We know that you'll develop health problems if you don't get the tiny amount you need, but we're still not sure why.

> ### Quack, Quack
>
> Some supplement pushers claim you need their super-duper (and expensive) mineral supplements because foods don't have enough minerals. Supposedly the soil they are grown in has been "depleted" of minerals by modern farming practices. These pushers are trying to confuse you by claiming that natural variations in soil minerals are caused by farmers—and that these variations have a bad effect on you. Don't be taken in.

RDAs and Adequate Intakes

In general, you need to be cautious about trace minerals. The toxic amount of a trace mineral often isn't that much higher than the safe amount. The adult RDA for selenium, for example, is 55 mcg. The toxic amount is about 600 mcg, or just more than 10 times the RDA. Likewise, too much iron can be more harmful than too little.

Most people get plenty of all the trace minerals from their food and don't need to take supplements. If you feel you need more of a particular trace element, try to get it from your food whenever possible.

Are You Deficient?

When was the last time you ever heard of anyone being deficient in copper? When was the last time you heard the word vanadium? As a rule, most people have all the trace minerals they need. With the exception of iron, you're not very likely to be deficient in any of them.

The bigger question is whether getting more of a trace mineral improves your health. Here, too, there just isn't a lot of solid evidence. In some cases—chromium, for example—it's possible that more is better. On the other hand, because we don't always know what too much might do, it's always best to be cautious and avoid super-large doses of trace minerals.

Eating Your Trace Minerals

Trace minerals are found in small amounts in a wide variety of foods. The amounts in your food generally come from the soil where the food is grown. Brazil nuts are high in selenium because the soil in the part of Brazil where they grow is high in selenium.

Trace minerals aren't evenly distributed around the world. To take selenium as an example again, parts of China have almost none—and some people there have a type of heart disease caused by severe selenium deficiency. Parts of the western United States, on the other hand, have very high selenium levels, and animals that graze on grass there sometimes get an overdose that causes illness and deformities.

Even if you eat a pretty unbalanced diet that's low in fresh fruits and vegetables, you're not very likely to be deficient in trace minerals. Some of them are inescapable. Iodine, for example, is added to almost all table salt—and as you know from reading Chapter 20, we all get more than enough salt every day. The water you drink gives you some of the trace minerals. Fluoride is often added to municipal water supplies, and chromium is found in "hard" water.

Getting the Most from Trace Minerals

Most good daily multi-supplements contain at least some of the trace minerals. The amounts vary—read the labels. A lot of multi-supplements contain at least the RDA for iron. As we'll discuss a little further on, this may not be a good idea for some people. Again, read the label carefully.

Sometimes combination supplements contain one or two trace elements that are especially important. For example, calcium supplements sometimes come with magnesium and boron, because these two minerals are needed to build healthy bones. These supplements are on the expensive side. Do you really need the trace minerals as well? Probably not, especially if you also take a daily multi-supplement.

There may be times when you want to take additional supplements of a particular trace mineral. Be very cautious here—take the smallest possible dose. Too much of a trace mineral could be as harmful as too little. Whenever possible, try to get your trace minerals from your food instead of pills.

Singling Out Sulfur

Okay, we lied in the chapter title—sulfur isn't a trace mineral at all. About one quarter of 1 percent of your body is made up of sulfur, so you have more than a teaspoon of the stuff in you. We're sticking it here because you need it and we don't know where else to put it.

Even though you need sulfur to make many amino acids and natural antioxidants (we'll talk more about this in Chapters 22 and 23) and the B vitamins thiamin, biotin, and pantothenic acid, there isn't much to say here. Sulfur is so common in your food that no one has ever been deficient in it, so no one has ever bothered to figure out an RDA or even an Adequate Intake for it. You also can't overdose on sulfur—you excrete any excess in your urine. Vitamin manufacturers don't generally make sulfur into supplements, and reference books that give the breakdown of nutrients in food don't bother listing it. Good food sources of sulfur include eggs (sulfur is the awful smell in rotten eggs), clams, fish, lean beef, milk, and dairy products. Sulfur is also found in smaller amounts in all plant foods, especially cabbage, beans, garlic, onions, and wheat germ.

Iron: Basic for Blood

Iron barely qualifies as a trace mineral, because you have less than a teaspoon of it in your body. You need it chiefly to carry oxygen in your blood. Every one of your red blood cells contains a protein called *hemoglobin*—and four atoms of iron are attached to every hemoglobin molecule. In your lungs, oxygen molecules attach to the iron atoms and are carried to your cells. When the oxygen reaches its destination, it's swapped for the waste carbon dioxide and carried back to your lungs. You get rid of it by exhaling.

def•i•ni•tion

Hemoglobin is the oxygen-carrying protein that gives your red blood cells their color. Every molecule of hemoglobin has four atoms of iron in it.

How much iron you have determines how much oxygen gets to the rest of your body. Not enough iron, and you start making fewer red blood cells. Not enough red blood cells, and you become anemic—weak, tired, pale, and short of breath.

Just how common is iron-poor blood? Not as common as all the advertising says, but common enough to be concerned—in fact, it's common enough to be the number one form of nutritional deficiency worldwide. You could be low on iron for a long time before you become anemic. An important 1997 study found that 1 out of 10 American women and small children were deficient in iron—or about 700,000 toddlers and 7.8 million women! Of those, about 240,000 toddlers and 3.3 million women were anemic. And according to the federal Centers for Disease Control (CDC), 12 percent of all American women aged 12 to 49 were iron deficient in 1999 to 2000. Among Mexican American women, some 22 percent were iron deficient.

Babies and toddlers need plenty of iron because they're growing so fast—and if they don't get it, they may fall behind in their mental development and never catch up. Teenaged girls need extra iron for growth, while women in general need extra iron to make up for the blood lost each month to menstruation. Pregnant women need plenty of iron to grow a healthy baby and prevent prematurity and low birth weight. In fact, pregnant women need iron so much that both the CDC and the Institute of Medicine recommend routine low-dose (30 mg) supplements. Nursing women also need extra iron, because they're passing a lot of their iron on to their babies. Anyone—male or female—who is very athletic also needs extra.

The RDA for Iron

The RDA for iron was changed in 2004; it was actually lowered a bit for adult men and raised a touch for adult women. Many nutritionists feel the new levels are really just bare minimums and far from ideal—especially for women. In general, a much larger dose—up to 75 mg a day—is quite safe for adults.

The RDA for Iron

Age in Years/Sex	Iron in mg
Infants	
0 to 0.5	0
0.5 to 1	11

Age in Years/Sex	Iron in mg
Children	
1 to 3	7
4 to 8	10
9 to 13	8
Young Adults and Adults	
Men 14 to 18	11
Men 19+	8
Women 14 to 18	15
Women 19 to 50	18
Women 51+	8
Pregnant women	27
Nursing women	10

Eating Your Iron

The average American diet has about 6 mg of iron for every 1,000 calories you eat. That means you need to eat about 2,500 calories a day to get enough iron. Because women generally eat less than 2,000 calories a day, you need to be certain you're getting enough iron by choosing iron-rich foods. Studies of food consumption show that only a quarter of women of childbearing age (ages 12 through 49) meet the RDA for iron through diet!

Iron is found in many common foods. It falls into two categories: *heme iron*, found in meat, and *nonheme iron*, found in plant foods. You absorb heme iron from your food better than nonheme iron, but vegetarians don't need to worry—many delicious plant foods are high in iron. The problem is that the fiber in those foods can decrease iron absorption. Vitamin C, however, increases nonheme absorption, so be sure to eat plenty of foods rich in this vitamin along with iron-rich foods. You can also increase the iron content of vegetable foods by using cast-iron cookware.

def•i•ni•tion

Heme iron is the iron found in hemoglobin—and because only animals have hemoglobin, heme iron is found only in meat. **Nonheme iron** is the iron found naturally in plant foods such as spinach and whole grains.

Rich sources of heme iron include organ meats, lean beef, chicken, oysters, and pork. Good sources of nonheme iron are whole grains, peas, beans, spinach, nuts, and blackstrap (unrefined) molasses. One of the best sources of iron is Cream of Wheat cereal—there's more than 7 mg in 6 ounces. Many cold breakfast cereals such as bran flakes also have plenty of iron, both naturally and from added supplements. You're sure to find iron-rich foods you like in the following chart.

The Iron in Foods

Food	Amount	Iron in mg
Almonds, dry-roasted	1 oz.	1.1
Barley	1 cup	2.1
Beef, ground	3 oz.	1.8
Black beans	1 cup	3.6
Bread, whole-wheat	1 slice	0.9
Broccoli, cooked	½ cup	0.6
Brussels sprouts	½ cup	0.9
Chicken	3 oz.	1.1
Chickpeas	1 cup	3.2
Kale	½ cup	0.6
Kidney beans	1 cup	3.2
Lima beans	½ cup	1.8
Liver, beef	3 oz.	5.8
Liver, chicken	3 oz.	7.3
Molasses, blackstrap	1 TB.	3.5
Oysters, raw	6 medium	5.6
Peanut butter	2 TB.	0.5
Pecans	1 oz.	0.6
Potato, baked	1 medium	2.7
Prune juice	8 oz.	3.0
Raisins, seedless	⅔ cup	2.1
Spinach, cooked	½ cup	3.2
Strawberries	1 cup	0.6
Tomato	1 medium	0.5

Food	Amount	Iron in mg
Tomato juice	6 oz.	1.1
Walnuts	1 oz.	0.7
Wheat germ	¼ cup	1.8
White beans	1 cup	6.6

Getting the Most from Iron

If you're anemic, your doctor will prescribe an iron supplement. If you want to get more iron by taking an over-the-counter supplement, look for one containing ferrous iron salts in the form of ferrous fumarate, ferrous sulfate, or ferrous gluconate. Time-release or enteric-coated iron tablets are a waste of money, because they'll pass through your system before you absorb much iron from them. Instead, space your iron supplements out over the day in two or three doses.

Iron supplements can cause nausea, constipation, or diarrhea, though, and they're not usually necessary. Get your extra iron by eating plenty of vegetables and other iron-rich foods, and take supplements only if your doctor has confirmed that you have iron-deficiency anemia or if your doctor prescribes them because you're pregnant.

> **Now You're Cooking**
>
> Foods cooked in cast-iron cookware absorb safe, tasteless amounts of extra iron. Acidic foods absorb the most. Tomato sauce simmered in a cast-iron pot could have as much as 300 times the iron as sauce simmered in an aluminum pot. In general, cooking vegetables makes more of their iron content available to be absorbed by your body.

It's Iron-ic

Iron deficiency is a major health problem worldwide, but too much iron is also a health problem for older adults. At least 10 percent of all Americans have an inherited condition called *hemochromatosis*, or iron overload, that makes them build up too much iron, which can damage your

def•i•ni•tion

> **Hemochromatosis** is an inherited condition that causes you to build up extra iron in your body. The symptoms don't usually appear until you're older than age 50.

Food for Thought

A study in 2004 showed that young women who were iron deficient did significantly worse on memory and attention tests than healthy young women. When the deficient took an iron supplement, their performance improved back to normal levels.

pancreas, liver, heart, and joints and put you at higher risk of a heart attack or stroke. The symptoms don't usually start to appear until you're older than 50 (if you're a man) or older than 60 (if you're a woman). If you have hemochromatosis, it's particularly important to avoid iron from multi-supplements or fortified foods. And because you can't tell whether you'll develop hemochromatosis as you get older, you might want to switch to a multi-supplement without iron if you're a man or a postmenopausal woman.

Iodine: Important for the Thyroid

You need iodine to make the *thyroid* hormones that regulate your body's metabolism. In fact, that's all iodine does for you, but it's a lot: those thyroid hormones play a big role in your growth, cell reproduction, and nerve functions, and how your cells use oxygen. One of the hormones, thyroxin, regulates how fast you use the energy from your food. If you don't have enough iodine, your thyroid swells up in an effort to make more hormones, a condition called *hypothyroidism*. The swelling is called a *goiter*.

def•i•ni•tion

Your **thyroid** is a small, butterfly-shaped gland found in your neck just below your Adam's apple. It produces hormones, including one called thyroxin that regulates your metabolism. A shortage of iodine can lead to **hypothyroidism,** or underactive thyroid. When that happens, your thyroid gland swells up and forms a lump called a **goiter** in your neck.

The RDA for Iodine

In total, you have between 20 and 30 mg of iodine in your body. The RDA is more than adequate to prevent a deficiency.

The RDA for Iodine

Age in Years/Sex	Iodine in mcg
Infants	
0 to 0.5	110
0.5 to 1	130

Age in Years/Sex	Iodine in mcg
Children	
1 to 3	90
4 to 8	90
9 to 13	120
Teens and Adults	
14+	150
Pregnant women	220
Nursing women	290

Until well into the twentieth century, iodine deficiency was a serious problem. People living in the Midwest and Great Lakes region, where the soil is very low in iodine, didn't get enough in their diets and often got goiters. Iodine deficiency during pregnancy causes a severe form of mental retardation called cretinism. To solve the iodine problem, in 1924 American salt producers began adding iodine to table salt at the rate of 400 mcg per teaspoon. Goiters and cretinism soon disappeared as public-health problems, and today iodine deficiency is very, very rare.

Iodine is added to a lot of daily multi-supplements, but it's not really needed, because most people get more than enough from the salt in their food. Too much iodine (more than 25 times the RDA) can also cause a goiter. More than 1,000 mg a day may also cause acne flare-ups in some people.

Warning!

Iron supplements in even small amounts can be toxic to young children. Keep iron supplements and multi-supplements containing iron out of the reach of children!

Chromium: Boon for Diabetics?

One of the most popular supplements today is chromium picolinate. Some people with diabetes swear it helps them control their blood sugar better. Some bodybuilders swear it helps them build muscle faster. Some people claim it helps lower high cholesterol, whereas others claim it boosts the production of the anti-aging hormone DHEA. And of course, some people claim it is the magic supplement that makes losing weight effortless.

Is chromium such a miracle mineral? Maybe, for some people with diabetes—but the other claims don't hold up.

The AI for Chromium

In 2001 the Institute of Medicine set an Adequate Intake standard for chromium for the first time.

The AI for Chromium

Age in Years/Sex	Chromium in mcg
Infants	
0 to 0.5	0.2
0.5 to 1	5.5
Children	
1 to 3	11
4 to 8	15
Boys 9 to 13	25
Girls 9 to 13	21
Young Adults and Adults	
Men 14+	35
Men 50+	30
Women 14 to 18	24
Women 19+	25
Women 50+	20
Pregnant women	30
Nursing women	45

Let's start with why you need chromium. In ways we still don't fully understand, chromium is involved with using fats, proteins, and carbohydrates. It's also needed to help the hormone insulin deliver glucose to your cells.

Because of the insulin connection, chromium is often touted as a way for people with diabetes to control their blood sugar. Chromium does seem to help some people with Type 2 diabetes get glucose into their cells better, but the research so far is inconclusive. We suggest you skip chromium supplements and try to get between 50 and 200 mcg a day from your food. If you decide to try supplements, talk to your doctor first and keep a close eye on your blood sugar.

What about all those other things chromium is supposed to do? There's not a lot of evidence to back up the cholesterol or DHEA claims (see Chapter 27 for more on DHEA). The bodybuilders may be disappointed, too. The studies that showed chromium helps you lose fat and build muscle were badly flawed, and researchers haven't been able to reproduce them.

What about chromium picolinate for weight loss? There's been a lot of hype in this area, of course, and not a lot of good research. If you take chromium supplements every day and also watch your diet and exercise regularly, you'll lose weight. Will it be because of the chromium? You decide.

It's relatively easy to get at least 50 mcg of chromium a day from your food. Apples, broccoli, barley, corn, beef, eggs, nuts, mushrooms, oysters, rhubarb, tomatoes, and sweet potatoes are all good food sources of chromium. Most good daily multi-supplements also have some chromium in them. If you decide to take a chromium supplement to help your diabetes, choose chromium polynicotinate or the patented type of trivalent chromium picolinate called Chromax-II GTF. (The GTF stands for glucose tolerance factor.) Skip supplements made with chromium chloride—the body doesn't absorb this form very well.

Selenium: An Essential Element

Your body's most abundant natural antioxidant is an enzyme called glutathione peroxidase. We'll talk a lot more about glutathione in Chapter 24, so for now we'll just mention that without selenium, you can't make glutathione. A major study in 1997 showed that selenium can be a powerful cancer-prevention supplement. People in the study took 200 mcg of selenium daily to see whether their skin cancer rate would drop. It didn't—but their rates of colorectal, lung, and prostate cancer went down sharply. A number of other studies have shown a similar protective effect for selenium against cancer, especially prostate cancer. A major study called the Selenium and Vitamin E Cancer Prevention Trial (SELECT) was started in 2001 and is looking at whether men at risk of prostate cancer can prevent it by taking supplemental selenium and Vitamin E. We won't know the results until 2011.

Selenium may also help protect you against heart disease. It also helps your immune system work effectively and helps remove heavy metals such as lead from your body.

Vitamin E works better and longer in your body when you have plenty of selenium. All that makes selenium pretty important for a mineral you need only in micrograms.

In 2000, selenium got a revised DRI. The amount you need is still quite low—you can easily get it from your food.

The RDA for Selenium

Age in Years/Sex	Selenium in mcg
Infants	
0 to 0.5	15
0.5 to 1	20
Children	
1 to 3	20
4 to 8	30
9 to 13	40
Adults	
14+	55
Pregnant women	60
Nursing women	70

Animal foods such as organ meats, seafood, lean meat, and chicken are all good sources of selenium. Whole grains such as oatmeal and brown rice are good plant sources of selenium, especially if they were grown in selenium-rich soil. The benefits of selenium for cancer prevention and other health problems seem to kick in only at 200 mcg a day, though, so you may want to consider supplements. Selenium supplements come in two forms. Yeast-based supplements are made from yeast grown in a selenium-enriched medium. "Organic" selenium is bound to an amino acid in the form of selenomethionine. Avoid inorganic forms of this mineral such as sodium selenite or selenate—you don't absorb them very well. You need to be very cautious with selenium supplements. In amounts greater than 400 mcg a day, selenium can be toxic, although up to 200 mcg a day seems to be safe.

Copper: Crucial for Your Circulation

Copper is involved in a lot of body processes, but its main functions are to help keep your heart and blood vessels healthy. You need copper to make an enzyme that keeps your arteries flexible—if you don't get enough, they could rupture. You also need copper to make the insulating sheath that covers your nerves. Copper works with iron to keep your red blood cells healthy. It's also very important for making the natural antioxidant superoxide dismutase (SOD)—we'll talk more about SOD in Chapter 24.

In 2001, the Institute of Medicine introduced an RDA for copper to replace the earlier Safe and Adequate Range.

RDA for Copper

Age in Years/Sex	Copper in mcg
Infants	
0 to 0.5	200
0.5 to 1	220
Children	
1 to 3	340
4 to 8	440
9 to 13	700
Young Adults and Adults	
14 to 18	890
19+	900
Pregnant women	1,000
Nursing women	1,300

Hardly anyone is ever deficient in copper—just about everyone gets plenty from their diet. There are some very rare inherited conditions such as Wilson's disease that make you store too much copper in your body, but on the whole, copper toxicity is also rare. You'd have to take in more than 10 mg a day to have any symptoms. The most common symptoms of copper overdose are nausea and vomiting.

Copper is found in a lot of common foods. There's more than 2 mg of copper in a single oyster; other shellfish, such as lobster, are also good sources. Other good foods for copper include nuts, avocados, potatoes, organ meats, whole grains, beans, and peas. You may also be getting some from your drinking water if it goes through copper pipes. Copper is also found in most good daily multi-supplements.

It's important to keep your zinc and copper levels in balance, because the two minerals compete with each other to be absorbed into your body. Most nutritionists recommend a ratio of 10 parts zinc to 1 part copper. In other words, if you're taking 30 mg of zinc, be sure to take 3 mg of copper as well—but don't take more than that.

Fluoride: Fighting Tooth Decay

Here's a trace mineral we know you *don't* need. Even so, fluoride is very valuable for preventing tooth decay and even repairing decay in its earliest stages. Fluoridated drinking water reduces cavities in children by 20 to 40 percent and in adults by 15 to 35 percent—and the effect is even greater if you also use fluoridated toothpaste.

Fluoride helps build strong bones and keep them that way. There's some solid evidence that people who live in areas with fluoridated water have less osteoporosis. New drugs that combine calcium and fluoride for treating osteoporosis are now being investigated and show a lot of promise.

There's no RDA for fluoride, but in 1998 an Adequate Intake level was established by the Institute of Medicine.

Adequate Intake for Fluoride

Age in Years/Sex	Fluoride in mg
Infants	
0 to 0.5	0.01
0.5 to 1	0.5
Children	
1 to 3	0.7
4 to 8	1.0
9 to 13	2.0

Age in Years/Sex	Fluoride in mg
Adults	
Men 14 to 18	3.0
Men 19+	4.0
Women 14+	3.0
Pregnant women	5.0
Nursing women	5.0

Today about 60 percent of the municipalities in the United States add fluoride to their water supplies at the rate of 1 mg per liter (which is another way of saying one part per million). That amount means the average adult will get between 1.5 and 4.0 mg a day just from drinking tap water.

The main reason water is fluoridated is that there really isn't any in food, with one exception: a cup of tea has about 0.3 mg. If you drink only bottled or filtered water or water from your own well, or if your community doesn't fluoridate its water, you and your family may not be getting the benefits of fluoride for your teeth and bones. Likewise, if you use "natural" toothpaste that doesn't have fluoride, you're not protecting your teeth fully.

There is no evidence at all that fluoride weakens bones or causes cancer, heart disease, kidney disease, Alzheimer's disease, or any other health problem.

Manganese: Mystery Metal

Until 1972, when the first case came up, we didn't even know you could have a shortage of manganese. This mineral is still pretty mysterious. It seems to do a lot of the same things as magnesium, such as help make your connective tissue, clot your blood, move glucose around your system, and digest your proteins. It may also be an antioxidant.

Most people take in anywhere between 2 and 9 mg of manganese a day. That seems to be enough, because manganese deficiency is extremely rare. There's no RDA, but we can tell you the Adequate Intake:

Adequate Intake for Manganese

Age in Years/Sex	Manganese in mg
Infants	
0 to 0.5	0.3
0.5 to 1	0.6
Children	
1 to 3	1.2
4 to 8	1.5
Boys 9 to 13	1.9
Girls 9 to 13	1.6
Young Adults and Adults	
Men 14 to 18	2.2
Men 19+	2.3
Women 14 to 18	1.6
Women 19+	1.8
Pregnant women	2.0
Nursing women	2.6

Foods that are high in manganese include tea, raisins, pineapple, spinach, broccoli, oranges, nuts, blueberries, beans, and whole grains.

Manganese can be very helpful for women with heavy menstrual flows. Eating more foods rich in manganese every day helps reduce the flow. Manganese is also an important mineral for building strong bones. If you don't get enough, you could be at greater risk for osteoporosis. Manganese also helps glucosamine work better (see Chapter 29).

The best way to get more manganese is to eat more foods that contain it. Many daily multi-supplements also contain manganese. Don't overdo it, though—too much manganese can interfere with your iron absorption.

Molybdenum: Making Enzymes

All your tissues contain tiny amounts of molybdenum. It's needed to make several enzymes, particularly one called xanthine oxidase. You need this enzyme to grow and develop normally and to use iron in your body properly.

The average adult gets between 45 and 500 mcg of molybdenum a day from food. Molybdenum deficiency is almost impossible.

Adequate Intake for Molybdenum

Age in Years/Sex	Molybdenum in mcg
Infants	
0 to 0.5	2
0.5 to 1	3
Children	
1 to 3	17
4 to 8	22
9 to 13	34
Young Adults and Adults	
Men 14 to 18	43
Men 19+	45
Women 14 to 18	43
Women 19+	45
Pregnant women	50
Nursing women	50

The amount of molybdenum in your food depends on where it was grown. The soil in some parts of the country is much higher in molybdenum than others. In general, good food sources include whole grains; lean meat; organ meats; beans; dark-green, leafy vegetables; and milk. Most people get plenty from their food and don't need extra, although molybdenum is often found in daily multi-supplements.

Other Trace Minerals

Did you know your body contains very tiny amounts of gold and silver? It does, but we have no idea why or what—if anything—would happen if you didn't have them. We do know why you have some other important trace minerals, though, so we'll run down the list and tell you the basics for each one.

◆ **Boron.** In the mid-1980s, researchers discovered that you need small amounts of boron to help you absorb calcium into your bones and keep it there. How much boron is still up in the air. There's no RDA or AI yet, but many nutritionists today suggest getting 3 mg a day. That's not a problem, because most people get 2 to 5 mg a day from their food. Good dietary sources of boron are fruits, especially apples, pears, peaches, grapes, dates, and raisins. Nuts and beans are also high in boron.

◆ **Cobalt.** Remember the chapter on cobalamin (Vitamin B₁₂)? You need cobalt to make this vitamin, which is essential for making red blood cells. In fact, that's *all* you need cobalt for. And because you don't need much cobalamin, you don't need much cobalt—a few micrograms is ample. If you're getting enough cobalamin from your food or supplements, you're getting plenty of cobalt.

Food for Thought

A careful study in one small region of China showed that people there had the world's highest rate of cancer of the esophagus—and also ate food grown in soil that was very low in molybdenum. The connection between cancer and low molybdenum seems clear, but so far there's no evidence that taking extra molybdenum prevents cancer.

Quack, Quack

Germanium is a mineral used to make computer chips. Can it do anything for humans? Probably not, although some people claim, on almost no evidence, that it boosts your immune system. This is one of the more expensive ways to waste your money—the capsules run about a dollar apiece.

◆ **Nickel.** We still don't know what nickel is doing there in your body, although it's probably involved with making some enzymes, hormones, and cell membranes. Too much nickel is associated with cancer, heart disease, and skin problems, but there are no known effects of too little nickel. Because you absorb very, very little nickel from your food, getting too much is almost impossible. Good food sources of nickel include chocolate, whole grains, nuts, beans, fruits, and vegetables.

◆ **Silicon.** You need silicon to make your bones, cartilage, and connective tissue. Nobody's ever been deficient in silicon because it's found in many foods, especially seafood, whole grains, root vegetables such as potatoes, and beans. Silicon supplements made from the horsetail plant are said to help your nails, hair, bones, and even arteries. Skip them—they're worthless.

◆ **Tin.** You've got this in your body, but we don't know what it does. This is one trace mineral you definitely don't have to think about.

◆ **Vanadium.** Recently a lot of vanadium products have come on the market, along with a lot of hype. Some of the ads even claim it "cures" diabetes. Don't believe it. Any possible benefit vanadium (it's sold in the form of vanadyl sulfate) might have on your blood sugar is outweighed by its possible dangers even in moderate doses. There's no known need for vanadium in your body.

Minerals You Should Miss

There are some minerals that are okay in trace amounts but definitely not okay beyond that. Here's the rundown:

◆ **Aluminum.** Too much aluminum can cause nerve and brain damage. The average person doesn't need to worry much about this, but if you're a heavy user of aluminum-based antacids you could have a problem.

◆ **Arsenic.** Believe it or not, you actually need this in very, very small amounts. Most people get about 140 mcg a day from their food. Doses larger than 250 mcg a day are toxic. Environmental arsenic from drinking water has been linked to cancer.

◆ **Cadmium.** Your body doesn't have any known use for cadmium, so it's never developed a way to get rid of it. Unfortunately, cadmium is found in cigarette smoke and air pollution, so you could accumulate a toxic amount over many years. High levels of cadmium have been linked to increased breast cancer risk. If you don't already have enough good reasons to stop smoking, cadmium is another.

> ### Quack, Quack
>
> A few years back, researchers found aluminum in the brains of people with Alzheimer's disease. This gave rise to the rumor that food cooked in aluminum pots and pans could cause Alzheimer's. Not so: aluminum cookware is perfectly safe.

◆ **Lead.** This stuff is really bad for you, even though your body normally has a tiny amount of it. Even small amounts of extra lead can cause nerve damage, anemia, mental impairment, and muscle weakness. Recent research also ties lead exposure to high blood pressure, cataracts, and osteoporosis in adults and learning and behavioral difficulties in children. Most cases of lead poisoning occur from exposure to lead-based paint and air pollution. Young children are especially at risk. According to the FDA, there's no safe level of exposure. High lead levels are sometimes found in imported herbal remedies and supplements—be cautious about using these products.

◆ **Mercury.** This is another mineral that you have naturally in very small amounts. In larger amounts, though, it can do real damage and should be avoided. Mercury is used in a lot of industrial processes, so it can end up in air and water pollution. Fish such as tuna and swordfish that swim in mercury-contaminated water and eat smaller fish that are also contaminated with mercury may accumulate high levels of it. If you then eat the fish, you'll also get the mercury that's in it. Experts suggest eating these fish no more than once a week—less if you're pregnant or breastfeeding. What about the mercury in your silver dental fillings? We're not sure whether this is really dangerous—it's an extremely controversial issue. If you want to replace your mercury-containing silver amalgam fillings, discuss it with your dentist.

How can you avoid all these dangerous minerals? To a degree, you can't in our industrial society. There are some simple steps you can take, though: have lead paint removed; stop smoking; and avoid contaminated food, water, and air.

Food for Thought _____

Nearly all shellfish and fish contain traces of mercury. For most people, the amount isn't cause for concern, but pregnant women need to be careful to avoid harming their unborn baby. The FDA and the EPA advise women who may become pregnant, pregnant women, nursing mothers, and young children to avoid eating swordfish, shark, king mackerel, and tilefish—these contain high levels of mercury. Shrimp, canned light and albacore tuna, salmon, pollock, and catfish have the least mercury and are safe to eat twice a week. Check local advisories for the safety of other fish from local waters.

The Least You Need to Know

◆ Your body needs very small amounts of some minerals.

◆ In almost all cases, you can get enough of the trace minerals from your food.

◆ Iron deficiency is fairly common, especially among toddlers and women. The RDA for iron is 11 to 18 mg.

◆ Other important trace minerals are iodine, chromium, and selenium.

◆ The trace minerals boron, cobalt, copper, manganese, and molybdenum are needed in very small amounts for good health.

Part 4

Exploring Other Supplements

There's a wide and wonderful world of supplements beyond vitamins and minerals. It's so wide and wonderful, in fact, that it's easy to get lost in it. We're here to help you stay on the right road. In this part we concentrate on the most valuable dietary supplements, such as amino acids, essential fatty acids, natural hormones, and flavonoids. These are safe, easy-to-take supplements that can help you with your everyday good health. We also discuss smart supplements, ways to relieve pain naturally, and discuss herbal supplements in depth.

New research and new products come along all the time in this fast-changing area. Not all of them deliver what they promise. We've tried to clear up the confusion so that you can set a straight course toward better health.

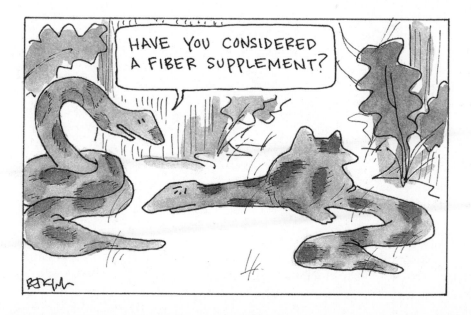

Chapter 22

Amino Acids: The Building Blocks of Life

In This Chapter

◆ What amino acids are

◆ Why amino acids are essential to life

◆ How your body uses amino acids to make hormones, enzymes, and antioxidants

◆ How individual amino acids can help health problems

Your body is a very busy place. Every second of every day, all around the clock, year after year, you make thousands of different enzymes, hormones, antioxidants, and chemical messengers. Every day millions of new cells replace old cells. Your taste buds, for example, last only a day or so, and you replace your entire skin every 30 days. Every day you make *millions* of red blood cells to replace the ones that wear out as they pound through your blood vessels.

The building blocks of everything that happens in your body are just 22 amino acids. All cells are made from them, and your body is regulated by them. Where do the amino acids come from? From the protein in the foods you eat, because proteins are nothing more than long chains of amino acids.

Why You Need Amino Acids

Pretty much all of you that's not bones and teeth is made up of *protein*. All that protein is made up of different combinations of *amino acids*. And all those amino acids are made just from atoms of hydrogen, oxygen, nitrogen, and carbon, with a little sulfur thrown in here and there.

def•i•ni•tion

A **protein** is an organic substance made up of hydrogen, oxygen, carbon, and nitrogen. Proteins are made from strings of amino acids. Every one of the 22 **amino acids** is a small molecule that has an amino group—a chemical fragment containing nitrogen, and an acid group—a chemical fragment containing carbon, oxygen, and hydrogen.

Amino acids are the building blocks of protein. The human body needs 22 different amino acids to make up the 50,000-plus proteins that make you, just as we can make all the words in the English language from just 26 letters.

The amino acids fall into two basic categories: essential and nonessential. Essential amino acids are the nine aminos you must get from your diet—like vitamins, you have to have them and, unlike vitamins, you can't get them any other way. (The amino acids arginine, histidine, and cysteine are essential for growing babies but not for adults.) Nonessential amino acids are the amino acids you can make in your body by combining two or more of the essential amino acids. Nonessential doesn't mean unnecessary. You don't have to get these aminos from your food (although they are found in foods), but you still need to have them. That means your food has to contain enough of the essential amino acids to build them.

Your body contains many other amino acids, such as carnitine and taurine, that don't fall into the essential/nonessential categories. We know that some of these aminos play important roles in your body. There are others that we still don't fully understand, but researchers are working on them. We believe there may be some exciting new developments in this area in the next few years.

Amino acids may have complicated names, such as phenylalanine, or confusingly similar names, such as glutamine, glycine, and glutamic acid. To make them easier to remember, we've listed them all in a chart. We're going to be talking about the different aminos by name, so refer back to the chart if you get mixed up.

The Amino Acids

Essential Amino Acids	Nonessential Amino Acids
Histidine	Alanine
Isoleucine	Arginine (essential for babies)
Leucine	Asparagine
Lysine	Aspartic acid
Methionine	Carnitine (essential for babies)
Phenylalanine	Cysteine
Threonine	Glutamic acid
Tryptophan	Glutamine
Valine	Glycine
	Proline
	Serine
	Taurine (essential for babies)
	Tyrosine

50,000 Proteins from Just 22 Aminos

You need all 22 amino acids to make the bigger protein molecules that keep you alive. Amazingly, those 22 aminos can be assembled into so many different three-dimensional combinations that your body can make more than 50,000 different proteins. That includes all the proteins that make up your tissues and form all the many enzymes, hormones, neurotransmitters, and other chemical messengers that keep your body working.

The instructions for making all these proteins are encoded in your genetic material—the DNA in the nucleus of every one of your cells. In a very complicated sequence of events, your DNA tells your cells to put together specific amino acids, anywhere from 2 or 3 to 1,000 or so, to make whatever protein happens to be needed at that moment. Amazingly, some cells in your body can produce as many as 10,000 different proteins! When exactly the right aminos are linked together in exactly the right order, they coil and fold up into exactly the shape of that protein and no other. That protein, folded into its particular shape, fits like a key into a lock with other proteins as it carries out its specific job in your body. When the job is done, other proteins come along and recycle it, breaking it back down so that its amino acids can be used again in another combination. The intricate complexity of your body is truly awesome!

def•i•ni•tion

Peptides are simple proteins that are easily absorbed into your body. A peptide is a very short chain of two or three amino acids.

When two or three amino acids combine into a short chain, they form a very simple protein called a *peptide*. You make a lot of different peptides. We're just starting to understand how many and how important they are. Most of your neurotransmitters, the chemical substances that send messages to and from your brain and help regulate your body, are peptides. They have complicated names only a biochemist could remember, such as bradykinin, leucine, enkephalin, and substance P.

The Recommended Intake for Amino Acids

Figuring out the Recommended Intake (RI) (the daily amount suggested by the Institute of Medicine, the same people who bring you the Recommended Dietary Allowances for vitamins and minerals) for amino acids gets complicated, because you really need to know two things: how much protein you need, and then how much of that protein should be made up of each of the nine essential amino acids. Bear with us as we work it out.

Food for Thought

A 1999 study of postmenopausal women found that the ones with the highest protein intakes had the lowest incidence of hip fractures from osteoporosis (thin, brittle bones).

First, the protein. How much do you really need? Probably a lot less than you're getting. The RI for protein is figured using a very complicated formula, but it basically comes down to this: you need 0.36 g of protein for every pound of body weight. So if you're that mythical 130-pound woman, you need about 46 g of protein (130 × 0.36) every day. In 2002, the Institute of Medicine set new standards for macronutrients such as protein. The following table gives the recommended protein intakes for everyone.

The Recommended Intake for Protein

Age in Years/Sex	Protein in g
Infants	
0 to 0.5	9
0.5 to 1	11

Age in Years/Sex	Protein in g
Children	
1 to 3	13
4 to 8	19
9 to 13	34
Boys 14 to 18	52
Girls 14 to 18	46
Adults	
Men 19+	56
Women 19+	46
Pregnant women	71
Nursing women	71

To put your protein needs in a different way, you need to get about 10 to 15 percent of your daily calories from protein. A gram of protein has about four calories, so our imaginary 130-pound woman gets about 188 calories a day from protein.

Let's get real with these numbers. There are about 28 g in an ounce. A quarter pound of hamburger has about 14 g of protein; a baked chicken leg has about 30 g. In an average American diet, you reach your daily protein quickly. In fact, you probably get way more of it than needed every day.

Now let's look at the amino acids. Animal proteins, such as meat, eggs, and milk, contain all nine of the essential amino acids, along with some of the nonessential ones. Nutritionists call these "high-quality" or "complete" proteins. The protein in eggs is such high quality that eggs are used as the standard to measure other proteins by (see the chart for the breakdown). So the proportions of the essential amino acids in an egg set the standard for how much of each essential amino acid you need. Looking at the following egg table, you can see that you need relatively little tryptophan, for example, compared to leucine.

Amino Acids in an Egg

Amino Acid	Amount in mg
Arginine	377
Cysteine	146
Histidine	149
Isoleucine	343
Leucine	537
Lysine	452
Methionine	196
Phenylalanine	334
Threonine	302
Tryptophan	76
Tyrosine	257
Valine	383

Now let's combine what we know about protein and what we know about amino acids. We know you need 0.36 mg of protein for every pound of your body weight. We know that protein needs to contain the different essential amino acids in roughly the same proportions as those found in an egg. Based on that, we can then figure out how much of each essential amino acid you need to get every day. The breakout is shown in the chart in terms of mg per each pound of your body weight. Checking the chart, you can see that a 130-pound woman needs 1,040 mg (130 × 8), or almost exactly 1 g of leucine every day. To put that in perspective, there are close to 2 g of leucine in a quarter pound of hamburger.

Adult Requirements for Essential Amino Acids

Amino Acid	Requirements in mg/lb
Histidine	5 to 7
Isoleucine	6
Leucine	8
Lysine	7
Methionine	8

Amino Acid	Requirements in mg/lb
Phenylalanine	8
Threonine	4
Tryptophan	2
Valine	6

Eating Your Aminos

Very few people in our modern society get less than the recommended amounts for high-quality protein. Most get more—vegetarians get about 50 to 100 g a day, and meat eaters get a lot more. Protein deficiency—and therefore amino acid deficiency—is almost unheard of. You'd have to be on a very weird and restrictive diet, or have a serious health problem, to be too low in protein.

It's important to get the right balance of amino acids though. If you're a strict vegetarian or vegan, you need to be sure you're getting enough variety in your food to give you plenty of all the essential aminos. Plant foods don't contain as much protein as animal foods, and they usually don't have enough of all the essential amino acids. Corn, for example, is very low in tryptophan and cysteine.

Most people get plenty of high-quality protein in their diets and don't need to worry about getting enough amino acids. You don't need to take amino acid supplements if you're in good health and eat a well-balanced diet.

> **Now You're Cooking**
>
> Vegetarian foods often pack an amino-acid extravaganza. In a 1-cup serving of red beans and rice (a traditional favorite in Latin America), the rice contains only 100 mg of lysine, but the beans are loaded with it—more than 450 mg a day. A 130-pound woman needs 910 mg a day, so one serving puts her halfway to the RDA for lysine.

Sometimes, though, you might want to be sure of having enough of the amino building blocks for a particular protein. For example, you need to have plenty of cysteine, glycine, and glutamic acid to make the antioxidant glutathione. If you need extra glutathione to fend off extra free radicals—because you have an infection, for example—you might need some extra amino building blocks. (Glutathione is so important to your health that we'll talk more about it in Chapter 24.) In that case, check out your

def•i•ni•tion

> Free-form amino acid supplements contain just those particular aminos in their pure form, not as part of a larger protein.

health-food store for *free-form* amino acid supplements. Read the label carefully. If it doesn't say free-form, the aminos you want are probably in there only as part of a protein chain made up of a combination of amino acids, usually in the form of a powder made from whey or soybeans. Your digestive system will have to break down the chain to release the amino acids. Free aminos are already in their simplest form, so they're absorbed into your body right away.

Watch out for amino acid formulas that claim to contain all the essential and nonessential amino acids. Read the labels carefully. Some of these formulas are really just protein powders with some added free amino acids. They're high in calories because they're designed for weight gain and building body mass.

Most people take their amino supplements by swallowing them in convenient capsules. If you'd rather take the powder form, just put a spoonful on your tongue and wash it down with a few swallows of a cold liquid. Aminos don't dissolve, so you'll have trouble stirring them into a drink.

Never add free-form amino acids to hot foods or use them in cooking. The heat changes their structure and makes them ineffective.

Amino Alert!

Some health problems can be made worse by amino acids. If you have kidney disease, you need to be very careful about how much protein you eat. Adding extra amino acids to your diet could cause problems, so be sure to discuss them with your doctor or nutritionist first.

In large doses, lysine can interfere with insulin production, so don't take supplements of this amino acid if you have diabetes or blood-sugar problems. (We'll talk about lysine for treating herpes a little later in this chapter.)

There are some rare genetic conditions that are worsened by amino acids. People with phenylketonuria (PKU), for instance, can't make the enzyme that converts the essential amino acid phenylalanine to the nonessential amino acid tyrosine. These people have to avoid phenylalanine in all forms—including aspartame, the artificial sweetener better known as Nutra-Sweet.

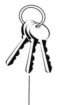

Food for Thought _____

Protein from animal foods such as meat, eggs, and milk is complete—it contains all nine essential amino acids. Protein from plant food is incomplete—one or more of the essential amino acids is present only in small amounts. People who don't eat animal foods can still easily get enough protein by eating a variety of different plant foods, especially beans and whole grains.

Arginine for Immunity

Arginine may be helpful for stimulating your immune system, healing wounds, and slowing the growth of cancer. One reason may be that arginine stimulates your thymus, the small gland in your upper chest that produces an important kind of infection-fighting white blood cell. There's also now evidence that arginine can help some patients with chronic heart failure and angina. It seems to work by helping the clogged arteries that nourish the heart open up more and let more blood through. If you have a heart condition, discuss arginine with your doctor before trying it.

For people with Type 2 diabetes, arginine may be helpful for improving insulin sensitivity. A study in 2001 showed that arginine helped, but the number of participants was small. Also, although they all had Type 2 diabetes, none were overweight. Most people with Type 2 diabetes are overweight, so it's not clear if this will work for them. If you want to try arginine to improve your insulin sensitivity, talk to your doctor first and keep a close eye on your blood sugar.

Arginine, along with methionine and glycine, forms the building blocks of creatine, a protein that is needed for making energy in your muscles and for muscle growth. Based on the logic that if you eat more of the building blocks you'll make more of the protein, some bodybuilders

Quack, Quack

An amino acid compound called arginine pyroglutamate is touted for improving memory problems, especially in older adults. It's also said to stimulate the release of human growth hormone. Does it? We don't know, but we tend to doubt it. Save your money on this one (until there's more evidence).

Quack, Quack

Supplement manufacturers know they can sell bodybuilders _anything_ if they claim it will bulk them up. Take HMB (beta hydroxy beta methylbutyric acid, also known as hydroxymethyl butyrate). There's very little evidence that this expensive supplement, related to the amino acid leucine, helps build muscles.

and athletes take supplements of all three. (We'll talk about creatine in more detail in just a bit.) What about avoiding foods high in arginine, such as nuts, whole grains, and chocolate, if you have herpes? We'll talk more about that a little later when we get to lysine.

Warning!

If you take a monoamine oxidase (MAO) inhibitor drug such as Nardil or Parnate to treat depression or anxiety, be sure to avoid foods and amino acid supplements containing phenylalanine, tryptophan, and especially tyrosine.

Carnitine for Cardiac Cases

Carnitine is an amino acid you make in your body from the essential aminos lysine and methionine. In foods, carnitine is found in meat, especially beef, pork, and lamb. There's virtually none in plant foods, so vegetarians should be sure they're getting enough foods that contain lysine and methionine, the building blocks for carnitine.

Your heart contains more carnitine than any other part of your body. It's there to help the mitochondria (the tiny power plants) in your heart cells produce energy. How? It helps by carrying fatty acids into the mitochondria, where they're converted to energy. Some researchers believe that taking supplemental carnitine may help people with heart problems by making their hearts work more efficiently. Extra carnitine can sometimes be very helpful for people with angina or heart failure. A study in Italy in 1995 suggests that giving carnitine to people who have had a first heart attack could help reduce their risk of heart failure later on. If you have a heart condition, discuss carnitine with your doctor before you try it (and read Chapter 26).

Carnitine may be helpful for people who have peripheral artery disease (PAD), a condition caused by blocked arteries in the legs. This can cause painful leg cramps and make it hard to walk even a short distance. Two good recent studies show that taking supplemental carnitine (2 g a day) significantly improved symptoms in patients with PAD. If you have this disabling disease, talk to your doctor about carnitine supplements before you try them.

More Reasons to Care About Carnitine

Recent research suggests that carnitine may help people with chronic fatigue syndrome (CFS), a mysterious illness that causes extreme tiredness, depression, loss of concentration, muscle pain, and other symptoms. In one study, 28 patients were given 3 g of carnitine a day. All the patients showed clear improvements in their well-being and mental outlook, and only one had any side effects. The researchers think carnitine works by improving energy production. Other studies have looked at carnitine to help the awful fatigue caused by chemotherapy treatment for cancer. Here, too, carnitine has been shown to help with fatigue.

Carnitine in the form of acetyl-L-carnitine (ALC) may be very helpful for relieving the pain of diabetic neuropathy, also known as diabetic nerve pain. This compound is widely used in Europe to relieve diabetic neuropathy and is just starting to be used in the United States. It seems to work best if you start taking at least 500 mg three times a day as soon as the first symptoms of neuropathy appear. ALC is expensive, but then again, diabetic neuropathy is very painful and hard to treat, so it may be worth trying. Talk to your doctor first.

The following paragraph contains material some parents might find unsuitable for children under 14. Carnitine can be helpful for older men with erectile dysfunction and low libido (sex drive). In fact, carnitine can be just as effective as the male hormone testosterone. In a 2004 study of 150 men with an average age of 66, carnitine improved sexual functioning by increasing bloodflow to the penis. It worked as well as testosterone—and it didn't cause the prostate enlargement that often goes along with testosterone treatment. Carnitine supplements may also help improve sperm quality in men with low sperm motility (sperm that don't "swim" well). Some studies show a benefit here; others don't. It's certainly worth a try; in the course of one study, 4 of the 30 infertile men taking carnitine got their wives pregnant.

Some people say carnitine improves athletic performance and endurance, helps Alzheimer's disease, improves memory, and treats depression. At this point, the research for athletes doesn't prove much, although it may help people who do endurance sports such as triathlons. The research on Alzheimer's and depression in the elderly is much more solid. Carnitine, in the form of acetyl-L-carnitine, is often helpful to these people, with no real side effects. We'll discuss this more in Chapter 30.

 Warning!

Some dieters try liquid protein diets as a fast way to lose weight. We strongly recommend against these because of possible heart failure. The FDA agrees and says they shouldn't be used even under your doctor's supervision.

Creatine for Muscles

Among athletes today, the nonessential amino acid creatine is one of the hottest nutritional supplements. It's said to be very effective for bulking up your muscles and helping you gain weight by adding lean body mass, not fat. (Yes, ladies, bodybuilders *want* to weigh more.) And, unlike anabolic steroids and other drugs often used by bodybuilders, creatine is legal and safe when used sensibly.

You make creatine in your liver and kidneys and get it from animal foods such as meat and milk. Creatine supplements may well enhance your ability to train hard and build muscle, mostly by increasing the water content of your muscle cells, which makes them not only bigger but able to work better. The supplements also help your body replenish adenosine triphosphate (ATP), which is where muscle energy comes from. Creatine is useful for athletes who perform short bursts of intense activity, such as weight lifting. It doesn't seem to do much for endurance athletes similar to runners.

Creatine isn't a magic pill. It helps only if you also work out. The usual dose is 20 to 25 g a day for a week or so to get your muscle cells loaded up with as much creatine as they can hold. After that, the maintenance dose is generally 2 to 5 g a day.

The big problem with creatine is that nobody knows whether it's safe to take over a long period. For this reason, some athletes cycle their creatine use, doing 2 weeks on and 1 week off. Also, it can cause water retention, which has led to some cases of kidney failure. Use this stuff cautiously in low doses; big doses are just excreted anyway. Teenaged athletes shouldn't take it at all. To avoid the chance of dehydration, don't take it right before you work out. And don't use creatine at all if you have any sort of kidney problem.

Cysteine for Pollution Protection

In Chapter 9 we talked about an amino acid called homocysteine and how too much of it can damage your heart. You naturally make homocysteine when you use cysteine, but that's no reason to avoid cysteine—this nonessential amino acid is very important to your health. Cysteine is one of the few amino acids to contain sulfur, so you need plenty of it to make glutathione, your body's most abundant natural antioxidant. We'll talk more about glutathione and cysteine in Chapter 24, so for now we'll discuss the role of cysteine in removing toxins from your body.

You're exposed every day to all sorts of toxins in the air you breathe and the foods you eat. All those toxins end up in your liver, where cysteine and glutathione corral them and escort them out of your body. In fact, cysteine is so good at protecting your liver that it's used in emergency rooms to treat overdoses of acetaminophen (Tylenol), which can cause serious liver damage.

A good way to keep your cysteine level high is to eat foods that contain cysteine or methionine, the essential amino acid your body needs to make cysteine. Good choices are eggs, meat, dairy products, and whole grains. If you want to try supplements, we suggest taking N-acetyl-L-cysteine (NAC), which is made naturally from cysteine. For reasons not fully understood, NAC is absorbed better than cysteine supplements.

Glutamine for the Gut

What's the difference between glutamine and glutamic acid? Not much. The two are very closely related, and your body converts them back and forth very easily. These amino acids are used to make many different neurotransmitters. Glutamine is particularly important for your brain and nerves.

Glutamic acid and glutamine are very abundant in foods. Some of the glutamine from your food is absorbed directly into the cells of your small intestine to nourish them, while the rest is absorbed into your bloodstream for use in other parts of your body. Some doctors and nutritionists believe that glutamine supplements may be very helpful for people with intestine problems such as ileitis and Crohn's disease. It's also possible that glutamine can help prevent peripheral neuropathy caused by chemotherapy for cancer, but there's not a lot of solid evidence for this. Talk to your doctor before you try glutamine supplements.

> ### Quack, Quack
>
> Based on one flawed study of mentally retarded people, some researchers claim glutamic acid can raise your IQ. We hope you're smart enough not to fall for this nonsense.

Lysine: Help for Herpes?

Some researchers believe that the balance of arginine and lysine in your body plays a role in treating the painful genital blisters and cold sores caused by the herpes virus. *Herpes* is the name of a group of viruses. Herpes simplex type 1 (HSV-1) is the virus that causes cold sores. Herpes simplex type 2 (HSV-2) is the virus that causes genital herpes. Herpes zoster is a related virus that causes chicken pox and shingles.

The thinking is that the virus feeds on arginine and is blocked by lysine. There really isn't a lot of solid evidence one way or the other for this, but many people with herpes swear that lysine works to stop an outbreak. Because not much else helps, it's certainly

Warning! _____

There is some evidence that lysine in large doses can slow growth. Do not give lysine supplements to children!

worth trying. Arginine-rich foods to avoid include chocolate, nuts, seeds, beer, coconut, grains such as oats, whole wheat, peanuts, soybeans and soy products, and wheat germ. Lysine-rich foods to load up on include fish, lean meats, chicken, soy products, milk, and cheese. You can also buy lysine supplements. Many patients say that taking 2,000 to 3,000 mg of lysine at the first sign of an attack helps ward it off or keep it from being as bad. Lysine is also suggested as a treatment for the pain of shingles and for post-herpetic neuralgia, a condition where the nerve pain from shingles lingers on even though the infection has cleared up.

Methionine and Taurine

Methionine and taurine, along with cysteine, are sulfur-containing amino acids. Methionine is an essential amino acid you have to get from animal foods such as eggs, fish, milk, and meat in your diet. Taurine is an amino acid that some researchers now believe should be listed in the nonessential category.

You make cysteine in your body only from methionine. You make taurine from methionine and cysteine and also get it from animal foods. Methionine may play a role in keeping your cholesterol down, but there's not enough evidence to make taking supplements worthwhile. Some researchers believe that taurine can help heart problems such as heart failure and arrhythmias. We're starting to realize that taurine is more important than we thought, but it's still too soon to recommend supplements—especially because they may have a depressing effect on your nervous system.

Recently a form of methionine known as SAMe (S-adenosylmethionine) has become very popular as a natural and very safe treatment for depression. There's some reasonably good scientific evidence to back this up. SAMe seems to work best if you take 400 mg three or four times a day and are sure to get enough of all the B vitamins every day. If you have bipolar disorder (manic depression), take SAMe only if your doctor recommends it.

Now You're Cooking

SAMe supplements are expensive—so expensive that some manufacturers are tempted to cheat by not including the amount claimed on the label. Be sure to buy this supplement only from a reputable manufacturer.

SAMe can be helpful for depression, but it's even more effective for treating arthritis pain. We'll talk more about this supplement in Chapter 29.

Tryptophan for Natural Sleep

You need the essential amino acid tryptophan to make serotonin and melatonin, both important body chemicals that help control your mood and sleep patterns. (We'll talk more about melatonin in Chapter 27.) *Serotonin* is a neurotransmitter—a substance you make to carry nerve impulses across the tiny gaps between nerves. Your body makes neurotransmitters from amino acids almost instantly, just when they're needed, and then breaks them down again very quickly to reuse the building blocks.

def•i•ni•tion

Serotonin carries impulses in the parts of your brain that control your mood and emotions. If you have plenty of serotonin to carry the impulses, you feel calm and confident. If you're short on serotonin, you might feel depressed, tense, angry, or anxious. You might also crave sugary carbohydrates and overeat. Too much serotonin, however, can be harmful to your heart—that's why some prescription drugs, such as phenfluramine (Redux), that raise your serotonin level were recalled by the FDA.

If you don't have enough tryptophan, you won't be able to make enough serotonin and melatonin, and you may start to feel depressed and have trouble sleeping. If you've been traveling through time zones, your melatonin levels may be off from jet lag, and tryptophan could help get them back in sync again.

If you want to get more tryptophan as a way to help insomnia, one simple way is to eat it. Good sources of tryptophan include turkey, peanuts, avocados, oranges, bananas, cottage cheese, fish, lean meat, and milk. A lot of unsweetened breakfast cereals, such as bran flakes, are also high in tryptophan. If you've been having insomnia, try having a snack of one of these foods—a turkey sandwich or a bowl of shredded wheat with milk—an hour before bedtime. It works surprisingly well for a lot of people.

In 1989, a contaminated batch of tryptophan supplements caused more than 1,500 cases of serious illness and 27 deaths. In 1990, the FDA banned pure tryptophan

Food for Thought

The migraine drug sumatriptan (Imitrex) works by mimicking serotonin, a neurotransmitter your body makes from tryptophan. The drug makes the small blood vessels in your brain contract, which relieves migraine pain. Sumatriptan pills work for about 60 percent of the people who take them; the injected form works 80 percent of the time. If you suffer from migraines, talk to your doctor about a prescription for sumatriptan.

supplements. In the late 1990s, a different form of tryptophan called 5-HTP (5-hydroxy-tryptophan), made by an entirely different process, became available. 5-HTP works as well as plain old tryptophan as a sleep aid, but the dose needed is smaller—usually 300 to 400 mg.

Phenylalanine, Tyrosine, and Migraines

Two amino acids, phenylalanine and tyrosine, are said to help depression, mostly because both are important for making the brain chemicals epinephrine, norepinephrine, and dopamine. In theory, if you're low on phenylalanine, you can't make tyrosine; and if you're low on either of these amino acids, you can't make enough of the brain chemicals. The upshot could be that you get depressed. The evidence for this chain of events is on the thin side, so we can't say for sure that taking supplements of these aminos will help.

There are some good reasons not to take them. Large doses of either amino or both together could raise your blood pressure. Don't use these supplements if you have high blood pressure. If you take an MAO-inhibiting drug such as Nardil or Marplan for depression, don't take these aminos—they could raise your blood pressure dangerously high. In fact, you should avoid foods high in phenylalanine and tyrosine, such as nuts, seeds, cheese, lima beans, avocados, bananas, and nonfat dried milk.

Both phenylalanine and tyrosine form tyramine, a substance that can trigger migraine headaches. If you get migraines, you should probably avoid supplements of these two amino acids and foods that are naturally high in tyramine. We list the worst offenders in the chart, but in general alcohol; many fruits; and all aged, dried, pickled, preserved, fermented, cured, or cultured foods are out.

Foods High in Tyramine	
Aged cheeses	Organ meats
Anchovies	Pickled herring
Avocados	Pineapple
Bananas	Prunes
Beans	Raisins
Beer	Raspberries
Chocolate	Sauerkraut
Nuts, including peanuts	Seeds such as sesame seeds or pumpkin seeds

Foods High in Tyramine	
Wine	Soy sauce
Sherry	Yogurt
Sour cream	

More than 23 million Americans get migraines, but studies show that only about 5 percent are prescribed drugs that can help prevent these awful headaches. There's been major progress in headache treatment in the last few years—if you're suffering, talk to your doctor.

The Least You Need to Know

◆ Amino acids are the building blocks of protein.

◆ Most people get all the amino acids they need from the protein in their food. Protein deficiency is very rare.

◆ You need all 22 amino acids to make the 50,000-plus proteins you need for life.

◆ Amino acids make the many enzymes, hormones, neurotransmitters, and other chemical messengers that regulate your body.

◆ Some individual amino acids can help health problems, including heart disease, insomnia, and herpes.

Essential Fatty Acids: When Is Fat Good?

In This Chapter

- What the essential fatty acids are and why you need them
- What foods are high in essential fatty acids
- How essential fatty acids can help your heart
- How essential fatty acids can help prevent cancer
- How you can help other health problems with essential fatty acids

Here's what we're *not* going to do in this chapter: we're not going to tell you how bad red meat is for you. We're not going to warn you about the dangers of high cholesterol. We're not even going to lecture you about going on a low-fat diet. If you ever read a newspaper, open a magazine, or watch television, you don't need us—you know already.

We're going to talk about the good fats—the ones you have to have for good health. Really, it's true: there are some fats you simply can't live without. Not only that, these same fats could help you live longer and better by keeping your heart healthy and possibly preventing cancer. All that, just from swapping that steak or burger for some shrimp or fish a few times a week. And after you feel the benefits of doing that, maybe you'll start thinking about that low-fat diet.

What's So Essential About Fat?

All that anti-fat information out there could make you think that all fat, no matter what, is just plain bad for you. As always, the truth is a lot more complicated. Bear with us as we explain a little about fats in general.

You definitely do need some fat in your diet and in your body. The fat you eat is a source of quick energy. And you have to have some fat in your diet to absorb and use Vitamins A, D, E, and K. You need fat to make your cell walls and many important hormones, enzymes, neurotransmitters, and other chemical messengers in your body. And you need some stored fat in your body to keep you warm and to cushion your organs.

Good Fat vs. Bad Fat

You need some fat for good health, but there are different kinds of fats. Which ones are best? The answer gets a little complicated, so hang in there as we get into some definitions. (If you don't want to read all of this, just skip down to the last line of this section.)

- **Fat.** A fat is an organic substance made from molecules of hydrogen, carbon, and a little oxygen. Fat doesn't dissolve in water.

- **Triglycerides.** Almost all the fat in our foods comes from triglycerides. These are fats made from a backbone of glycerol (carbon atoms linked together) and three (that's where the *tri-* comes from) fatty acids. Your body stores fat in the form of triglycerides.

- **Fatty acids.** A fatty acid molecule is made from a chain of carbon atoms bound to hydrogen atoms. At the tail end of the chain is a carbon atom attached to two oxygen atoms—that's what makes the fat an acid. There are different kinds of fatty acids (and we'll talk about them later in this chapter), but for now you need to remember that the chains of carbon and hydrogen atoms vary in length. They're usually from 12 to 24 carbon atoms long.

- **Saturated fats.** If every carbon atom in the fatty acid is matched up with a hydrogen atom, the fat is saturated—it can't hold any more hydrogen. Saturated fats are bad fats, because they've been shown to raise your cholesterol. They're usually solid at room temperature, such as butter and lard, and come from animals—meat, poultry, and whole-milk dairy foods. Some vegetable oils, such as palm oil and coconut oil, are also saturated.

◆ **Monounsaturated fats.** In monounsaturated fats, there's a missing hydrogen atom. An extra carbon atom takes its place. Monounsaturated fats are good fats, because they can help lower your cholesterol. Good examples of monounsaturated fats include olive oil, canola oil, and peanut oil.

◆ **Polyunsaturated fats.** These fat molecules have several missing hydrogen atoms, so they have several extra carbon atoms in their place. Polyunsaturated fats are also good for you, because they can help prevent heart disease. Good examples are corn oil, safflower seed oil, sunflower seed oil, and fish oil.

◆ **Tran fatty acid.** If you force an extra hydrogen atom into an unsaturated fat such as corn oil, it changes from a liquid to a soft solid—such as margarine, for example. The process is called hydrogenation, as in partially hydrogenated vegetable oil, a major ingredient in a lot of worthless processed foods such as cookies and potato chips. Tran fatty acids, or trans fats for short, aren't good for you at all. In fact, they're so bad that starting in 2007 the FDA will require food processors to list the trans fat content of their products on the label. Trans fats have been shown to be a major contributor to clogged arteries and high cholesterol.

Here's what it all comes down to: mono and poly fats—good; saturated fats—bad; trans fats—really bad.

The Good Fats

Let's get back to those fatty acids. You have 20 different fatty acids in your body, but they're all made from just two: *linoleic acid* and *linolenic acid*. These two fatty acids are *essential.* You must get them from your food because your body can't make them. (Some experts feel only linoleic acid is essential, because you can make some linolenic acid from it.) Similar to essential amino acids for proteins, essential fatty acids are the building blocks for all the other fats in your body

def•i•ni•tion

Linoleic acid is a fatty acid found in many plants and also in fish. **Linolenic acid** is a fatty acid found in many seeds, including corn. Both linoleic and linolenic acids are **essential**—you can't make them in your body, so you have to get them from your food. Many foods, such as vegetable oils of various sorts, contain both kinds of fatty acids.

(although you also get the other fats from foods). Essential fatty acids are also the building blocks for your cell membranes and for many of the important hormones and other chemical messengers that tell your body what to do.

Omega-3 and Omega-6

Researchers divide the fatty acids into four separate groups, depending on where their double carbon bonds fall relative to the acid tail of the chain. The tail end is called the omega end (from the last letter of the Greek alphabet). If we start counting from the omega end of linoleic acid, the first double carbon bond we come to is at the sixth carbon atom. So another name for linoleic acid is *omega-6;* the fatty acids made from linoleic acid are in the omega-6 family. The double carbon bond for linolenic acid comes at the third atom, so linolenic acid is also called *omega-3,* and the fatty acids made from it are in the omega-3 family. Sometimes the letter *n* is substituted for omega. An n-3 fatty acid is the same as an omega-3; ditto for n-6 and omega-6. In this book, we follow the style used in major medical journals and use the omega system.

Omega-3 and omega-6 essential fatty acids are especially important for making prostaglandins in your body. Prostaglandins are hormonelike substances made from fatty acids. They regulate many activities in your body, including inflammation, pain, and swelling. They also play a role in controlling your blood pressure, your heart, your kidneys, and your digestive system. Prostaglandins are important for allergic reactions, blood clotting, and making other hormones.

Prostaglandins are a double-edged sword: some cause swelling and others relieve it. You use omega-3 fatty acids to make some kinds of prostaglandins and omega-6 fatty acids to make others. By changing the amounts of omega-6 and omega-3 fatty acids in your body, you may be able to change your prostaglandin levels.

Why You Need Omega-6

Omega-6 fatty acids (linoleic acid) are the most common polyunsaturated fatty acids in food. The omega-6 family actually has three members: *gamma-linoleic acid (GLA)*, *arachidonic acid (AA)*, and *dihomo-linoleic acid.* Of the three, GLA is probably the most useful for helping health problems. Arachidonic acid, on the other hand, is needed to make some prostaglandins that cause unpleasant symptoms, such as swelling.

Omega-6 fatty acids are found in all foods that have polyunsaturated fats in them. Especially good sources are cooking oils such as corn oil, safflower oil, sunflower oil, and soybean oil. Nuts and seeds, such as walnuts, peanuts, almonds, and sunflower seeds, are also good sources. The tiny seeds of the borage, black currant, and evening primrose plants are very rich sources of omega-6 fatty acids in the form of GLA, so they're often used to make supplements.

Why You Need Omega-3

Omega-3 fatty acids (linolenic acid) are found in the leaves and seeds of many plants, in egg yolks, and in cold-water ocean fish. The omega-3 family has three related members: *alpha linolenic acid* (*LNA*), *eicosapente-noic acid* (*EPA*), and *docosahexanoic acid* (*DHA*). LNA is found in plant foods, especially nuts, soybeans, canola oil, and flaxseed oil. EPA and DHA are found in fish oil.

Fish oil has been shown to have a lot of very good effects on your health. It can lower your triglyceride and cholesterol levels, reduce your high blood pressure, prevent blood clots, and help prevent sudden death from heart rhythm problems. It may even prevent cancer. In fact, fish oil is so helpful for some medical problems that we'll discuss it separately later in this chapter.

> **Now You're Cooking**
>
> According to studies from the Harvard Medical School, eating nuts frequently—more than 5 ounces a week—could reduce your chances of having a heart attack or dying from one by more than 30 percent. The reason may well be the linolenic acid in the nuts. To give you an idea of how many nuts you need to eat, those little airline nut packets contain only 1 ounce.

Getting the Most from Omega-3s

Omega-3s in the form of EPA and DHA are found in all fish and seafood—the oilier the fish, the more it has. As you can see from the chart, cold-water fish such as salmon, bluefish, herring, and tuna are excellent sources. So are cod, flounder, mackerel, and shrimp. Canola oil, soybean oil, and walnut oil are also good sources of omega-3 fatty acids. Another good way to get omega-3s is by taking flaxseed oil. Your body converts the LNA in the oil into EPA and DHA.

Fish Oil Supplements

If you don't like to eat fish or want to get larger amounts of fish oil than you can get from eating fish, you can try fish oil supplements. In large amounts, fish oil capsules can give you gas, diarrhea, and heartburn. If you take a lot of them, you get fish breath and a fishy body odor. (You'll be very popular with the neighborhood cats, but not with anybody else!) You can avoid the fish-breath problem by taking slow-release capsules, but these are more expensive.

Read the label carefully when you buy fish oil supplements. The amounts of EPA and DHA are less than the size of the supplement. For example, a 1,000-mg capsule might have only 180 mg of EPA and 120 mg of DHA, or 300 mg of combined omega-3s. To get 1 g of EPA/DHA, you'd have to take four capsules. Store your fish oil capsules in a cool, dark place—the refrigerator is ideal. Spread out your dose over the day.

The Omega-3s in Fish

Fish	Omega-3 in g
Bass	0.6
Bluefish	1.2
Catfish	0.6
Crab, Alaskan king	0.6
Flounder	0.3
Herring	1.1 to 1.7
Mackerel	2.2 to 2.6
Mullet	1.1
Salmon, canned Chinook	3.0
Salmon, pink	1.0 to 1.9
Salmon, sockeye	1.3
Sardines	2.9
Shrimp	0.3 to 0.4
Swordfish	0.2
Trout	1.1 to 2.0
Tuna, canned	1.5 to 1.7

Note: Amounts are for 3.5-ounce (100 g) servings.

If you're a vegetarian or don't like the side effects of fish oil, you can get your omega-3s from flaxseed oil (also sometimes called linseed oil). Enzymes in your body convert the linolenic acid in the flaxseed oil into EPA and DHA—the fatty acids that are best for your heart.

The Omega-3s in Vegetable Oils

Oil	Omega-3 in mg
Canola	111
Flaxseed	533
Soybean	68
Walnut	104
Wheat-germ	69

Note: Amounts are for 1 g (1,000 mg).

Fat Becomes Official

In 2002, the Institute of Medicine set DRIs for linoleic and linolenic acids for the first time. The Recommended Intakes are in the chart below.

The Recommended Intake for Linoleic Acid and Linolenic Acid

Age in Years/Sex	Linoleic in g	Linolenic in g
Infants		
0 to 0.5	4.4	0.5
0.5 to 1	4.6	0.5
Children		
1 to 3	7.0	0.7
4 to 8	10.0	0.9
Boys 9 to 13	12.0	1.2
Girls 9 to 13	10.0	1.0
Young Adults and Adults		
Men 14 to 18	16.0	1.6
Men 19 to 50	17.0	1.6
Men 51+	14.0	1.6
Women 14 to 18	11.0	1.1
Women 19 to 50	12.0	1.1

continues

The Recommended Intake for Linoleic Acid and Linolenic Acid   (continued)

Age in Years/Sex	Linoleic in g	Linolenic in g
Women 51+	11.0	1.1
Pregnant women	13.0	1.4
Nursing women	13.0	1.3

True deficiencies of essential fatty acids are quite rare. Even so, some nutritionists believe that today we eat so many saturated and trans fats that many of us don't get enough essential fatty acids for optimal health. The essential fatty acids we do eat tend to be unbalanced. We eat too many omega-6s, mostly from the corn and sunflower-seed oils used in many processed foods, and not enough omega-3s. This imbalance, some researchers believe, causes many health problems by getting your prostaglandins and other body chemicals out of whack. Our recommendation? Avoid trans fats, cut back on omega-6 foods, and try to get at least 1,000 mg (1 g) of omega-3s every day. Checking the chart, you can see you can easily get that much from just one small serving of canned tuna, sardines, or salmon.

Omega-3 Helps Your Heart

In the 1930s, Danish researchers studied the Eskimos of Greenland. They found that the Eskimos ate very large amounts of fatty fish and seal meat (seals eat nothing but fish), yet they almost never got heart disease. The researchers decided that the omega-3 fatty acids EPA and DHA kept the Eskimos' hearts healthy. Can they do the same for you?

Several long-term studies have shown that men who eat fish several times a week have less heart disease than men who don't eat fish regularly. The most convincing is the DART (Diet and Reinfarction Trial) study of 1989, which looked at men who had already had heart attacks. The men who were told to eat lots of fish had 29 percent fewer second heart attacks than those who continued with their preheart-attack diets. Some other studies, though, haven't really shown any differences in the overall heart disease rate. In 1995, for example, the ongoing Physicians' Health Study showed that there was no association between the amount of fish oil the men in the study ate and their chances of having a heart attack. But in 2002, the female counterpart to the Physicians' Health Study, the Nurses' Health Study, found that the women who ate fish 5 times a week had a 45 percent lower risk of dying from heart disease than the women who only rarely ate fish. Other studies over the years have shown that overall, the people with the most omega 3s in their diet from any source have the lowest risk of death from heart attacks.

When it comes to another heart problem, the benefits of fish oil are clearer. We're pretty sure that fish oil supplements can help prevent sudden death from heart-rhythm problems (arrhythmias). In one important study, there were eight sudden deaths in the control group that didn't take fish oil supplements and none in the group that did—even though the fish oil group didn't lose any weight or improve their cholesterol levels. Later studies have shown that if you already have a heart rhythm problem, fish oil doesn't seem to help. But every year some 250,000 Americans die suddenly from heart rhythm disturbances—and only about half of them had any earlier symptoms of heart disease.

Fish oil supplements may also reduce heart attacks by preventing blood clots from blocking the arteries leading to your heart. The fish oil makes your platelets—the tiny cells in your blood that form blood clots—less "sticky," so they're less likely to lump together and form a clot. "Thinner" blood also helps prevent strokes.

If you take fish oil on a regular basis, you may thin your blood to the point where it takes you a just a little bit longer to stop bleeding. This sounds scary, but actually fish oil doesn't thin your blood any more than a daily low-dose aspirin tablet does—and today most doctors recommend aspirin for all older patients, even if they don't have heart problems. On the other hand, if you have any sort of bleeding problem or are taking a blood-thinning drug such as coumadin or warfarin, skip the fish oil supplements. If you want to try fish oil supplements for your heart, discuss them with your doctor first.

Stopping Strokes

The more fish and foods high in omega-3 fatty acids you eat, the less likely you are to have a stroke. In 2002, results from those nice women of the Nurses' Health Study showed that women who eat fish 5 or more times a week cut their risk of stroke by a bit more than 50 percent compared to women who eat fish less than once a month. Eating fish just once a week cuts the risk by 22 percent. Very similar results were found in 2002 among the nice guys of the Physicians' Health Study. The benefit is most notable for preventing ischemic strokes, the kind where a blood clot blocks an artery in the brain.

Fish Oil and Fat Levels

Taking fish oil or flaxseed supplements can lower your triglyceride level if it's too high. One drawback is that the supplements might lower your overall triglycerides, but raise your LDL ("bad") cholesterol. There's a way around this problem. Combining fish oil or flaxseed oil with garlic supplements seems to lower your triglycerides *and* lower your LDL cholesterol. You need a lot of both for the treatment to work: about 5 to 15 g of fish or flaxseed oil and 1 g of garlic (we'll talk more about garlic in Chapter 25). If you want to take big doses of fish or flaxseed oil, talk to your doctor first.

Food for Thought _____

Eating fish is good for you, but if you eat fish often, you need to be aware of the mercury that's in it. Nearly all shellfish and fish contain traces of mercury. The highest levels are swordfish, shark, king mackerel, and tilefish. Shrimp, canned light and albacore tuna, salmon, pollock, and catfish have the least mercury and are safe to eat twice a week.

A lot of studies show that fish or flaxseed oil lowers your cholesterol level. It does, but *only* if you also lower the amount of saturated fat you eat. If you take the capsules but continue with a high-fat diet, your cholesterol won't go down. In fact, it might even raise your LDL level, which you definitely don't want.

Some researchers believe that the GLA in evening primrose oil can reduce your LDL cholesterol. You need to take a fair amount—up to 3 g a day.

Helping High Blood Pressure

Fish and flaxseed oil can lower your blood pressure, but not by much and only if it's pretty high to begin with. The effect isn't really worth the trouble. There are better, natural ways to lower your blood pressure (check back to Chapter 17 on calcium and Chapter 18 on magnesium for more information).

Warning! _____

Don't take fish oil supplements if you have a clotting disorder or take blood-thinning drugs such as warfarin!

Fish Oil and Diabetes

People with diabetes used to be told to avoid fish oil supplements, because they were thought to raise blood sugar. In fact, this isn't the case—the supplements will probably have no effect on your blood sugar, but they may lower your blood pressure and triglycerides. If you want to try fish oil, talk to your doctor first.

GLA, an omega-6 fatty acid, is sometimes helpful for nerve damage caused by diabetes (diabetic neuropathy). The doses needed are low—less than 500 mg a day. Talk to your doctor before you try this—and also read about lipoic acid in Chapter 24.

Calming Crohn's Disease

Fish oil supplements can be very helpful for keeping Crohn's disease, a chronic inflammation of the colon, under control. In one study, patients who took fish oil supplements were able to keep their symptoms from coming back much longer than patients who didn't. They did just as well on the fish oil as patients who were taking a powerful drug, and they didn't have the drug's side effects. The patients in the study took a slow-release form of fish oil capsules that kept them from getting unpleasant side effects such as gas and fishy breath.

Helping Rheumatoid Arthritis

Rheumatoid arthritis is a serious and very painful disease that causes inflammation and stiffness of the joints. It's not the same as the ordinary sort of wear-and-tear arthritis some of us get. Some of the pain and swelling of rheumatoid arthritis comes from "bad" prostaglandins that are made from arachidonic acid—which is an omega-6 fatty acid. For some patients, omega-3 oils seem to help counteract the "bad" prostaglandins and relieve the symptoms. The doses needed are fairly high, in the range of 3 grams of fish oil or flaxseed oil a day. Because rheumatoid arthritis is usually treated with powerful anti-inflammatory drugs that can have nasty side effects, omega-3 oils are certainly worth a try. Be sure to discuss them with your doctor before you try them.

Fish Oil Fights Cancer

Fish oil may play a role in preventing cancer and slowing tumor growth. In a 1999 study in Italy, the people who ate the most fish had the lowest rates of colorectal cancer and other cancers of the digestive tract. The amount of fish needed to lower the risk of these cancers by up to 50 percent? Just two servings a week.

Flaxseed oil may help prevent breast cancer, especially in older women past menopause.

Food for Thought

You get more than just fish oil from eating fish. Here's what else you get from one 3.5-ounce can of sardines: 382 mg calcium (1 cup of milk has 297 mg); 8.9 mcg cobalamin (3.5 ounces of beef has 2 mcg); 297 IU Vitamin D (1 cup of milk has 100 IU); .23 mg riboflavin (equal to ½ cup of spinach).

They seem to work by keeping estrogen, the female hormone, from helping the cancer get started and grow. (This is such an important area of research that we'll discuss it separately in Chapter 27.) Some recent studies suggest that omega-3 fatty acids from fish or flaxseed can help prevent prostate cancer or slow it down if it does occur.

Brain Food

That old saw about fish being brain food may have some real truth to it. There's mounting evidence that the omega-3 fatty acids found in fish oil—and also flaxseed oil and in nuts—can help fight depression and ward off Alzheimer's disease.

The link between low levels of DHA and EPA and depression has been extensively studied. A 2001 study in Finland found that the less fish people ate, the more likely they were to have depressive symptoms. A study in 2003 of elderly people in Holland found that those who were depressed had much lower levels of omega-3 fatty acids in their blood than those who weren't. Later studies have borne this out. This is a promising area for treating depression safely without powerful drugs—stay tuned.

> **Now You're Cooking**
>
> To get the most from the omega-3 oils in fish, steam, bake, or broil it, but don't fry it. The high temperature needed for frying destroys the oils. For fish-haters and vegetarians, flaxseed oil is a good way to get your omega-3s. Try using it in salad dressings, but don't cook with it—heat destroys the omega-3s. Store flaxseed oil in the refrigerator.

Omega-3s may help keep your brain functioning well as you age. A 2003 study of older residents of Chicago, funded by the National Institutes of Health, found that those aged 65 or older who ate fish once a week had a 60 percent lower risk of Alzheimer's disease than those who ate fish only rarely or never. Here's another area where the research is both promising and ongoing.

GLA: The Promise of Evening Primrose Oil

The GLA in evening primrose oil may be helpful for relieving PMS symptoms, especially breast tenderness and swelling. It seems to work best if you take 500 to 1,000 mg every day (not just in the days before your period), along with 50 mg of pyridoxine. (For more on how pyridoxine helps PMS, check back to Chapter 8.)

Many people claim that taking GLA supplements helps their skin, hair, and nails look better. Supplements seem to work best if you have dry skin or hair—it probably won't do much for you if your skin or hair are normal or oily. Brittle nails seem to improve if you take GLA supplements. GLA also often helps people with mild eczema.

Other Good Fats

Omega-6s and omega-3s aren't the only good fats. There's also the omega-9 or oleic acid group, for example. Oleic acid is found in olive oil, peanut oil, avocados, and nuts. These monounsaturated fats seem to play a role in keeping your heart healthy, keeping your blood pressure normal, and preventing cancer. We don't have space here to go into the many advantages of the Mediterranean diet (lots of olive oil, grains, fresh fruits and vegetables, and fish), but we urge you to look into it.

Fat to Lose Fat?

Conjugated linoleic acid (CLA) is just one of the latest in a long line of supplements that are supposed to magically help you lose weight. If you're a gym rat, you've probably heard that CLA can help you lose body fat and bulk up on muscle. The problem is that the studies that suggest this might be possible have only been done on lab rats. There's very little evidence for humans. Likewise, there's very little to show that CLA helps lower cholesterol, treat arthritis, or fight cancer. Stay away from this one.

The Least You Need to Know

- You need essential fatty acids to make your cell membranes.

- Essential fatty acids are also needed to make many body chemicals, including hormones and prostaglandins.

- Good sources of essential fatty acids in food oils are flaxseed oil, canola oil, soybean oil, walnut oil, corn oil, safflower oil, and wheat-germ oil.

- Fish, especially cold-water fish such as salmon, tuna, and sardines, and flaxseed are good food sources of omega-3 essential fatty acids.

- Fish oil or flaxseed supplements can help prevent heart attacks and strokes, lower cholesterol, and treat some intestinal problems.

- A diet high in omega-3 fatty acids from fish and other foods can help prevent Alzheimer's disease and treat depression.

Chapter 24

Super Antioxidants

In This Chapter

- ◆ Why you need glutathione
- ◆ Which foods are high in glutathione
- ◆ The antioxidant powers of cysteine and selenium
- ◆ What lipoic acid can do for you

Antioxidants, antioxidants, antioxidants. By now you've gotten the message: you need plenty of antioxidants to corral those damaging free radicals before they can wreck your body. The best antioxidant of all is the one you make naturally in your body: an amazing substance called glutathione. This super antioxidant is everywhere in your body.

But glutathione does more than just mop up free radicals similar to a very thirsty sponge. It also rounds up all sorts of dangerous toxic wastes in your body and whisks them quickly away, before they can do any harm. The best news of all about glutathione? You can easily get more of it into your system just through the foods you eat.

The Crucial Role of Glutathione

Every second of every day, your body makes damaging free radicals. And every second of every day, your body makes a powerful substance called *glutathione* (abbreviated *GSH*) that grabs hold of those free radicals and smothers them. Glutathione also picks up any toxic substances (from air pollution, say) that have found their way into your body and escorts them out.

What is this amazing stuff? Glutathione is a tripeptide—a small protein made from just three amino acids. Molecules of cysteine, glycine, and glutamic acid combine in your cells to make glutathione. Of the three aminos needed to make glutathione, cysteine is the most important, because cysteine contains sulfur, which is also needed to make glutathione. You also need the trace mineral selenium to make glutathione. Your body generally has plenty of glycine and glutamic acid (or its close cousin glutamine), but sometimes the cysteine and selenium are in short supply. When that happens, you could end up without enough glutathione to defend your body.

def•i•ni•tion

Glutathione (GSH) is your body's most abundant and most important natural antioxidant. It's an enzyme found inside and outside of every cell in your body.

Are You Deficient?

Your glutathione level naturally drops as you get older. That's bad, because this lowers your defenses against free radicals and toxins and leaves you open to disease. The higher your glutathione level, the less likely you are to get heart disease, diabetes, high blood pressure, and a whole range of other problems. Glutathione protects your eyes against free radicals and helps prevent cataracts and other blinding eye conditions. Most important of all, glutathione boosts your immune system and helps it work at top efficiency—and that keeps you healthy no matter what your age.

You might be low on glutathione for a lot of reasons aside from just getting older. We could write a whole book about why (in fact, we did—it's called *Glutathione: The Ultimate Antioxidant*), but for now, let's just give a few good reasons:

◆ **You're sick with a bad cold or flu or have an injury of some sort.** You're making a lot of extra free radicals that need to be squelched, and your immune system needs glutathione to make white blood cells, so you're using up glutathione faster than you can make it.

◆ **You're exposed to a lot of toxins.** Glutathione finds toxic wastes in your body and carts them off. If you're exposed to a lot of toxins every day—air pollution, exhaust fumes, or dry-cleaning chemicals, for example—your glutathione is very, very busy. You're using so much of it to eliminate toxins that there's not a lot left to fight free radicals.

◆ **You have a chronic disease such as asthma or rheumatoid arthritis.** You need extra glutathione to boost your immune system and fend off the extra free radicals your disease creates—and a shortage of glutathione makes your symptoms worse by letting free radicals attack. This gets very circular. It's even possible that a shortage of glutathione is why you're sick to begin with.

◆ **You're an alcoholic.** Chronic alcohol abuse sharply lowers the amount of glutathione in your lungs and leaves them vulnerable to damage from illness.

You can easily see why it's so important to be sure you have enough glutathione in your system.

Glutathione and Your Health

There's a lot of very interesting research going on about glutathione. We'll just hit some of the highlights. A 2006 study of nearly 2,000 men and women found that those who ate a lot of fruits and vegetables that are high in glutathione (avocados and grapefruit, for instance) reduced their risk of oral and throat cancer. Research in 2005 showed that autistic children have much lower levels of glutathione in their blood. Exactly what that means and why their levels are low isn't understood, but it's a promising clue in this very puzzling disease.

Finally, there's also now some evidence that glutathione may help people with the genetic lung disease cystic fibrosis (CF). People with CF get a thick mucus buildup in their lungs that makes it hard to breathe and makes them vulnerable to infection. Ordinarily, you have a lot of glutathione in your lungs, because your lungs, especially in the tiny airways, need the antioxidant protection. People with CF have far less glutathione in their lung secretions than normal—and this lack may play a role in the chronic inflammation and infection they get. It's possible that inhaling glutathione could help. It's safe and seems to show a benefit, but the medical jury is still out.

Boosting Your Glutathione Level

It's easy to raise your glutathione level—some glutathione is found in almost all fruits and vegetables. We've listed some of the best sources in the chart. Cooking destroys a lot of the glutathione, so eat these foods raw or just lightly steamed.

Some vegetables contain substances that naturally make your body make more gluta-thione. The best choices here are broccoli, cabbage, Brussels sprouts, cauliflower, kale, and parsley. Recent research shows that fish oil also makes you produce more glutathi-one (see Chapter 23 for more information about fish oil).

Foods High in Glutathione

Food	Glutathione in mg
Acorn squash	14
Asparagus	26
Avocado	31
Broccoli	8
Cantaloupe	9
Grapefruit	15
Okra	7
Orange	11
Peach	7
Potato	13
Spinach	5
Strawberries	12
Tomato	11
Watermelon	28
Zucchini	7

Note: Amounts are for 3.5-ounce (100 g) servings.

Now You're Cooking

Eggs are a good way to boost your glutathione level. One egg has 146 mg of cysteine and 196 mg of methionine. Both of these amino acids contain sulfur, which your body needs to make glutathione.

You can also take glutathione supplements. This doesn't always work well for everyone. Remember, glutathione is a tripeptide, a small protein made from three amino acids. Some of the glutathione you swallow in a supplement gets broken down into its amino acids by your digestive juices, and some gets absorbed straight into your body through your small intestine. If you're low on glutathione to begin with, you'll probably absorb a lot. For maximum protection against free radicals and toxins, we suggest getting at least 100 mg a day of glutathione. This could be hard to get from your food alone, so you might want to take supplements. Glutathione supplements are extremely safe—even taking several grams at a time is harmless. Take your glutathione supplements with meals to absorb the most from them.

Supplements to Boost Glutathione

If you don't want to take glutathione supplements, you can eat foods high in cysteine or take cysteine supplements instead. You have to have plenty of cysteine to make glutathione, because cysteine has that all-important sulfur molecule in it. By taking supplements, you make sure you've got enough. We recommend cysteine supplements in the form of *N-acetyl cysteine* (*NAC*). This form is easily absorbed by your body.

Most people have plenty of the other two aminos—glycine and glutamic acid—needed to make glutathione. Even so, taking extra glutamine (your body converts glutamine to glutamic acid very easily) helps raise your glutathione level. This seems to work not because you're short on the glutamine building block, but because glutamine stimulates your liver to make more glutathione. Glutamine is found in almost all foods. The best sources are lean meats, eggs, wheat germ, and whole grains.

def•i•ni•tion

N-acetyl cysteine (NAC) is a form of the amino acid cysteine. Your body can easily absorb NAC from supplements. NAC supplements can do more than just boost your glutathione level. Raising the level of cysteine in your blood seems to stimulate your immune system and make you produce more infection-fighting T4 white blood cells.

If you want to take extra glutamine, we recommend the less-expensive powder form over tablets. The powder is tasteless and odorless and dissolves easily in water. Drink it down or sprinkle it on cold foods such as your breakfast cereal. Don't mix it with acidic liquids such as orange juice or put it on something hot—you'll destroy the glutamine.

The usual dose for extra glutamine is anywhere from 1,000 mg to 5,000 mg.

Riboflavin (Vitamin B_2) helps your body combine amino acids into proteins, so be sure you're getting enough. The RDA for riboflavin is just fewer than 2 mg a day. If you want to boost your glutathione level, though, you'll need more. We suggest 25 to 50 mg a day—a dose that's perfectly safe. Vitamin C also helps boost your glutathione level. We suggest taking 500 mg a day.

You also need to be sure you've got enough selenium in your system. That's because you need selenium to make one of the vital enzymes needed to make glutathione in your cells. We suggest getting 25 mcg a day. (See Chapter 21 to learn more about why you need tiny amounts of this mineral.)

Finally, lipoic acid helps you make glutathione and use it more efficiently. Lipoic acid is so important that we're going to discuss it separately.

Lipoic Acid: The Vitamin That's Not a Vitamin

When researchers in the 1950s isolated a sulfur-containing fatty acid, they thought at first they had found a new vitamin. The new substance, which they called *lipoic acid*, turned out to be essential for helping your mitochondria—the tiny power plants in your cells—turn glucose into energy. The researchers thought you got your lipoic acid from your food, especially animal foods. If you have to have something, and you can get it only from your food, it's a vitamin, right? After some more study, the researchers found that your body makes the very small amounts of lipoic acid you need for producing energy.

def•i•ni•tion

Lipoic acid, also sometimes called alpha-lipoic acid or thioctic acid, is needed to help your cells turn glucose into energy and to recycle glutathione. Lipoic acid is also a powerful antioxidant.

That's not the end of the story, though. In the late 1980s, researchers found that lipoic acid is also a very powerful antioxidant—one that's both water-soluble and fat-soluble, so it can work everywhere in your body. They also realized that you use lipoic acid as part of the complicated process that recycles your glutathione so that it can capture more free radicals. Because almost all the lipoic acid you make naturally is busy being used in your mitochondria, there's not a lot left over for your glutathione—and there's none left over to act as an antioxidant.

Lipoic acid helps boost your glutathione level by helping you recycle it better. But because you naturally don't have a whole lot of lipoic acid, you can recycle only so much glutathione and no more—unless you take lipoic acid supplements. The usual dose is fairly small, just 200 mg a day.

Lipoic acid supplements can also give you extra free-radical protection throughout your body. This could help prevent a lot of health problems, including atherosclerosis and cataracts. Lipoic acid could also be useful for people with liver disease.

Helping Diabetic Neuropathy

People with diabetes sometimes get a painful nerve condition called *diabetic neuropathy*. We still don't know exactly what causes the problem, but free radicals are the main suspect. Because lipoic acid is fat-soluble, it can enter into nerve cells and help prevent free-radical damage there. The doses needed are fairly high. In Europe, where doctors can—and often do—prescribe lipoic acid, the usual dose is 600 to 1,200 mg a day. It has been widely used in Germany for decades for treating diabetic neuropathy. Lipoic acid has been extensively studied in Europe, but America has lagged behind. In 2006, however, a collaborative study between the Mayo Clinic and a medical center in Russia found that intravenous ALA worked extremely well. A large, multicenter trial of oral lipoic acid called Neurological Assessment of Thioctic Acid in Neuropathy (NATHAN I) is still ongoing. Early results show a definite benefit from oral lipoic acid as well, although the improvements take much longer to be felt—several months instead of several weeks.

> **def•i•ni•tion**
>
> **Diabetic neuropathy** is a fairly common problem for diabetics. This condition causes unpleasant tingling, numbness, and pain in the nerves of your feet and legs, and can sometimes spread to the nerves of your arms and trunk.

There's some good evidence that lipoic acid can also help with another nerve-damaging complication of diabetes called autonomic neuropathy. When this happens, the nerves that control internal organs such as your heart or kidneys are damaged, with predictably serious consequences.

The usual treatment for diabetic neuropathy is analgesics such as ibuprofen, or in more severe cases, narcotic painkillers or the antiepileptic drug gabapentin. All these drugs can have serious and even dangerous side effects. Lipoic acid is very safe and has no side effects at all. If you have diabetes and want to try lipoic acid, be sure to talk to your doctor first. Lipoic acid in doses up to 1,800 mg daily seems to be quite safe. Lipoic acid may also improve your blood-sugar level, so you'll have to check your blood often and adjust your medication if needed.

The Least You Need to Know

◆ Glutathione is your body's most abundant natural antioxidant.

◆ You can boost your glutathione level by eating foods high in glutathione and by taking glutathione supplements.

◆ You also can raise your glutathione level by taking supplements of cysteine, selenium, and glutamine—the building blocks for glutathione.

◆ Lipoic acid is another powerful antioxidant you make in very small amounts. Lipoic acid supplements can help raise your glutathione level.

◆ Lipoic acid can be very helpful for diabetic neuropathy, a painful nerve condition.

Chapter 25

Flavonoids for Humanoids

In This Chapter

◆ What flavonoids are

◆ Which foods are high in flavonoids

◆ How flavonoids mop up free radicals

◆ How flavonoids protect against cancer and heart disease

◆ How to protect your eyes with flavonoids

Everywhere you go, people are telling you to eat lots of fresh fruits and vegetables. Why? It's not just that these foods are crammed with vitamins and minerals. It's not just that they're low in calories, low in fat, and high in fiber. It's because they're packed with flavonoids—the stuff that gives them their color and taste. And it's the flavonoids, as much if not more than the other stuff, which makes fruits and vegetables so good for you.

There are so many flavonoids and they're so good for you that we're still trying to figure them all out. So far, we've managed to identify some really important ones, such as alpha carotene, but there are plenty more we haven't pinned down yet. We know they're in there, though, and that you should get as many of them as possible. How? By following the advice everyone's giving you: eat lots of fresh fruits and vegetables—five to nine servings a day.

What Are Flavonoids?

Flavonoids—also called bioflavonoids—give fruits and vegetables their characteristic flavors and bright colors. These chemically complicated substances make oranges orange, red peppers red, and blueberries blue. But flavonoids do more than just give color and flavor to plant foods—they also give powerful antioxidant protection to the people who eat them.

Flavonoids are part of a much larger family of plant substances called phytochemicals. So far, scientists have discovered more than 4,000 different phytochemicals in plants. More than 600 are flavonoids or carotenoids, and of those, about 50 to 60 stay active after you've eaten them and are valuable for your health. Most flavonoids are great antioxidants that can help prevent heart disease and cancer. Others may be helpful for their ability to relieve swelling, pain, and allergic reactions. Some may even help you fight off viruses.

There's a lot we still don't know about flavonoids. When you get right down to it, our lack of knowledge is the best reason of all to be sure you eat plenty of fresh fruits and vegetables every day. Somewhere in that big mix of flavonoids are the ones that keep you healthy—and that's not even counting the vitamins, minerals, and fiber in fruits and veggies.

Food for Thought

Flavonoids were discovered in the late 1930s by Albert Szent-Györgi, discoverer of Vitamin C. He gave a friend a crude sample of Vitamin C made from lemons to help his bleeding gums. The bleeding stopped temporarily. Later, Szent-Györgi gave him a purer form of Vitamin C—and it didn't work. In purifying it, he had removed the flavonoids. When his friend used just the "impurities," the bleeding stopped completely. Szent-Györgi looked more closely at what he had taken out. He called it Vitamin P for vascular permeability (a fancy way to say blood vessels that bleed easily). Vitamin P turned out not to be absolutely essential in your diet—so technically, it's not a vitamin.

There are so many different flavonoids that it's hard to sort them all out. One reason is that plant foods have lots of different flavonoids in them. Broccoli, for example, is a good source not just of cancer-fighting indoles but also of the antioxidants sulforaphane, quercetin, and lutein—and also of Vitamin C, calcium, potassium, folic acid, chromium, and boron. Oranges have more than 40 different flavonoids, including almost all the ones we'll talk about in this chapter. On top of all that, flavonoids are what make many medicinal herbs work—but describing all that would take a whole other book. In this chapter, we stick to explaining the major flavonoid groups and discussing some of the food groups that are good flavonoid sources. And here's a tantalizing hint to keep you reading: chocolate is a good source of flavonoids!

Carotenoids: Orange You Glad You Know?

Carrots, sweet potatoes, squash, and other orange and red foods get their color from substances called *carotenoids*. The carotenoids are such a large and important family that we need to break them down into two main branches:

- ◆ **Carotenes** contain only carbon and hydrogen atoms. They're found in carrots, squash, and many other orange- or red-colored foods. Your body can convert alpha and beta carotene into Vitamin A; the carotenes are also very powerful antioxidants.

- ◆ **Xanthophylls** contain carbon, hydrogen, and oxygen atoms. These carotenoids are found in many dark-green, leafy vegetables and in egg yolks. They're also orange or yellow (*xantho* means "yellow" in Greek), but the color is covered up by the green chlorophyll in these foods. Xanthophylls are great antioxidants, but they have no Vitamin A activity.

All the carotenoids are fat-soluble. To get the most carotenoids from these foods, eat them with a little dietary fat. Supplements containing mixed carotenoids usually contain mostly beta carotene, along with alpha carotene, lutein, lycopene, and other carotenoids in varying combinations. These supplements are often made from a type of algae called *Dunaliella salina*. They're a good insurance policy if you don't eat many fruits and vegetables.

Top 20 Antioxidant Foods

Okay, it's pretty clear that fruits and vegetables are good for you because they're high in antioxidants. But which fruits and veggies are the best choices? According to a 2004 study by the U.S. Department of Agriculture, small red beans pack the most antioxidant power; other beans, such as red kidney beans, pinto beans, and black beans are also rich sources of assorted antioxidants. Among the other top 20 are blueberries, cranberries, blackberries, raspberries, and strawberries. Red Delicious, Gala, and Granny Smith apples are in there; as are prunes, cherries, black plums, red plums, artichokes, and—surprise—russet potatoes.

But what about all those vegetables, such as broccoli, kale, and cabbage, that we keep hearing are such great sources of antioxidants? They just miss the top 20 cut-off in the study, but that's no excuse to skip them. They're still excellent overall sources of antioxidants, and of some specific ones we'll talk about later in this chapter.

Now You're Cooking

Flavonoids in fruits and vegetables aren't hurt much by cooking. In fact, cooking breaks down tough cell walls in vegetables and makes flavonoids easier to absorb. Don't peel fruits and vegetables—many flavonoids are in the skin. Steam, sauté, or stir-fry fresh vegetables lightly or use frozen vegetables. Canned produce has very little left in the way of flavonoids, vitamins, minerals, or taste.

The Carotenes

No, these aren't adolescent carrots. They're flavonoids found in many orange- and red-colored fruits and vegetables. The most important member of the carotene family is beta carotene. Because you convert some of the beta carotene you eat into Vitamin A, we talked a lot about it in Chapter 3, so check back there to find out more. In this section, we focus on three other very important carotenes: alpha carotene, beta-cryptoxanthin, and lycopene.

Alpha Carotene

Although beta carotene is the most abundant carotene in foods, its close cousin alpha carotene is a much stronger antioxidant, especially for quenching those destructive singlet oxygen free radicals. Alpha carotene is found in all the same foods as beta carotene, including carrots, sweet potatoes, cantaloupe, broccoli, kiwi, spinach, mangos, and squash. As a rough rule of thumb, the amount of alpha carotene in a food is about 10 to 20 percent of the amount of beta carotene.

Beta-Cryptoxanthin

Sounds like a character from a horror movie about zombies, doesn't it? Actually, cryptoxanthin is a carotene found in oranges, mangoes, papayas, cantaloupes, peaches, prunes, and squash. You may not realize it, but you eat some every time you eat butter, because cryptoxanthin is also used to color butter. It's a very good quencher of singlet oxygen free radicals.

Lycopene

Pizza lovers, rejoice! Lycopene is a cancer-fighting antioxidant found in large amounts in tomatoes—it's one of the things that makes them red. (Watermelon and pink grapefruit have lycopene, too, but in much smaller amounts.) Lycopene is the most abundant carotene in your body. Surprisingly, most people have levels that are far higher than their beta carotene levels. Lycopene has about twice the antioxidant power of beta carotene.

A major study in 1995 showed that men who eat lots of tomato-based foods are much less likely to get prostate cancer. In general, lycopene seems to protect against cancer of the digestive tract, including colon cancer, and against lung cancer. New research suggests that lycopene may also help ward off heart disease. In 1997, a major European study showed that men who eat the most lycopene are only half as likely to have a heart attack as the men who eat the least. And in 2002, results from the Health Professionals Follow-up Study showed that the men who had the highest intake of lycopene had a 16 percent lower risk of prostate cancer than men who had the lowest intake of lycopene.

> **Now You're Cooking**
>
> You absorb lycopene well only if you eat it with dietary fat—such as the olive oil in tomato sauce or the cheese on your pizza. Cooked tomatoes are better, because cooking breaks down the cell walls and releases the lycopene. To get the most lycopene from fresh tomatoes, eat them with an oil-based salad dressing.

Lycopene may also help prevent colorectal cancer, according to a German study in 2004. The men who had the lowest lycopene levels were also the most likely to have precancerous polyps.

In 2003, researchers at the Harvard School of Public Health reported that lycopene may help stave off heart disease in women. Among the 40,000 or so participants in the ongoing Women's Health Study, the ones who ate 7 or more servings of tomato-based foods a week had a nearly 30 percent reduction in their risk of heart disease compared to the women who ate 1.5 servings or less a week. That's a pretty substantial benefit for eating pizza! It also suggests that a daily dose of something made with tomatoes is a good idea. The amount of lycopene you need every day to get its protection is around 6.5 mg. Any sort of tomato-based food gives you lycopene—check out the chart for some good choices.

The Lycopene in Food

Food	Serving Size	Lycopene in mg
Canned tomatoes	1 cup	24
Chili sauce	1 tablespoon	2
Cocktail sauce	¼ cup	7
Pink grapefruit	½ medium	2
Raw tomato	1 medium	5
Spaghetti sauce	½ cup	20
Tomato juice	1 cup	23
Tomato ketchup	1 tablespoon	3
Tomato paste	2 tablespoons	9
Tomato sauce	¼ cup	10
Tomato soup (condensed)	1 cup prepared	13
Watermelon	1 cup cubed	13

The Xanthophylls

Xanthophylls are carotenoids that are mostly found in dark-green, leafy vegetables. They aren't converted in your body into Vitamin A. In general, all xanthophylls are valuable antioxidants. The xanthophylls lutein and zeaxanthin also protect your eyes against free radical damage.

Food for Thought

In the 1830s and 1840s, Dr. Miles's Compound Extract of Tomato was a popular remedy for just about everything. The firm's slogan was "Tomato Pills Cure Your Ills." Dr. Miles and his many competitors were on to something, even if they didn't know what it was—the vitamins, minerals, and lycopene in tomatoes are indeed good for you, although we can't say they cure anything. And even if they didn't help, tomato pills didn't hurt—which is more than can be said for many of the standard medical treatments of the time.

Lutein and Zeaxanthin

Your macula—the part of your retina you use for acute vision—is crammed with lutein and zeaxanthin. They help protect the delicate cells of your macula from the harmful effects of ultraviolet light in sunshine. A major study at Harvard Medical School showed that older people who ate the most high-carotenoid foods had the lowest rates of age-related macular degeneration—which is one of the major causes of blindness in the elderly. They may also help prevent cataracts, where the lens of the eye becomes cloudy, robbing you of your vision. Nearly 20 million Americans have cataracts; every year some 1.5 million cataract operations are done, at an estimated cost of $3.4 billion. Lutein and zeaxanthin probably work to protect your eyes because their yellow color blocks light from the ultraviolet (blue) end of the spectrum.

Both lutein and zeaxanthin are also effective antioxidants that may help fight heart disease, colon cancer, and lung disease. The research here is ongoing—we expect more good evidence in the future.

All dark-green, leafy vegetables are good sources of these xanthophylls; kale, turnip greens, collard greens, and spinach are especially good choices. So are yellow and orange foods, such as corn, acorn squash, oranges, tangerines, and peaches. Egg yolks are also an excellent source. Lutein is available as a standalone supplement, but if you are concerned about your vision, we suggest you try a supplement that contains lutein as part of an eye-health formula. Today many eye doctors recommend these formulas for patients. Zeaxanthin isn't available as a supplement—which is another good reason to make sure your diet has plenty of fresh fruits and vegetables.

Capsanthin

This antioxidant xanthophyll is found in red peppers—the redder the better. Redder doesn't mean hotter, though. Capsanthin is found in hot peppers, of course, but capsanthin supplements are made from paprika, which is made from sweet red peppers. Another flavonoid called capsaicin is found in hot peppers. It's used in nonprescription pain-relieving skin creams such as Zostrix (don't swallow this stuff or get it in your eyes or an open wound). The creams are often recommended for nerve pain from shingles and diabetic neuropathy. They seem to work by countering the pain from the nerves with the mild burning sensation from the cream—this jangles up the affected nerves and blocks the pain impulse. Some people take cayenne capsules, but we're not quite sure why.

Have a Nice Cup of Tea

When you brew yourself a nice cup of tea, you're actually brewing a potent antioxidant mix. Tea has two polyphenol substances in the catechin family—epigallocatechin gallate and epicatechin gallate—that are the most potent antioxidants of all the flavonoids. That makes tea into more than just a relaxing hot drink—it protects against heart disease, stroke, and cancer. Not only that, tea may also help keep your bones strong and may even help you lose weight.

I ♥ Tea

Catechins help make your platelets, the tiny cells in your blood that make it clot, less "sticky." When your platelets are less sticky, they're less likely to clot, which means you're less likely to have a heart attack or stroke from a clot in an artery. A number of good studies, starting in the 1990s, have backed this up. In one study of older people in Holland, those who drank three or more cups of black tea a day had about half the risk of a heart attack as those who didn't drink tea at all. And if they did have a heart attack, the heavy tea drinkers were much less likely to die from it. That tallies with studies in the United States. In one study of men and women in the Boston area, for instance, the participants who drank at least one cup of tea a day had a 44 percent lower risk of a heart attack than those who drank no tea. Another study showed that among people who have had a heart attack, the ones who regularly drank the most tea were the least likely to die during the three or four years after. Moderate tea drinkers (up to 14 cups a week) had a 28 percent lower death rate; heavy tea drinkers (14 or more cups a week) had a 44 percent lower death rate.

Another study in Holland showed that men who drank four cups of tea a day had a much lower risk of stroke than those who didn't—whether or not they also took vitamins. Other studies around the world have shown that regularly drinking tea can reduce your risk of high blood pressure and lower your LDL ("bad") cholesterol level. And a 2006 study of more than 40,000 men and women in Japan found that heavy tea drinkers had a lower death rate from all causes.

Catechins and Cancer

The catechins in tea act as powerful antioxidants that can keep cancer from getting started and may help slow it down if it does. That doesn't mean tea is some sort of magic bullet against cancer or a substitute for standard medical treatment. It does mean that enjoying tea as a refreshing, inexpensive, calorie-free beverage at least a couple of times a week is probably a good idea.

The evidence that tea has a protective effect against cancer is good and getting better. There are way too many studies to go into them here. For now we'll just say that tea may help prevent breast cancer, oral cancer, colon cancer, prostate cancer, stomach cancer, and esophageal cancer. That's a lot of protection!

Tea and Your T-Score

Your T-score is a measure of bone density as determined by a DEXA bone scan—a quick, painless test every woman older than age 65 should have. If you're a long-term tea drinker, it's likely that your T-score will be higher, meaning your bone mineral density is high. According to a 2000 study in England of older women, those who drank at least one cup of tea a day had higher bone mineral density than those who didn't drink tea. Similar results were reported in a 2002 study in China. People who drink tea at least once a week over 6 to 10 years have higher bone mineral density than those who don't drink tea. (Actually, the most remarkable results of these studies may be that they show there are people in England and China who don't drink tea.) It's unclear what exactly in tea accounts for the improvement in bone density. It may be the catechins, but it could also be the fluoride or any number of other substances in tea. Of course, just drinking more tea isn't a guarantee you won't get osteoporosis. You still need to get adequate calcium, Vitamin D, and Vitamin K, eat enough protein, get plenty of weight-bearing exercise, and quit smoking. (Check back to Chapter 17 for more on this.)

Sip the Pounds Away

Green tea is yet another herb that's promoted as a way to lose weight painlessly. As with any other weight-loss elixir, the hype is based on just a shred of science. Some intriguing evidence suggests that green tea could increase your metabolic rate ever so slightly and help speed up your weight loss a tiny bit. The results are nowhere near as dramatic as all the hype makes them sound—in fact, you probably won't notice any results at all—but there's no reason not to add a daily cup or two of green tea to your weight-loss program. The studies have shown that it's not the caffeine in the tea that causes the metabolic effect, so decaffeinated tea would work as well.

Which Tea?

The benefits of tea are found mostly in green tea, the kind used in China and Japan, because green tea has the most catechins. Green tea is made by steaming and then drying the fresh tea leaves. The steaming removes an enzyme that oxidizes the catechins and makes them less potent. Oolong tea (the kind served in Chinese restaurants) and black tea (the kind used in typical tea bags) aren't steamed. Instead, they're exposed to the air for a few hours and then allowed to ferment. The process oxidizes the catechins and makes them less potent. Even so, these teas are nearly as powerful as green tea. One cup of green tea has about 375 mg of catechins; a cup of black tea has 210 mg. Adding milk to your tea can keep the catechins from being absorbed as well. Sugar and other sweeteners—natural or artificial—have no effect.

You probably need to drink at least two and possibly five cups of tea a day to get any real benefit. Decaffeinated tea works as well as regular. If you don't want to drink that much, try supplements containing green tea extract. Look for capsules that contain at least 30 percent catechins.

Health in a Coffee Cup

If you don't like tea, try some coffee for your health instead. It turns out that there's more in your java than just the caffeine jolt. That cup of joe is filled with antioxidants. And because at least half of us drink at least one cup a day, coffee is actually the main source of dietary antioxidants for most Americans. (In case you're interested, the next four most common sources are, in descending order, black tea, bananas, beans, and corn.)

The rap against coffee used to be that it could harm your heart. The reasoning was that the caffeine in the coffee raised your blood pressure and increased your heart rate, making you more susceptible to a heart attack. Recently, several major epidemiological studies have shown, however, that coffee consumption doesn't raise your risk of heart disease. Among the participants in the Iowa Women's Health Study, drinking coffee reduced the risk of death from cardiovascular disease by a remarkable 24 percent compared to those who didn't drink coffee. Even if you've already had a heart attack, there's no reason to cut back—a study of nearly 2,000 heart attack patients showed no increased risk of death among the coffee drinkers. A 2006 study showed, however, that people with a particular gene that makes them metabolize the caffeine in coffee more slowly than normal may be at slightly higher risk of a heart attack if they regularly drink coffee.

The other big rap against coffee used to be that it raised your risk of Type 2 diabetes. The controversy over this has gone on for decades, but it seems to have finally been ended with several excellent recent studies showing that regularly drinking coffee actually *reduces* the risk. The caffeine in coffee may have an effect on your blood sugar if you have Type 2 diabetes, but this tends to be very individual—it raises blood sugar for some people but not others.

Other possible health benefits of coffee include lowering your risk of liver cancer, colon cancer, Parkinson's disease, and gallstones.

The caffeine in coffee may be responsible for some of the health benefits, but the antioxidants and other substances, such as magnesium, also seem to play a role. In the diabetes studies, for instance, people who drank decaf got the same protection—but only if they drank several cups a day.

Food for Thought _____

Caffeine is what gives coffee—and also tea, cola drinks, and the herbal drinks maté and guarana—their characteristic jolt. Too much caffeine can temporarily raise your blood pressure and increase your heart rate, make your hands tremble, and keep you from sleeping, but in smaller doses it's very safe. In fact, caffeine is the only drug that can legally be added to food. And added it is—many soft drinks such as Mountain Dew contain added caffeine.

Quercetin: The Flavonoid from Onions

The flavonoid quercetin is very active—it's the important ingredient in a lot of medicinal plants. Quercetin helps reduce inflammation and swelling, blocks allergies, kills viruses, and acts as an antioxidant.

Quercetin is found in many different plant foods, but ordinary onions are the richest source. Their high quercetin content explains why onions are widely used in folk medicine as a treatment for allergies and asthma—the quercetin slows or prevents allergic reactions and relaxes swollen bronchial tubes. A recent study showed that middle-aged men who ate five or more apples a week had better overall lung function than men who didn't. The most likely explanation is that apples contain a lot of quercetin.

Quercetin also blocks your production of an enzyme that changes glucose into a damaging sugar alcohol. If you have diabetes, high sugar-alcohol levels can cause cataracts, diabetic neuropathy, and other complications.

Quercetin can help prevent cancer by blocking the growth of cancer cells. In a major Chinese study, people who ate the most onions had the least stomach cancer. A lot of the research on this is still in the test-tube stage, though, so we can't really be sure about how—or even whether—quercetin helps prevent cancer in people.

There are more than 500 plants in the big *Allium* family, including onions, scallions, chives, leeks, shallots, and garlic. The highest quercetin levels are in red onions, yellow onions, and shallots. Apples are another good dietary source of quercetin. In fact, according to a study published in 2000, people who eat an apple a day have a lower risk of stroke than those who don't. There are goodly amounts of quercetin in apples, black tea, grapefruit, and red wine. Dark green vegetables such as broccoli also have some quercetin. Quercetin isn't absorbed all that well in your digestive tract. You absorb more from cooked onions than raw ones. (You'll also have better breath.)

Garlic: It's Good for You

Garlic is a member of the extended onion family, but it stands out from all the others because of one phytochemical: alliin. This sulfur-containing compound is what gives garlic its pungent smell and taste. In folk medicine, garlic is used for everything from athlete's foot to influenza (to say nothing of its ability to ward off vampires). There's some truth to garlic's antibiotic activity, but recent research has concentrated on garlic as an antioxidant, a way to lower cholesterol, and a way to prevent cancer.

Garlic is one of the most potent antioxidant foods around—it's especially good for capturing peroxyl free radicals. The antioxidant effect of garlic could be why people who eat a lot of it tend to be healthier in general.

Until very recently, researchers believed garlic really did help cholesterol. They had good reasons: several solid studies backed them up. But recently a number of studies have shown that garlic supplements don't lower cholesterol. In the studies that showed it did, it now seems more likely that the heart-healthy diet the participants followed is what did the trick. Garlic supporters argue that the patients in the recent studies just weren't taking enough.

What if you don't follow a healthy diet? In that case, research suggests garlic may indeed help keep your cholesterol down. Also, there's more to heart health than just cholesterol. A chemical in garlic called ajoene (*ajo* is Spanish for garlic) seems to thin your blood and prevent your platelets from forming clots that can lead to a heart attack. Ajoene (methyl allyl trisulfide) may also help dissolve clots after they form. Other garlic compounds may help your heart by lowering your blood pressure.

The news on the cancer front is better. Several different compounds in garlic can slow or prevent the growth of tumor cells. The evidence is particularly good for a link between eating a lot of garlic and a reduced risk of prostate and stomach cancer. However, the studies haven't been backed up by clinical trials yet. The benefits of garlic come from eating one to three fresh cloves every day. Not too many people like to eat that much garlic, though—and not too many people like to be around people who do. Raw garlic, cooked garlic, and even garlic powder from the spice shelf all give you the complete benefits of garlic. Because too much garlic can cause stomach upsets and garlic breath, you might want to try garlic supplements. These fall into two categories: dried garlic pills (the most popular brand is Kwai, imported from Germany) and aged garlic in pills or liquid form (the most popular brand is Kyolic, imported from Japan). Dried garlic (Kwai) has a compound called alliin; aged garlic (Kyolic) doesn't. Because nobody really knows which compounds in garlic are the most important, it's hard to say which type of supplement is better. Try them both and go with your personal preference.

A Berry Good Idea

Did you ever notice that not too many foods are blue? If more of them were, we might all have sharper eyesight—and also have lower cholesterol and sharper brains as we age. That's because blue fruits such as blueberries, blue grapes, and plums are high in a group of flavonoids called anthocyanins. The anthocyanins are very effective free-radical fighters, especially in the tiny blood vessels of your eyes. They're valuable for preventing eye problems, especially those affecting your retina, such as macular degeneration and night blindness.

Just eating a lot of blueberries probably won't help protect your eyes, though. Supplements made from bilberries (a Scandinavian plant very similar to blueberries) are available. To help protect against macular degeneration, you'll need to take one or two 40-mg capsules a day of an extract standardized to contain 25 percent bilberry anthocynanins. And don't forget the lutein and zeaxanthin, as explained earlier in this chapter.

Bilberry can really help with another common vision problem: night blindness, or difficulty seeing in dim light and recovering from glare, such as from oncoming car headlights. Taking a dose of bilberry extract helps reduce night blindness symptoms for about 2 hours. The effect wears off, however, and taking supplements on a regular basis won't do anything to improve the problem permanently. If you're having trouble driving at night, give bilberry a try—it could make a big difference. The usual dose is 120 to 240 mg of an extract standardized to contain 25 percent bilberry anthocyanins.

Eating a lot of berries may be a smart move. Overall, berries such as blueberries, raspberries, strawberries, and cranberries are loaded with antioxidants. Lab studies suggest that something in berries helps protect brain cells against the effects of aging.

A compound called pterostilbene in blueberries may help lower cholesterol. It does in lab rats, anyway, although it remains to be seen if it has the same effect in people. Compounds in strawberries and raspberries may help prevent cancer, but so far, the studies are only in rats.

Resveratrol: Red Wine Rescuer

The French ignore all the things we Americans do to stay healthy. They eat foods high in fat and calories. They smoke cigarettes. They wouldn't dream of going to the gym to work out. They also live longer and have less heart disease than anyone else in Westernized society. What's going on here?

It's what scientists call the French paradox. What seems to save the French from their bad habits is what some might consider another bad habit: they drink a lot of red wine. And red wine is high in healthful flavonoids, including catechins and antho-cyanins. As we've already explained, these flavonoids are great antioxidants that help protect your heart. Resveratrol, another substance in red wine, lowers your cholesterol and helps prevent artery-clogging blood clots. Resveratrol has an extra benefit: it can help prevent cancer, particularly prostate and colon cancer. This only works when you drink wine in moderation, however—too much alcohol is associated with an increase in cancer risk.

Many doctors recommend a glass of red wine with your evening meal as a way to lower your risk of heart disease. That's because Frenchmen who drink 2 to 3 glasses of wine a day have about a 30 percent reduction in their risk of heart-related death compared to those who don't drink alcohol at all. But is it the resveratrol in the wine or the alcohol that does the trick? Studies show that alcohol-free red wine works just as well—which suggests that resveratrol or perhaps something else in wine provides the protection. On the other hand, moderate consumption of alcohol of any sort (one drink daily for a woman, two for a man) has been shown to reduce the risk of heart disease, so maybe it's the alcohol after all. Whichever it is, the heart risk reduc-tion from red wine is real but small. It's much more important to stop smoking, lose weight, exercise regularly, and watch your diet.

If you don't want to drink alcohol, you can still get the benefits of resveratrol by drinking alcohol-free red wine (but don't even think of asking for it in France!) or purple grape juice, or by eating plenty of red or purple grapes. You'd have to drink three times as much grape juice to get the equivalent of one glass of red wine, and you'd have to eat a lot of grapes. Resveratrol supplements are available, but there's no real evidence to show they're helpful.

Chocolate: Chockfull of Health

Chocolate is good for your heart. Sounds too good to be true, but the evidence in recent years has been mounting steadily. Chocolate, especially dark chocolate, is an excellent source of antioxidants, particularly the group known as flavanols. It's the flavonols that are probably responsible for chocolate's ability to help lower your blood pressure and keep your blood flowing smoothly through your arteries. In a 2006 study of older Dutch men, the ones who ate the most foods made from cocoa beans, such as chocolate bars, cocoa beverages, and chocolate pudding, had the lowest blood pressure—and their risk of death was 50 percent lower than those who ate little or no chocolate. If you eat a lot of chocolate, the extra calories may outweigh any benefit from the antioxidants, but in moderation, chocolate every day is starting to sound like a good health idea.

Broccoli to the Rescue

You keep hearing that broccoli is good for you, but what exactly is it supposed to do? Crunching on *cruciferous* vegetables such as broccoli, cabbage, Brussels sprouts, and cauliflower is a very good way to reduce your risk of cancer. These vegetables contain a class of chemicals known as isothiocyanates, which are known to help prevent cancer, especially lung cancer. To take just one good example, a study of more than 18,000 men in China found that those who had the highest levels of isothiocyanates in their blood from eating cruciferous vegetables had a 36 percent lower risk of developing lung cancer over a 10-year period—even though most of them smoked and they lived in an area with high air pollution.

def•i•ni•tion

Cruciferous vegetables are members of the cabbage family, including arugula, bok choy, broccoli, Brussels sprouts, cabbage, cauliflower, chard, collard greens, kohlrabi, kale, mustard greens, Napa cabbage, radishes, turnips, turnip greens, and watercress. They're called cruciferous because they all have four-petaled flowers arranged in the shape of a cross.

Unexpected Health from Unlikely Plants

Many, many plant foods contain valuable flavonoids. So do parts of plants we don't normally eat. And so do some plants that we don't think of as food at all. Here's a run-down of some of the other flavonoids:

- **OPCs.** Oligomeric proanthocyanidins (you can see why we prefer the abbreviation) are flavonoids found in many plants and in red wine. Supplements are made from grape seeds or pine bark. (The commercial mixture from pine bark is called pycnogenol.) OPCs are very active free-radical scavengers, especially for trapping hydroxyl free radicals. Enthusiasts also claim that OPCs help problems caused by poor circulation, such as easy bruising, varicose veins, hemorrhoids, and intermittent claudication. Do they? Yes—OPCs and pycnogenol can be very helpful, especially for varicose veins. Try them and see whether they work for you. The usual dose for general antioxidant protection is 50 mg a day. For circulation problems, the dose is between 150 and 300 mg daily.

Warning!

Flavonoids in grapefruit juice can cause dangerous drug interactions by increasing the potency of some prescription drugs, including statin drugs. Talk to your doctor about possible interactions.

- **Citrus flavonoids.** Several flavonoids found in citrus fruits, including hesperidin, quercetin, rutin, and naringin, can help lower cholesterol and may help improve circulation in your tiny blood vessels.

- **Pomegranate juice.** This increasingly popular beverage—and supplements made from pomegranates—is very high in antioxidants. Polyphenols in pomegranate may help lower your cholesterol and could help prevent prostate cancer.

There's a lot of research into flavonoids going on right now. All sorts of other foods turn out to have flavonoids that could help your health. It's the proanthocyanidins in cranberry juice, for instance, that make it useful for treating urinary tract infections.

The Least You Need to Know

- Flavonoids are the substances that give color and flavor to plant foods.
- To get the most flavonoids, eat a variety of fresh fruits and vegetables every day.
- Most flavonoids are powerful antioxidants. Many are also helpful for preventing or treating specific health problems such as asthma or eye problems.

◆ Carotenoids, including beta carotene and lycopene, are powerful antioxidants. Lycopene may help prevent prostate and lung cancer.

◆ Other important flavonoids include quercetin, found in onions, and catechins, found in tea.

◆ Garlic contains many flavonoids and other valuable substances, as do onions, red wine, citrus fruits, grapes, vegetables in the cabbage family, and many other fruits and vegetables.

◆ Coffee, chocolate, and berries are all high in flavonoids.

26

Coenzyme Q_{10}: Cellular Spark Plug

In This Chapter

- What coenzyme Q_{10} (ubiquinone) is
- How coenzyme Q_{10} makes energy in your cells
- Which foods are high in coenzyme Q_{10}
- How coenzyme Q_{10} can help protect your heart
- How coenzyme Q_{10} can lower your blood pressure
- How coenzyme Q_{10} can help people with Parkinson's disease

What makes you tick? At the most basic level—inside your cells—it's something called coenzyme Q_{10}. You need this special stuff to release energy in your cells. Without it, you come to a stop.

Coenzyme Q_{10} acts similar to the spark plugs in your car engine. Spark plugs convert gasoline to energy inside the pistons of the engine. The energy drives the pistons, which drive the car. Coenzyme Q_{10} in your cells works the same way. If one of your spark plugs isn't working right, your car engine stops running well. If all the spark plugs aren't working, your car sputters to a stop, even if the gas tank is full. Something very similar happens in your body if you run low on coenzyme Q_{10}—you can't produce enough energy to keep your body running.

Co Q What?

Back in 1957, researchers at the University of Wisconsin found something in beef hearts that seemed to be basic for making energy in living cells. They analyzed it and found it was a *quinone*, one of a group of substances that are found in all living plants and animals that use oxygen. Early researchers called the substance *ubiquinone*, meaning a quinone that was found everywhere.

The basic structure of quinone differs slightly among living things. In humans, the quinone has 10 units in a side chain of molecules. In the 1960s, researchers discovered that ubiquinone in humans is a very important *coenzyme*, so they started calling it coenzyme Q_{10}, or CoQ_{10} for short.

def•i•ni•tion

Quinones are brightly colored organic substances found in all living plants and animals that need oxygen to survive. **Ubiquinone** is one name for a quinone that is found in all human cells. Its name comes from the prefix *ubi-*, meaning "everywhere," combined with quinone.

Ubiquinone is a **coenzyme**—a substance, usually a vitamin or mineral, which attaches as a sort of tail to a complex *enzyme*. An enzyme is a chain of amino acids that makes a chemical reaction happen in your body without being changed itself. The coenzyme completes the enzyme; without it, the reaction can't happen.

CoQ_{10} works in the mitochondria of your cells. These mini power plants provide the energy that runs your body. In a very complex process, CoQ_{10} shuttles tiny, electrically charged particles back and forth in the mitochondria among the three essential enzymes that are needed to generate energy. Without CoQ_{10}, the whole process grinds to a halt.

Starting in the 1960s, coenzyme Q_{10} research really took off in Japan. It was approved there as a treatment for heart failure in 1974. Today it is one of the most widely prescribed drugs in Japan. It's also widely prescribed in Italy, Sweden, Denmark, Israel, and Canada. In the United States, though, coenzyme Q_{10} is not considered a drug. Instead, it's a food supplement that you can buy in any health-food store.

CoQ₁₀ for Cardiac Cases

So far, the most exciting news about coenzyme Q_{10} is that it can be helpful for some types of heart disease. In a number of serious studies, coenzyme Q_{10} has been shown to be especially good for people with heart failure. One good study found that coenzyme Q_{10} helps protect the heart against the harmful effects of the drug doxorubicin, which is used to treat breast cancer.

The biggest benefit seems to come from the way CoQ_{10} improves energy flow in your mitochondria. Your heart muscle has the most mitochondria of any muscle in your body, and it also has—or should have—the highest level of coenzyme Q_{10}. People with *heart failure*, though, frequently have low coenzyme Q_{10} levels, which is probably why they often improve when they start taking CoQ_{10}. Their hearts start to pump harder and circulate their blood better.

Coenzyme Q_{10} has no side effects and doesn't cause any bad drug interactions. Best of all, studies show that heart failure patients who take coenzyme Q_{10} feel better overall and spend less time in the hospital.

In early studies of CoQ_{10}, heart patients were given just 30 mg a day and showed some improvement. Today the usual dose for heart disease is anywhere from 100 to 300 mg a day. Because you can't overdose on coenzyme Q_{10}, these doses are quite safe.

def•i•ni•tion

When your heart is damaged or weak and can't pump blood to the rest of your body very well, you have **heart failure.** Symptoms of heart failure include extreme tiredness, breathlessness, and swelling in the ankles and legs. Drugs such as digitalis, diuretics, and blood thinners are often used to treat heart failure.

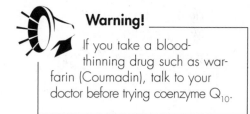

Warning!

If you take a blood-thinning drug such as warfarin (Coumadin), talk to your doctor before trying coenzyme Q_{10}.

If you have heart failure or any other sort of heart disease and want to try coenzyme Q_{10}, you *must* talk to your doctor first. The sooner you start taking CoQ_{10} after your heart disease has been diagnosed, the better it will work, but it will still take several weeks to start helping. You *must* continue to take your medication—coenzyme Q_{10} should be taken along with, not instead of, any drugs your doctor prescribes. A few months after you start taking coenzyme Q_{10}, your symptoms may get a lot better. You may even want to take less of your prescription medicines. *Never* try to change your heart drugs on your own—you *must* talk to your doctor.

CoQ_{10} may give you another heart benefit as well. It seems to reduce the "stickiness" of your platelets, the tiny cells that form blood clots. If your platelets are less likely to clump together to form an artery-blocking clot, you're less likely to have a heart attack. This is a promising area of research, but it's far too soon to recommend CoQ_{10} as a blood thinner or as a way to prevent heart attacks. That's because some studies show that coenzyme Q_{10} might interact with blood-thinning drugs and make them less effective.

Lowering Your Blood Pressure

Coenzyme Q_{10} could help lower your blood pressure, especially if it's high because of a heart problem or diabetes. The benefit seems to come from the way coenzyme Q_{10} helps your blood vessels open wider, which reduces the pressure inside them. (For more information about your blood pressure, look in Chapter 2 for basic information; also check Chapters 17 and 18.)

If you want to try coenzyme Q_{10} for your blood pressure, talk to your doctor first. CoQ_{10} takes a while to start helping. You'll have to take about 200 mg a day for several months before you see a drop. In the meantime, you *must* keep taking your high blood pressure medicine—*coenzyme Q_{10} should be taken along with, not instead of, any drugs your doctor prescribes.* After you start taking CoQ_{10}, your blood pressure may drop and you may need less of your prescription drugs. *Never* try to change your high blood pressure medicine on your own—you *must* talk to your doctor.

Cholesterol and CoQ$_{10}$

Artery-clogging cholesterol deposits are made in part when the LDL ("bad") cholesterol in your blood reacts with oxygen. Coenzyme Q_{10} may help keep your cholesterol from oxidizing, which in turn keeps it from plugging up your arteries. The studies here are inconclusive, although they do show that coenzyme Q_{10} doesn't make high cholesterol worse. If you have high cholesterol, your doctor may prescribe a statin drug such as lovastatin (Mevacor), pravastatin (Pravachor), or simvastatin (Zocor) to bring it down. These drugs work well, but they may also block your production of coenzyme Q_{10}, because some of the processes blocked by the drug are the same steps needed to make coenzyme Q_{10}. If you need to take medicine to lower your cholesterol, talk to your doctor about taking coenzyme Q_{10} supplements as well.

Helping Parkinson's Disease

In 2002, a major study of coenzyme Q_{10} showed that it has value as a way to delay the disabling effects of Parkinson's disease. The participants were all in the early stages of Parkinson's disease. They had the tremor, slowness of movement, and stiffness characteristic of this degenerative brain disorder, but they were not yet taking levodopa, the standard medication. The participants who took the largest dose of coenzyme Q_{10}—1,200 mg per day for 16 months—had 44 percent less decline in mental function, movement, and ability to perform daily living activities than those who took the placebo. More research is needed, but overall, this is very encouraging news. If you'd like to try coenzyme Q_{10} for Parkinson's disease, discuss it with your doctor first.

> **Quack, Quack**
>
> Does skin cream with CoQ_{10} in it prevent wrinkles or firm your skin? You've read this far in this book, so you've probably already correctly guessed that the answer is "no."

Getting Your Coenzyme Q₁₀

About half the coenzyme Q_{10} in your body comes from the foods you eat; almost all the rest is made in your liver. Many foods have at least some coenzyme Q_{10} in them, so the average person eats about 5 mg a day. Good sources of coenzyme Q_{10} in food include oily, cold-water fish such as tuna, mackerel, and sardines. Organ meats, beef, and vegetable oils such as soy or canola oil are also good sources. Wheat germ, rice bran, and soy foods such as tofu all have some coenzyme Q_{10}.

You have to eat a lot of these foods to get any real amount of coenzyme Q_{10}. To get 30 mg of CoQ_{10} in one sitting, for instance, you'd have to eat a whole pound of sardines or more than 2 pounds of peanuts. The process of making coenzyme Q_{10} in your body is very complicated—it takes at least 15 steps and needs plenty of Vitamin C, Vitamin E, selenium, and the B vitamins.

All things considered, we suggest raising your CoQ_{10} level by taking supplements. CoQ_{10} comes in a variety of forms, but we recommend taking only an oil-based gelcap. That's because CoQ_{10} is absorbed better when it's taken with dietary fat. Doses range from 30 to 300 mg daily. You'll get the most benefit if you divide your doses over the day. Coenzyme Q_{10} supplements are extremely safe. They don't cause any drug interactions or side effects and you can't overdose on them. Bear in mind, though, that they're on the expensive side and they won't do anything for you if your coenzyme Q_{10} level is normal—the supplements help only if your level is low.

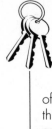

Food for Thought _____

Every day you hear about "natural" remedies for health problems—remedies your doctor says don't work or aren't proven. Should you try them, even though they're not part of mainstream medicine? We can't say. We can tell you to carefully consider the source. Advertisements, word-of-mouth recommendations, or the advice of a part-time clerk at the vitamin counter aren't good enough. The information you get this way is often distorted or just plain wrong. Before you start taking vitamins, minerals, and other supplements to treat a health problem, seek qualified help from a nutritionally oriented physician or other professional who can give you rational advice based on solid scientific evidence.

The Least You Need to Know

- Coenzyme Q_{10} is a vitaminlike substance essential for making energy in your cells.

- You get some coenzyme Q_{10} in your food and make the rest in your body.

- Coenzyme Q_{10} supplements are sold in drug stores and health-food stores. They are very safe and unlikely to interact with other drugs.

- Coenzyme Q_{10} can be helpful for protecting your heart.

- Coenzyme Q_{10} can help lower your blood pressure.

- Coenzyme Q_{10} can be a helpful treatment for the early stages of Parkinson's disease.

Chapter 27

Help from Natural Hormones

In This Chapter

- ◆ How hormones help regulate your body
- ◆ How your diet can help your hormones
- ◆ How melatonin can help jet lag and insomnia
- ◆ How natural hormones can help relieve hot flashes from menopause
- ◆ How you can prevent heart disease with soy

Women have them. Men have them. Teenagers *really* have them. What are they? Hormones—chemical messengers that control and coordinate what goes on in your body. Hormones regulate your blood pressure and heartbeat. They control your growth, your sleep cycle, your blood sugar, your sexuality, and lots of other things in your body. They even play a role in your emotions. And when your hormones get out of whack, a lot of things can start to go wrong.

The good news is that sometimes you can help your hormones get back in sync safely and easily. Insomnia and jet lag, for instance, are really helped a lot by natural hormones—there's no need for dangerous sleeping drugs. And just changing your diet to include small amounts of soy foods every day can help solve some of the problems of menopause.

What's a Hormone?

Hormones are the chemical messengers your body makes in your endocrine glands—your thyroid or pancreas, for example. Hormones coordinate what goes on in your body, making all your tissues and organs work together smoothly. Your endocrine system and the hormones it makes are marvelously complex—far too complex to explain in detail here. Diabetes or an underactive thyroid, for example, are hormone problems that you need to work with your doctor to treat. In this chapter, we focus on insomnia, jet lag, and menopause symptoms—hormone-related problems you can do a lot to help through diet and supplements.

Melatonin: From A to Zzzz

Melatonin is a hormone made by your *pineal gland* (a small gland inside your brain). Your pineal gland controls your sleep/wake cycle and your body's internal clock—what scientists call your *circadian rhythm*. Melatonin's main function is to help you fall asleep, but today all sorts of other claims are made for it. Can melatonin cure insomnia, prevent jet lag, block cancer, restore immune function, improve your sex life, and even retard aging? Let's look more closely at what melatonin can really do.

A Good Night's Rest

Melatonin does help you sleep. When your eyes notice it's getting dark, that information is sent to your pineal gland, which then starts to make melatonin, which makes you drowsy. That's why melatonin is sometimes called the Dracula of hormones—it only comes out at night. Most people begin making melatonin at sunset, reach a peak at around 2:00 in the morning, and then gradually taper off toward sunrise. During the day, your melatonin levels are so low they're barely detectable. Until you're about 40, you make plenty of melatonin. After that, you make less as you get older, which may be one reason many elderly people don't sleep well.

def•i•ni•tion

Your **pineal gland** is a small, pea-sized structure found in the center of your brain. Its primary role is to control your **circadian rhythm.** This is your body's 24-hour internal clock, which controls your cycles of sleeping and waking.

Taking melatonin supplements on a regular basis a few hours before bedtime does help many people with frequent sleep problems get to sleep faster and stay asleep longer. If you have only occasional nights where you just can't seem to get to sleep, melatonin probably won't do much for you, especially if you're younger than age 40. On the other hand, melatonin isn't addictive, you don't build up a tolerance or dependency, and it has no side or morning-after effects (unlike most over-the-counter sleep medicines). In fact, it's so safe it's the only hormone you can buy without a prescription. If you have occasional insomnia, melatonin is worth a try. The dosage for getting to sleep varies hugely from person to person. Some people need just 100 mcg, while others take several milligrams. For most people, 100 to 400 mcg taken 2 to 4 hours before bedtime works very well. In most scientific studies, the doses range from 0.3 mg up to 5 mg.

> ### Quack, Quack
>
> Melatonin can make you very drowsy. Take it only if you're planning to go to sleep soon. Most of the other claims for melatonin, including its use as a drug to fight cancer, are based on lab research or very limited human testing. There's just not enough information yet to recommend it for anything except getting to sleep.

Relieving Jet Lag

Recent clinical studies have shown that melatonin as a sleep aid is most effective for sleep disturbances due to jet lag and swing-shift or night-shift work, and that it works best for people who have to get to sleep during daylight hours. To deal with jet lag, take a 3 mg dose of melatonin the first night you're at your destination. Be sure you have nothing else to do but nod off at that point, because the melatonin could make you very sleepy. You should sleep well and wake up feeling pretty close to normal. If you have trouble getting to sleep the next few nights, keep using the melatonin. Don't use it for more than five days in a row—by then, you should be adjusted to your new time zone. If you're adjusting to a change in shifts or a switch to night work, follow the same schedule.

Melatonin Magic?

Researchers have looked at melatonin for a lot of different health problems, including asthma, breast cancer, and seasonal affective disorder (SAD), but so far it hasn't turned out to be a magical cure for anything. As for claims that melatonin is a miracle anti-aging medicine, or that it improves your immunity or your sex life, our advice is to spend the money on a gym membership instead.

Maximizing Your Melatonin

Important as melatonin is, your body produces it only in very small amounts—you make no more than about 300 mcg a night. Taking larger doses of melatonin supplements doesn't seem to do any harm, though. Even in doses as large as 6 g, melatonin isn't toxic. If you're pregnant or nursing, skip the melatonin—we don't know whether you pass it on to your baby, or what happens if you do. And don't give melatonin to kids—they already make plenty of it. We recommend synthetic (also called pharmacy-grade) melatonin. "Natural" melatonin is made from the pineal glands of slaughtered cows and could contain dangerous viruses and impurities. Buy your melatonin from a reputable supplier to be sure of getting a high-quality product.

Soy Meets Girl

Soybean foods such as soy milk, tofu, and miso may be the best foods around for protecting women against breast cancer, relieving the symptoms of menopause, and protecting you against osteoporosis. Soy can also help protect men and women against heart disease.

Soybeans are naturally very high in isoflavones, substances found in many plant foods. In particular, soybeans are high in *phytoestrogens*, isoflavone compounds similar to the female hormone *estrogen*. Two isoflavones found abundantly in soy, *genistein* and *daidzein*, have been shown to help relieve menopause symptoms and to help prevent breast cancer. Another isoflavone in soy called ipriflavone may help prevent osteoporosis.

Let's start with ways isoflavones help women. To do that, we need to discuss estrogen first. Estrogen is a *steroid* hormone—in other words, it's a hormone your body makes in your adrenal glands and your ovaries. Your breasts, ovaries, and uterus all have special receptors for estrogen—the estrogen fits into them just like a key into a lock. Estrogen also plays an important role in keeping your bones strong, especially in the years immediately following menopause. Too much estrogen, however, is just as bad as too little, because estrogen can trigger breast, ovarian, and uterine cancer in older women. And when the cancer starts, estrogen can make it grow faster.

In the case of cancer, what if you could block the estrogen receptors? That would slow down the cancer or even stop it—and that's exactly what successful cancer-fighting drugs such as tamoxifen do. What if you could block the receptors *before* the cancer starts? That's exactly what soy isoflavones, especially genistein, can do. Genistein and daidzein act like very weak estrogen—just strong enough to beat your real estrogen to the receptors, but not strong enough to trigger cancer.

Soy foods have lots of other valuable anti-cancer substances as well. Soy foods are good sources of natural chemicals, such as protease inhibitors, saponins, phytosterols, and phytates, which may block cancer cells and keep them from developing.

Soy isoflavones can also help menopause symptoms, especially hot flashes. Nearly half of all American women have this annoying problem as they go through menopause, but only about 10 percent of Japanese women get them. Again, soy foods seem to make the difference. The average Japanese woman eats a pound of tofu (bean curd) a week.

Food for Thought _____

Although we think of estrogen as the main female hormone, men make it in small amounts as well. Estrogen may play a role in triggering prostate cancer. Among Japanese men, who eat a lot of soy foods, prostate cancer is much less common. The cancer protection seems to come from the soy in their diet.

As part of the normal aging process, women gradually stop producing the female hormone estrogen and stop menstruating, a process known as menopause. The process can take several years, usually starting in the late forties or early fifties; the average age of menopause in the United States is 52.

For decades, doctors routinely prescribed hormone replacement therapy (HRT) using a combination of estrogen and another female hormone, progesterone (usually in the synthetic form progestin), for menopausal and postmenopausal women. The thinking was that the hormones helped relieve some of the unpleasant symptoms of menopause, such as hot flashes, and also helped protect against osteoporosis and heart disease.

Unfortunately, the thinking turned out to be wrong. In 2002, results from the long-running Women's Health Initiative (WHI) study showed that while combined HRT did help relieve hot flashes, it increased the risk of breast and endometrial (uterine) cancer. It did help prevent osteoporosis, but not as well as the new drugs for this condition do. And as for protecting against heart disease, the opposite turned out to be the case. The results of the WHI's four-year Heart and Estrogen/Progestin Replacement Study (HERS) found that overall, taking the hormones didn't do anything to protect the hearts of the women in the study. In fact, among the women who already had heart disease, the number of heart attacks went up when they started taking HRT. In 2004, further results from the HERS study showed that estrogen alone increased a woman's risk of stroke and blood clots, although it did protect from hip fractures. In 2003 and 2004, additional results from the WHI Memory Study (WHIMS) showed among women aged 65 and older, taking estrogen and progestin doubled the risk of dementia. Taking estrogen alone still raised the risk, though not as severely.

Today hormone replacement therapy (HRT) for menopausal and postmenopausal women usually involves taking only supplemental estrogen, not a combination of estrogen and progestin. Estrogen-only HRT is still widely used, but the chief reasons are for relieving severe hot flashes and vaginal dryness. Most doctors suggest the smallest possible dose for the shortest possible time, and most women who use HRT today take it only for a few years during and after menopause. The decision to use HRT is a very individual one that each woman has to make for herself after discussing her overall health and family history with her doctor.

For many women with unpleasant menopause symptoms such as hot flashes and vaginal dryness, taking soy isoflavone supplements or eating plenty of foods high in soy are a reasonable alternative to hormone replacement therapy. Soy isoflavones are weaker in their effect than estrogen and don't seem to trigger cancer. If you already have heart disease, soy isoflavones make even more sense. As for preventing heart disease, your best bets are still to stop smoking, improve your diet, lose weight if you need to, exercise more, and talk to your doctor about ways to lower your cholesterol and blood pressure if they are high.

If you decide to try soy isoflavones, you may have to experiment a bit to find the dose that works for you. Doses of up to 200 mg a day are within the safety limits, but most women feel positive benefits from just 50 mg of mixed isoflavones (genistein and daidzein) a day. To be sure of getting a good product with enough active isoflavones, choose supplements from a reliable manufacturer. Be sure to tell your doctor you are taking soy supplements, and don't take them if you are also taking estrogen.

Bones from Beans

If you're concerned—as we think you should be—about the risks of HRT, but you're also at risk for osteoporosis, consider ipriflavone. This is a synthetic derivative made from natural soy isoflavones (mostly daidzein) that may help slow down bone loss. Ipriflavone doesn't seem to have any other estrogenic effects, so women who are at risk of breast or uterine cancer can take it.

Ipriflavone is sold in health-food stores under brand names such as Ostivone and Iprical. Ipriflavone probably works even better if you also take supplemental calcium and Vitamin D.

Soy for Your Heart

In 1999, the FDA began allowing food manufacturers to claim that foods containing soy may lower your risk of heart disease. There's some solid research behind this—and it helps both men and women. Taking in 25 g of soy protein a day—the equivalent of 4 cups of soy milk—could reduce your LDL "bad" cholesterol by as much as 5 to 7 percent if it's already high. That might not sound like much, but even a small reduction in your LDL has a big payoff in heart health. Soy protein isn't a magic bullet, however—you still have to lose weight, watch your diet, stop smoking, and exercise.

Eating Your Soy

You can get the natural benefits of genistein, daidzein, and all the other good stuff in soy just by eating more soybean foods. The best choices are tofu (bean curd), soy milk, miso (fermented soybean paste used in soups), tempeh (a chewy cake made from fermented soybeans), and textured soy protein (TSP—also called textured vegetable protein or TVP). Fermented soy foods have the most genistein. Soy sauce and tamari don't have much in the way of isoflavones, though, even though they're also fermented.

Tofu is so popular today that you can find it in just about any supermarket—check the produce section. It's just as nutritious as meat, but when you eat tofu you get the soy isoflavones along with far fewer calories, almost no saturated fat, and a good dose of calcium. Soy milk is also easy to find in supermarkets. You can use the unflavored kind just like regular milk—drink it, put it on your breakfast cereal, or make it into a shake. The flavored versions are tasty and low in fat and calories. They're great on their own or in shakes.

> **Now You're Cooking**
>
> Soy protein powder, available at your health-food store, is another way to get the benefits of soy in your diet. Mix the powder with juice or use it in shakes and smoothies. As little as 30 to 40 g a day—roughly 3 to 4 tablespoons—may be enough to help your hot flashes.

To claim a soy food is heart-healthy, the FDA says it has to have at least 6.25 g of soy protein per serving. You'll see the claim on a lot of foods, but be wary. Soy burgers, soy hot dogs, soy cheese, and soy ice cream, which all taste a lot like the real thing, are very popular now. They're low in calories and fat, but these foods are highly processed and have a lot of additional ingredients, so they don't have much in the way of isoflavones left, even if they can claim they contain soy protein. Soybean oil, which is the primary ingredient in vegetable cooking oil, doesn't have many isoflavones, either.

How much soy do you need to eat to relieve menopause problems and get cancer protection? Most researchers believe that anywhere from 20 to 50 mg of soy isoflavones every day will help, depending on how severe your symptoms are. There are about 30 to 40 mg of isoflavones (about 80 percent of it genistein) in a typical serving of soy food. What's a typical serving? Half a cup of tofu or tempeh, one cup of soy milk, or a quarter cup of textured soy protein. Based on that, you don't really need to eat large servings of soy foods—just 12 ounces of soy milk a day could be enough to help cool off your hot flashes. You'll get the isoflavones along with lots of other useful nutrients, such as protein, calcium, boron, lecithin, folic acid, and omega-3 fatty acids—and you'll get additional protection against artery-clogging cholesterol.

Help from Herbal Hormones

Black cohosh and red clover are herbs that are traditionally recommended as natural treatments for menopause symptoms. A traditional Native American remedy, black cohosh has been extensively studied. In some but by no means all studies, a standardized extract (Remifemin) seems to help hot flashes. Black cohosh doesn't seem to have any effect on estrogen levels, so it's probably safe for women who are at risk for breast and endometrial cancer. If you want to try black cohosh, talk to your doctor first and choose a high-quality product from a reputable manufacturer. Some supplements sold as containing black cohosh are actually made with a cheaper related herb imported from China.

Red clover is another traditional Native American remedy. This herb contains isoflavones, so it may have an effect on your estrogen levels. The problem is that a number of studies have shown that taking red clover doesn't help hot flashes any more than taking a dummy pill does. Red clover is also recommended for men with benign prostatic hypertrophy (BPH). Here, too, dummy pills work as well.

I Yam What I Yam—Not

The original birth-control pills were made from a substance called diosgenin, first discovered in Mexican wild yam roots. Diosgenin is chemically similar to the female hormone progesterone, but there's no evidence that using a cream or tincture made from wild yam (also called Mexican yam) will help PMS or menopause symptoms. And wild yam is most definitely *not* an effective birth-control method. Despite the rumors, sweet potatoes contain no progesterone or estrogen, so you won't get any natural hormones by eating them. The confusion arises because we use the words *yam* and *sweet potatoes* interchangeably to mean the sweet, orange-colored tuber traditionally served at Thanksgiving. Scientifically, though, yams are the tuberous roots of a tropical vine in the *Dioscorea* family.

DHEA: Fountain of Youth or Hype?

You have two adrenal glands, each about the size of a grape. Your adrenals sit on top of your kidneys and produce a number of different steroid hormones. The hormone they make the most is *dehydroepiandrosterone*, or *DHEA* for short. Your body converts DHEA into other steroid hormones, including testosterone and estrogen, as you need them. For that reason, DHEA is sometimes called the "mother" hormone.

Studies suggest that people with high DHEA levels live longer and have less heart disease and cancer. Other studies hint that DHEA helps prevent Alzheimer's disease, autoimmune diseases such as lupus, osteoporosis, depression, chronic fatigue syndrome, and other problems. The ads for DHEA supplements promise that it builds muscle, burns fat, stimulates your sex drive, and, of course, slows aging. If you think this all sounds too good to be true, you're right. DHEA may have some genuine value, but it's not a fountain of youth or a cure-all. A lot of the studies that claim it can help with assorted health problems aren't very conclusive: they're too small, or they're only on lab animals, or they're seriously flawed in some other way.

Although we know that DHEA won't improve athletic performance or somehow restore your youthful energy levels, there is one intriguing study from 2004 that suggests it could help you lose weight. In a 6-month double-blind study of 56 elderly people, half took 50 mg DHEA supplements daily and half took dummy pills. The DHEA half lost abdominal fat and improved their insulin sensitivity; the dummy half had no change. Does this mean DHEA is the magic weight-loss drug we've been looking for? Not so fast—one study of 56 old folks is hardly conclusive, though that hasn't stopped the hype from unscrupulous supplement marketers.

Other Hormones

Several other over-the-counter natural hormones have been touted a lot recently. In fact, you can't open a health magazine these days without reading something about them. Let's home in on these hormones.

Androstenedione for Athletes

Androstenedione is the hormone slugger Mark McGwire says helped him hit his record-breaking 70 home runs in 1998. Did it? Well, andro (to use the short name that's much easier to type) does get converted by your body into testosterone, and there are some studies suggesting that taking andro can raise your testosterone level, which in turn can help you build more muscles if you work out a lot. On the other hand, other studies show it doesn't do anything positive and might be harmful, causing a serious drop in your HDL ("good") cholesterol, prostate enlargement, and breast enlargement in men. So, guys, unless you want to be called "Chesty" for the wrong reason, stay away. Another good reason to stay away from andro is that it was added to the federal list of banned anabolic steroids in 2004—using this hormone is now illegal.

Pregnenolone for Hormone Power

If DHEA, as previously discussed, is the "mother" hormone, then pregnenolone is the "grandmother." Your body makes this hormone from cholesterol. In an intricate series of steps, pregnenolone gets turned into all your steroid hormones, including androstenedione, DHEA, estrogen, progesterone, and testosterone. So, the reasoning goes, why take supplements of all those hormones? Why not just take extra pregnenolone and let your body convert it into the other hormones? That makes sense, as far as it goes. The problem is that there's no evidence taking extra pregnenolone actually does raise your levels of steroid hormones. There's also no evidence that pregnenolone helps Alzheimer's, menopause, rheumatoid arthritis, or memory loss. As with the other over-hyped, under-researched hormones, pregnenolone won't help you lose weight, feel more energetic, build muscle, or magically restore your body to its youthful glory.

Help from Human Growth Hormone

We can say without question that human growth hormone (hGH) is one hormone that definitely does help—and that there's plenty of scientific evidence in its favor. It's not a do-it-yourself hormone, however. Human growth hormone is made in labs. It can be obtained only by prescription, it has to be injected daily, and it's *extremely* expensive. The only medical reason for taking hGH would be if your levels of your own growth hormone (GH) were very low, as they can be in some elderly, frail people, and some children with diseases that cause stunted growth.

Because hGH is so expensive and needs a doctor's prescription, a lot of supplement manufacturers have been pushing formulas containing the amino acids arginine, ornithine, lysine, and glutamine. Your body needs these aminos, sometimes called precursors, to make its own growth hormone. There's no evidence, however, that taking the precursors does anything at all to raise your GH level. Some companies push an arcane assortment of precursor amino acids "stacked" together, claiming these will naturally help your body produce more growth hormone. They won't, but they will add to the stack of money the supplement makers have.

The Least You Need to Know

◆ Hormones are chemical messengers your body makes in your endocrine glands, including your pineal gland, adrenal glands, and sex organs.

◆ Hormones regulate your body and control many functions.

◆ The hormone melatonin controls your body's internal clock. Melatonin supplements can help you cope with insomnia from jet lag or shift changes.

◆ Soy isoflavones and soy foods such as tofu (bean curd) contain genistein and daidzein—plant estrogens that can help relieve hot flashes from menopause.

◆ Eating soy foods every day may help protect men and women from heart disease.

Chapter 28

Fiber: Moving Things Along

In This Chapter

- ◆ Needing fiber from your food
- ◆ Discovering the different kinds of fiber
- ◆ Learning about foods that are high in fiber
- ◆ Lowering your risk of heart disease with fiber
- ◆ Helping bowel problems with fiber
- ◆ Helping diabetes with fiber

You're giving yourself all sorts of good nutrition whenever you chomp through a juicy piece of fresh fruit or a nice, crunchy vegetable. You're getting vitamins, minerals, flavonoids, and antioxidants of all sorts. You're also getting one more fabulous nutritional benefit: lots of fiber.

What's so great about this stuff? Why do you hear about it all the time these days? It's because fiber has been shown to lower your cholesterol, cut your risk of a heart attack, and help prevent bowel problems. It's also very helpful for people with diabetes—it could even help you lose weight.

The best thing about fiber, though, is that it's in those same fresh fruits and vegetables we've been telling you about all through this book. It's just one more really good reason to eat them.

Why Fiber Is Fabulous

Back in the 1970s, two British doctors, Denis Burkitt and Hugh Trowell, were studying disease in Uganda. They realized that their patients got very few of the digestive problems the doctors often saw in their patients back in England. Their African
patients hardly ever had constipation, diverticulitis, colon cancer, or hemorrhoids.
They also hardly ever got fat or had diabetes. Their cholesterol levels were low and
they hardly ever had heart disease or high blood pressure. Why not? These patients
ate mostly unprocessed foods that were very high in dietary fiber. Because of that, they
had large and frequent bowel movements. The doctors drew the logical conclusion: a
high-fiber diet can help prevent certain diseases, especially the digestive problems that
people who eat a typical low-fiber, high-fat Western diet often get. Ever since, we've
been learning more and more about the importance of fiber in keeping you healthy.

How Much Fiber Is Enough?

In 2002, the Institute of Medicine created a DRI for fiber and determined the
Recommended Intake (RI) for individuals. As the following chart shows, it's pretty
much the same as the recommendations organizations such as the American Heart
Association, the National Institutes of Health, and the American Cancer Association
have been making for years. They all say that adults should aim for 20 to 30 g of
dietary fiber a day. Most of us get far less than that—the average American eats only
12 g of fiber a day.

The RI for Fiber

Age in Years/Sex	Fiber in g
Infants	
0 to 0.5	No data
0.5 to 1	No data
Children	
1 to 3	19
4 to 8	25
Boys 9 to 13	31
Girls 9 to 13	26

Age in Years/Sex	Fiber in g
Young Adults and Adults	
Men 14 to 50	38
Men 51+	30
Women 14 to 18	26
Women 19 to 50	25
Women 51+	21
Pregnant women	28
Nursing women	29

Insoluble and Soluble Fiber

Dietary fiber is a general term for the indigestible parts—mostly cell walls—of plant foods. There are basically two kinds of dietary fiber: insoluble and soluble.

Insoluble Fiber

Insoluble fiber is cellulose, the main fiber in the cell walls of all plant foods. Insoluble fiber absorbs water, but it doesn't dissolve in it. As we'll discuss a little further on, the ability to absorb water makes insoluble fiber very helpful for your colon and bowel problems. Bran of any sort is an excellent source of insoluble fiber.

Soluble Fiber

Most of the fiber in plant foods is soluble fiber of one sort or another. Soluble fibers dissolve in water to form a soft gel in your intestines. As the gel moves through your intestines, it can help a lot of health problems, including high cholesterol and diabetes (we'll explain how later). Here's a breakdown of the different kinds of soluble fiber:

- **Pectin.** If you've ever made jam, you know that pectin forms a gel. Pectin is found in all plant cell walls, but it's most abundant in the skins and rinds of fruits and vegetables. Apple peel, for example, is about 15 percent pectin.

- **Mucilage.** Sounds really gross, doesn't it? Mucilage is a general term for the gumlike soluble fiber found in seeds, beans, grains, and nuts. Guar gum is the most common mucilage. It's found in beans, and it's also widely used in processed foods as a thickener. Guar gum is used to make cream cheese, for example, and it's also used in salad dressings, ice cream, soup, and even toothpaste.

def•i•ni•tion

In any discussion of fiber, your bowel movements have to be mentioned. There are a lot of words for your body's solid waste, but because this is a family book we'll use the word **stool**.

Both soluble and insoluble fibers are important for your health. Insoluble fiber helps keep your *stool* soft, bulky, and easy to pass, so you have regular bowel movements and avoid some problems of the large intestine—possibly including colon cancer. Insoluble fiber also may help prevent heart attacks. Soluble fiber can help lower your blood cholesterol, remove wastes and toxins from your body, and help you control your blood sugar if you have diabetes. (We'll talk more about the health benefits of different kinds of fiber later in this chapter.)

Eating More Fiber

Imagine yourself eating six chocolate-chip-pecan cookies in a row. All too easy, isn't it? Now imagine yourself eating six apples in a row. Impossible. The sugar in fruit satisfies your sweet tooth, while the fiber in it fills you up quickly—with far fewer calories and none of the fat from cookies or candy. (Actually, because fiber is by definition indigestible, it doesn't really have any calories at all.) This chart gives you the fiber and calorie counts for some favorite fruits and vegetables. All plant foods—fruits, veggies, nuts, grains, and seeds—contain both soluble and insoluble fiber in varying amounts.

The Fiber in Fruits and Vegetables

	Serving Size	Calories	Fiber in Grams
Fruits			
Apple, with skin	1 medium	81	3.0
Applesauce	½ cup	97	1.5
Banana	1 medium	105	1.8
Blueberries	1 cup	82	3.3
Cherries	10	49	1.1
Kiwi	1 medium	46	2.6

	Serving Size	Calories	Fiber in Grams
Nectarine	1 medium	67	2.2
Orange	1 medium	65	2.3
Peach	1 medium	37	1.4
Pear	1 medium	98	4.3
Raisins	⅔ cup	296	5.3
Strawberries	1 cup	45	3.9
Vegetables			
Broccoli	½ cup	22	2.0
Brussels sprouts	½ cup	30	3.4
Carrots	½ cup	35	1.5
Cauliflower	½ cup	12	1.2
Chickpeas	1 cup	269	5.7
Corn kernels	½ cup	89	3.0
Green beans	½ cup	22	1.1
Kidney beans	1 cup	225	6.4
Lima beans	1 cup	217	13.5
Lettuce, iceberg	1 leaf	3	0.2
Lettuce, romaine	½ cup	4	0.5
Navy beans	1 cup	259	6.6
Parsnips	½ cup	63	2.1
Peas	½ cup	67	2.2
Potato, with skin	1 medium	220	3.3
Spinach	½ cup	21	2.0
Sweet potato, with skin	1 medium	118	3.4
Tomato, raw	1 medium	26	1.6
Turnip	½ cup	14	1.6
White beans	1 cup	253	7.9

Note: Fiber content in vegetables assumes food is lightly steamed or baked.

It's not that hard to add 5 or 10 g of fiber to your ordinary diet every day. Look at what you eat for lunch, for instance. One slice of ordinary white bread has much less than 1 g of fiber, while a slice of whole-wheat bread has 1.6 g. Just switching to whole-wheat instead of white bread for your sandwich adds about 2 g of fiber. Have an apple instead of (or along with) some cookies and you add another 3 g—now you're up to 5 g without even noticing! You can easily find other ways to add fiber to your diet. If you do, you may discover one of the unsung benefits of fiber. As you eat more high-fiber foods, you'll probably lose weight, gradually and painlessly, because you'll feel full sooner. You lose weight because you're eating fewer calories, but you don't feel hungry or deprived.

Food for Thought

According to a 1999 study in the *Journal of the American Heart Association*, people who rank in the top 20 percent in terms of fiber intake weigh on average 8 pounds less than those in the lowest 20 percent.

As you add more fiber to your diet, you may have some problems with gas, bloating, and diarrhea. To avoid this, don't suddenly start eating a lot more fiber. Instead, add it to your diet gradually—one extra piece of fruit a day, for example. If you have any discomfort, cut back until the problem stops, then gradually begin adding more fiber again. It could take you a couple of months to get up to 30 g a day without any unpleasant or embarrassing side effects.

Which Type of Fiber?

Food labels today list the amount of fiber per serving, but they don't always break it down by type. The fiber in most plant foods is about 35 percent insoluble fiber and about 45 percent soluble fiber (the rest is miscellaneous other stuff). In general, you don't need to think too much about the type of fiber because plant foods always have some of each kind. As a rough guide to the best sources of insoluble and soluble fiber, though, take a look at the following table.

Good Sources of Fiber

Insoluble Fiber	Soluble Fiber
Artichokes	Apples
Broccoli	Carrots
Carrots	Cauliflower
Dried beans and peas, cooked	Citrus fruits

Insoluble Fiber	Soluble Fiber
Nuts	Corn
Parsnips	Dried beans, cooked
Popcorn	Lentils
Potatoes, with skin	Oat bran
Seeds	Oatmeal
Sweet potatoes, with skin	Pears
Wheat bran	Rice bran
Whole grains	Sweet potatoes

Food for Thought

Not all "high-fiber" breakfast cereals, breakfast bars, and snacks are as good for you as they seem. Some of these cereals contain added oil and sugar and don't really have much in the way of whole grains—although they do have a lot of calories. Likewise, some breakfast bars and granola bars are very high in calories from fat and sugar but low in fiber. Read the labels carefully and don't be fooled by labels that say "natural." These products can be just as full of sugar and fat as the others.

Federal regulations now allow food producers to make claims for the health benefits of fiber on the labels. To claim that a food is "high-fiber," it must contain at least 5 g or more per serving. These foods must also meet the definition for low fat (3 g or less per serving), or the level of total fat must appear next to the high-fiber claim. To claim that a food is a "good source of fiber," it must contain 2.5 to 4.9 g per serving. To claim that a food has "more" or "added fiber," it must have at least 2.5 g more fiber per serving than that food would ordinarily have.

What about all those food packages announcing that they contain whole grains? Well, whole grains are an excellent way of getting more fiber into your diet, but so far there's no official FDA or USDA definition of what a food high in whole grains is. This may well change over the next few years, however, as the benefits of whole grains become clearer.

Fiber Supplements

It's not always easy to get enough fiber from your food. Sometimes you may want to take a fiber supplement to make sure you're getting enough. Fiber supplements are also useful if you're suffering from constipation and some colon problems.

Fiber supplements come in several different forms. The most popular is a powder (you have a choice of flavors) made from psyllium. There are about 3.4 g of soluble fiber in 1 rounded teaspoon (7 g) of *psyllium powder*. Psyllium also comes in capsules and in chewable wafers. Each dose has about 3 g of fiber. You can also buy psyllium seeds in your health-food store. They're often called flea seeds or natural vegetable powder. Flaxseeds are another good natural-fiber supplement.

def•i•ni•tion

Psyllium powder is actually the husks of tiny seeds from the plantago plant. Also called plantain, this is the same weed that grows on your lawn. It's available in any drugstore. Metamucil is a popular brand; generic brands are also available.

Other fiber supplements are made from calcium polycarbophil (Equalactin, FiberCon) or methylcellulose (Citrucel). They, too, come in a variety of forms and flavors. Of all the supplements, though, doctors recommend psyllium the most because it's the least likely to cause gas or diarrhea.

To use the powder, flea seeds, or flaxseeds, stir a teaspoon or so into eight ounces of water or juice and drink it down immediately before it gets too sludgy. If you use the capsule or wafer form, you must immediately drink eight ounces of liquid. If you don't, the fiber will swell up in your stomach and could form a blockage.

Warning!

Don't use fiber supplements in pill form if you have any sort of problem with your esophagus!

Most people find they get the most predictable benefit from fiber supplements if they take them in the early evening—you should see results in about 12 to 24 hours. Don't use a larger dose or take fiber supplements more than three times a day unless your doctor recommends it. As with any fiber, taking too much could cause gas, bloating, or diarrhea. If fiber supplements cause problems for you, cut back on the dose until the problem goes away, and then gradually increase the dose.

Do fiber supplements keep you from absorbing vitamins and minerals in your intestines? We're not sure. To be on the safe side, take your vitamin and mineral supplements at a different time from your fiber supplements.

Now You're Cooking
Juice is a great way to get extra fiber—but only if you make your own. Commercial juices have the fiber strained out. Home juicing machines remove some of the fiber, but a lot of it stays in the juice. If you want, you can stir the removed fiber back in before drinking the juice.

Water, Water Everywhere

We can't stress the importance of water enough. Every single cell in your body has water in it—in fact, half your body is nothing but water. Your kidneys and large intestine are responsible for conserving the water you take in from your food and drink, but you lose a lot of water when you breathe and in your sweat, urine, and stool. If you don't drink enough water, your large intestine will try to make up the difference by absorbing more from your stool—and that leads to constipation and other bowel problems.

In 2002, the Institute of Medicine came out with a DRI for total water. By total water they mean all water contained in food, beverages, and drinking water, so the table below doesn't mean that you need to drink the recommended amount of water—the liquid you get from your food and other beverages also counts toward the Recommended Intake (RI).

The RI for Total Water

Age in Years/Sex	Total Water in Liters Per Day
Infants	
0 to 0.5	0.7
0.5 to 1	0.8
Children	
1 to 3	1.3
4 to 8	1.7
Boys 9 to 13	2.4
Girls 9 to 13	2.1

continues

The RI for Total Water   (continued)

Age in Years/Sex	Total Water in Liters Per Day
Young Adults and Adults	
Men 14 to 18	3.3
Men 19+	3.7
Women 14 to 18	2.3
Women 19+	2.7
Pregnant women	3.0
Nursing women	3.8

Note: One liter equals 0.95 quarts.

Fiber in your intestines absorbs a lot of water and carries it out of your body. There's a lot of water in fresh fruits and vegetables, but you still need to be sure you're drinking enough as you increase your fiber intake.

Fiber and Heart Health

People who get plenty of fiber in their diet are less likely to have heart disease. The evidence for this is strong—it's based on numerous very solid studies. What's most interesting about the studies is that it doesn't take much extra fiber to get the heart-healthy benefits. Overall, the people in the studies who got the most fiber (more than 20 grams a day) had significantly less heart disease than those who got the least fiber. In one study of older women, the highest intake was only eight grams more than the lowest intake—that's the amount in just one serving of a high-fiber breakfast cereal. In a study of middle-aged and older men, the ones who got the most dietary fiber from whole-grain foods had an 18 percent lower risk of heart disease than those who got the least. And in a major 2004 analysis of 10 studies that looked at dietary fiber and the risk of heart disease, the researchers found that every 10 gram increase in fiber led to a 14 percent decrease in the risk of having a heart attack and a 27 percent decrease in the risk of dying from heart disease. Likewise, a 2005 analysis of 24 studies that looked at fiber and high blood pressure showed that adding fiber to your diet helps lower blood pressure, especially if it's already high.

It's Official: Oatmeal Lowers Cholesterol

In 1997, the FDA decided that oatmeal makers could make this health claim on their packages: "May reduce the risk of heart disease." That's because eating oatmeal, oat bran, or foods that are high in oats helps lower your cholesterol. Most important, it lowers your LDL ("bad") cholesterol without also lowering your HDL ("good") cholesterol. How do oats accomplish this miracle? Through their unique soluble fiber. Here's why. Your liver uses cholesterol to make digestive juices called bile acids. The bile is squirted out from your gall bladder into your small intestine to help you digest your foods, especially fats. If you eat a low-fiber diet, a lot of the bile acid gets reabsorbed into your blood through your intestinal wall. Because bile acids have a lot of cholesterol in them, that can raise your blood cholesterol level. If you could keep the bile acids from being reabsorbed, your cholesterol would go down. That's exactly what oats do. Oats are full of a soluble fiber called beta glucan. When you eat oat bran, oatmeal, or oat flour, the soluble fiber forms a gel that traps the bile acids and carries them out of your body. Your liver reacts to all this by making more bile acids. To do that, it pulls cholesterol out of your blood. Because you're not reabsorbing the cholesterol from your bile acids, and because you're also using up blood cholesterol to make more of them, your cholesterol level drops.

> **Now You're Cooking**
>
> To claim that it helps lower cholesterol and prevent heart disease, an oat food must contain at least 0.75 g of soluble fiber in a serving. You need to eat at least 3 g a day of soluble fiber to lower your cholesterol.

If your cholesterol is on the high side, try having any sort of oat cereal for breakfast (see the following table for the fiber in some popular choices). After a few months of devoted oatmeal-eating, you could see a real drop in your cholesterol level. If you also eat a lot of beans, it could drop even further. And if your cholesterol is only borderline high (200 to 240 mg/Dl), lowering it by just 10 percent could cut your risk of a heart attack by 50 percent.

The Fiber in Oat Cereals

Cereal	Serving Size	Fiber in Grams
Cheerios	1¼ cup	2.0
Honey Bunches of Oats	⅔ cup	1.6
Oat bran, cold	½ cup	3.0

continues

The Fiber in Oat Cereals   (continued)

Cereal	Serving Size	Fiber in Grams
Oat bran, cooked	⅓ cup dry	4.2
Oat Flakes	⅔ cup	2.1
Oat Squares	½ cup	2.4
Oatmeal, instant	1 packet	2.0
Oatmeal, quick	1 cup	2.7
Oatmeal, rolled	1 cup	3.0

Food for Thought

In a major recent study of male health professionals, the men who ate the most fiber had the lowest risk of heart attack. Interestingly, it was insoluble fiber that seemed to provide the most protection against a heart attack—the amount of soluble fiber the men ate didn't seem to matter. The lesson? Eat a variety of fruits and vegetables to get both kinds of fiber.

Oatmeal for Breakfast

Oatmeal is an inexpensive and delicious way to get more fiber into your diet. One reason oats are such a good choice is that only the inedible outer hull of the oats is removed in processing. The oat bran stays on the kernel, so you always get some bran whenever you eat oat foods. The oatmeal shelf at the supermarket can be a little confusing. Here's a rundown:

◆ **Steel-cut oats.** The most expensive kind, these are oat grains that have been cut very roughly. They take a long time to cook (20 to 30 minutes—plus you have to stir them a lot), but the extra-chewy, nutty flavor is worth it. Tip: save some money by buying your steel-cut oats in bulk at a health-food store.

◆ **Rolled oats.** Also called "old-fashioned" oats, these are the oats that come in the familiar round carton. You can also buy "table-cut" oats in bulk at health-food stores. To make these oats, raw oats are steamed, rolled into flakes, and dried. Rolled oats cook in just 5 minutes; table-cut oats take a few minutes longer.

◆ **Quick oats.** Basically the same as old-fashioned oats, but the flakes are rolled thinner so the oats cook faster. They have slightly less fiber, but take only 3 minutes to cook.

◆ **Instant oats.** These oats are flaked into such tiny pieces that all you have to do is add boiling water and stir. The processing reduces the fiber content a little, but the real problem is that these products almost always have added sugar and artificial flavorings.

There are only 145 calories in a bowl of oatmeal, but the traditional toppings of sugar and cream add a lot of calories. Skip them and get an extra nutrition boost by topping your morning oatmeal with some sliced fresh fruit, wheat germ, raisins, dried fruits, or nuts.

> **Now You're Cooking**
>
> Oatmeal isn't just for breakfast. Try using rolled oats instead of bread crumbs—in meat loaf or on top of fruit crisps, for example. With a little experimentation, you can oat up breads, muffins, cookies, and even pancakes.

Fiber and Colon Cancer

For a long time, it was just a given that a high-fiber diet would help prevent colon cancer. Then, in 2000, a four-year study looked at whether a high-fiber diet could keep polyps in the colon, which can lead to cancer, from coming back in people who had already had some removed. It turned out that the high-fiber diet didn't help—and this result was confirmed in 2005 by a study that combined the results of 13 other studies. Does that mean you can go back to cheeseburgers and fries and skip the salads? Nope. The truism turns out to be wrong, but as the heart studies we talked about earlier show, there are still plenty of good reasons to eat lots of fiber.

Help for Bowel Problems

In this section we talk about your bowel movements. The only way to do that is to speak frankly, but if that embarrasses you, feel free to skip ahead to the next section.

Let's start with constipation. Constipation ("irregularity") happens when you have fewer bowel movements than normal for you, or when your stool is hard, dry, and difficult to pass. Too little fiber in your diet is almost always the culprit here. If you gradually increase your daily fiber intake to 30 grams a day, and also increase your water intake, your constipation problems will almost certainly disappear. That's because insoluble fiber helps give bulk to your stool and keeps water in it; soluble fiber forms gels that soften the stool. In combination, they help you form a large stool that's easy to eliminate. If you eat plenty of fiber each day, you'll be able to go regularly and have a full and complete bowel movement with no trouble at all.

def•i•ni•tion

Hemorrhoids (also called "piles") are a very common problem—some 25 million Americans have them. A hemorrhoid happens when a vein in your rectum (the last portion of your digestive tract) becomes swollen, itchy, and painful—in severe cases, it may bleed. Hemorrhoids are almost always a result of straining during bowel movements.

Straining for a bowel movement is one of the major causes of *hemorrhoids*—enlarged veins in and around your anus. By eating more fiber, you'll pass your stool easily and quickly. That helps keep hemorrhoids from getting started. If you already have them, it keeps them from getting worse. And if you're having a painful flare-up, you may need to use a fiber supplement containing psyllium—the soluble fiber will make your stool much easier to pass. If you have hemorrhoids, talk to your doctor about eating more fiber, drinking more water, and other self-help steps you can take.

Fiber can also help diarrhea by slowing down the time it takes for food to pass through your intestines. Diarrhea is the frequent passing of loose, watery stools. It's often caused by eating something that disagrees with you, overeating, or by a stomach bug or stomach flu. Fiber often helps soak up the liquid and slow things down. If you've got a stomach bug that's giving you diarrhea, go for the soluble fiber, especially pectin. Pears, bananas, blueberries, and apples (grate them with the peel) are good choices. On the other hand, the sorbitol (a type of sugar) in high-pectin fruits and juices causes diarrhea for some people, so be cautious. If your diarrhea doesn't go away in a few days, call your doctor.

A number of other serious bowel problems, including Crohn's disease, ulcerative colitis, diverticulitis, and irritable bowel syndrome, are helped a lot by fiber. If you have any of these bowel problems, discuss dietary fiber and fiber supplements with your doctor before making any changes.

Food for Thought

A traditional Scandinavian remedy for diarrhea is dried blueberries (check your health-food store). Soak a teaspoonful of the berries in one cup of boiling water until the berries are softened, about five minutes. Drink the liquid and then eat the berries. Repeat three to seven times daily for up to three days. Most doctors recommend a few days on the BRAT diet: bananas, rice, applesauce, and toast. Drink plenty of plain water, mild tea or herbal tea, or diluted fruit juice (the sugar in undiluted juice could make the diarrhea worse). Avoid milk and carbonated drinks.

Beneficial Bacteria

Fiber also helps you keep a good balance of friendly bacteria in your colon. It's perfectly normal to have literally trillions of bacteria in your colon. Most of the bacteria are beneficial, but sometimes the unfriendly ones can get the upper hand, especially if you've been taking antibiotics. When that happens, you can start having problems with cramps, diarrhea, gas, and other bowel upsets. A low-fiber diet makes it easier for the unfriendly bacteria to take hold. Eating more fiber makes conditions in your colon ideal for the friendly bacteria and not so great for the unfriendly ones. The friendly bacteria multiply faster and crowd out the bad guys—and the balance tips back in your favor.

Sometimes the bad bacteria can really take hold, though, and don't want to give up. If you have frequent gas and bloating and alternating diarrhea and constipation, along with general feelings of tiredness or depression, it could be because an overload of unfriendly bacteria is giving off waste products that make you feel sick. Just getting more fiber may not help. In mild cases, sometimes just eating live-culture yogurt, which contains beneficial acidophilus bacteria, will help restore a better balance. (Look for live-culture yogurt in your health-food store—commercial brands don't have live bacteria.)

In more severe cases, you may need to take supplements of beneficial bacteria to help the good guys get back in charge. Three good guys are especially helpful: acidophilus, bifidobacteria, and boulardii. The usual dose for a mild overgrowth of bad bacteria is 1 to 2 g (about ½ teaspoon) of acidophilus and 250 mg (about ⅛ teaspoon) of bifidobacteria, mixed with 3 ounces of cold water. Also swallow one or two 300-mg capsules of boulardii. Take it all on an empty stomach. For a more severe overgrowth, you may need to increase the doses to up to 10 g of acidophilus, 6 g of bifidobacteria, and up to 6 boulardii capsules, spread out over the day before meals. Clearing up the problem could take several weeks or even longer.

To help the good bacteria get a foothold in your colon, you can also take supplements containing *fructooligosaccharides* (*FOS*). These provide a sugary fuel for the good guys. FOS comes as a syrup or powder you can use as a sweetener on foods or stir into drinks. Start with 1 g a day and gradually work up to 3 or 4 g daily.

def•i•ni•tion

> **Fructooligosaccharides** (FOS) are natural sugars that help feed beneficial bacteria. Small amounts of FOS are found in honey, garlic, and artichoke flour. Supplements of syrup or powder are much more concentrated—they contain 95 percent FOS.

Fiber for Diabetes

Eating a high-fiber diet—at least 30 g a day and preferably 50—can help people with diabetes better control their blood sugar. This seems to work because soluble fiber—especially the guar gum in beans—slows down your digestion of carbohydrates. If the carbs enter your bloodstream more slowly, your blood sugar doesn't jump up as sharply after you eat a meal. If you have diabetes, eating more fiber may help even out your blood sugar highs and lows and improve your A1C number (a measure of blood sugar over several months). It may also help improve your cholesterol levels. The National Diabetes Association now recommends a high-fiber diet of at least 8g soluble fiber and 16g insoluble fiber for all people with diabetes. If you have diabetes, discuss adding fiber to your diet with your doctor before you try it.

The Least You Need to Know

◆ Dietary fiber is found in all plant foods, including fruits, vegetables, beans, whole grains, nuts, and seeds.

◆ Soluble fiber forms a soft gel in your colon. Insoluble fiber absorbs water in your colon. Plant foods contain both kinds of fiber.

◆ Most people eat too little fiber. Many doctors now recommend 30 g of fiber a day.

◆ Eating more fiber can help lower your cholesterol and prevent heart attacks.

◆ A high-fiber diet can help prevent digestive and bowel problems.

◆ Eating more fiber helps people with diabetes control their blood sugar better.

Chapter 29

Natural Pain Relief

In This Chapter

- ◆ Helping pain with natural treatments
- ◆ Relieving arthritis pain the natural way
- ◆ Helping relieve aches and pains
- ◆ Helping relieve migraines

You know that old expression, "No pain, no gain?" Well, forget it. When it comes to the pain of arthritis and migraine headaches, there's no need to suffer. In this chapter, we discuss supplements that can not only relieve pain, but also help fix the underlying problem that causes the pain. Best of all, these remedies work without the side effects of conventional pain medication. They're gentler and safer—but they're not always fast-acting. For sudden or severe pain, talk to your doctor. It's important to know what's causing the pain before treating it.

Arthritis: The Unavoidable Ache

It's a sad fact of life: live long enough, and you're almost certain to get *arthritis*—pain and inflammation (swelling) in one or more of your joints. There are more than 170 types of arthritis, but the most common by far is *osteoarthritis.* Nearly two thirds of all Americans in their 60s and 70s have osteoarthritis of the knees, for example. In all, this form of arthritis affects anywhere from 16 to 20 million adults in the United States.

def•i•ni•tion

Arthritis (sometimes also called *rheumatism*) is a general term for pain and swelling in a joint. The word comes from the Greek *arthro,* meaning "joint," and *-itis,* meaning "inflammation" (pain and swelling). **Osteoarthritis** is the most common form of arthritis. If you have osteoarthritis, the *cartilage* that lines and cushions your joints gradually deteriorates, causing pain, swelling, and stiffness. **Cartilage** is the super-smooth, tough tissue attached to the ends of your bones. It forms your joints and cushions your bones.

The first-line medical treatment for osteoarthritis is nonsteroidal anti-inflammatory drugs (NSAIDs) such as aspirin, acetaminophen (Tylenol), ibuprofen (Advil), and naproxen (Aleve). These drugs, both over-the-counter and by prescription, relieve arthritis symptoms, but are also very likely to have nasty side effects, including stomach ulcers and intestinal bleeding. In 1999, a new group of prescription NSAIDs called COX-2 inhibitors was approved. These drugs, including celecoxib (Celebrex), work about as well as older NSAIDs, but are less likely to cause stomach upsets, gastritis, and ulcers—at least when taken regularly for less than six months. COX-2 inhibitors have been implicated in some cases of heart attacks, however, and they're also on the expensive side, so doctors today prescribe them cautiously. Many NSAIDs affect your ability to absorb folic acid, so if you take these drugs, consider taking a supplement. (For other good reasons, check back to Chapter 9.)

Ulcers and heart attacks aside, the real problem with NSAIDs is that they don't do anything to solve the underlying cause of arthritis. They do relieve the pain, stiffness, and swelling caused by damaged cartilage; however, the damage is not only still there, but it will also gradually get worse. In fact, the NSAIDs may actually damage arthritic joints further by blocking your body's natural repair process for cartilage. In addition, long-term use of these drugs can cause kidney disease.

Glucosamine: Help for Arthritis

There's a better way to help osteoarthritis: a safe, nonprescription dietary supplement called glucosamine sulfate. Here's how we think it works. Your body normally builds up and breaks down your cartilage. It's a complex process, and for reasons we don't have space to go into here, you need glucosamine sulfate as one of the raw materials.

Taking glucosamine supplements seems to give your body the crucial raw material it needs to repair damaged cartilage. The supplements also seem to stimulate the repair process.

Glucosamine doesn't always work for everyone, and it can take a few weeks to start kicking in, but many arthritis sufferers call it a wonder drug. Their pain and stiffness improve markedly, and they can sometimes cut back on or even stop the powerful drugs they've been taking for pain and swelling. Several studies have shown that glucosamine works as well as NSAIDs such as ibuprofen and piroxicam (Feldene), and

an important study in 1999 showed that glucosamine can definitely protect your joints. In 2006, the long-awaited results of a major study, the Glucosamine/Chondroitin Arthritis Intervention Trial (GAIT), were released. The study showed that glucosamine with chondroitin (we'll explain that one a little further down) didn't help much more than a placebo for people with mild arthritis knee pain. But for people with moderate to severe pain, the combo helped quite a bit—nearly 80 percent of the participants got relief. They reported very few side effects.

Food for Thought

The best way to avoid osteoarthritis is to keep your weight down. Studies show that obesity is the single most important—and most preventable—risk factor for arthritis. The more you weigh, the more stress you put on weight-bearing joints, such as your knees and hips, and the faster the cartilage in those joints will break down.

No foods contain glucosamine, so if you want to try it you'll have to take supplements. These are made from chitin, the processed shells of shrimp, crabs, and lobsters; vegetarian versions of glucosamine are also now available. We strongly recommend glucosamine sulfate over other forms, because the sulfur is important for building cartilage. The usual dose is 500 mg two or three times a day, preferably with meals. Glucosamine is very safe and has no side effects. You can't overdose on it, but taking more than 1,500 mg a day won't help your arthritis more.

You'll probably have to take glucosamine for anywhere from three to six weeks before it really starts to kick in. It's okay to continue with NSAIDs while you're taking glucosamine—but you'll probably be able to lower your dose or even stop when you start feeling the improvement.

Glucosamine is even more effective if you're getting enough Vitamin C and manganese (see Chapters 13 and 21). And, as we'll discuss in the next section, it may work better if you combine it with another supplement called chondroitin.

Chondroitin: The Other Half

Just as the cartilage in your body naturally contains glucosamine, it also contains another substance called *chondroitin*. The role of chondroitin in your joints is complex. It helps protect your cartilage from enzymes that can damage it, and it also stimulates the production of new cartilage. Chondroitin seems to work synergistically with glucosamine to give you a one-two punch of cartilage protection. As with glucosamine, chondroitin supplements are very safe and have virtually no side effects.

What about all those products made from cow or shark cartilage that are supposed to help arthritis? They contain some chondroitin sulfate, and some people claim they work, but we're skeptical. Stick to combined glucosamine and chondroitin in a high-quality supplement from a reputable manufacturer.

ASU for Arthritis

An effective new supplement for arthritis called ASU (avocado soybean unsaponifiables) has come onto the market recently. Made from avocado and soybean oil, this supplement has been a prescription treatment for arthritis in France since the 1990s. In the United States it's a supplement you can buy on your own. The evidence for the effectiveness of ASU is based on serious studies and holds up well. The supplements are safe and have no side effects. If you want to try this one, take 300 mg daily. Just taking soybean or avocado oil won't help arthritis. Buy a high-quality product containing only pure ASU from a reputable manufacturer.

Not the SAMe Old Thing

The supplement SAMe (S-adenosylmethionine) is another effective natural treatment for arthritis. As with glucosamine and chondroitin, SAMe reduces pain and swelling just as well as NSAIDs, but without the side effects. One study suggests that 1,600 mg a day of SAMe works as well as 750 mg a day of naproxen (Aleve).

A lot of good studies support using SAMe to treat arthritis, but there's also one big problem: this stuff is very expensive. Not only that, but the doses needed are fairly high. In general, you need to take 1,200 mg a day for it to work.

If you decide to try SAMe, buy your supplements only from a reliable manufacturer. Independent testing has shown that some products said to contain SAMe either didn't have the amounts the labels claimed or had none at all!

Oiling the Joints

Remember the Tin Man in *The Wizard of Oz?* All it took to get his joints moving smoothly again was a few squirts from the oilcan. Well, it's not quite so simple for people with rheumatoid arthritis (RA), but solid evidence shows that fish oil and GLA can definitely help this very severe form of arthritis. (We discussed the basics of these essential fatty acids back in Chapter 23.)

The evidence is strongest for fish oil. Several good studies have shown that the omega-3 fatty acids in fish oil (but not flaxseed oil) reduce inflammation in people with rheumatoid arthritis. The doses needed are fairly large—about 6 g or more a day. These amounts are safe, although they may cause mild digestive upsets. It can take anywhere from 6 to 12 weeks for fish oil to take effect.

GLA, an essential fatty acid found in evening primrose oil, borage oil, and black-currant oil, may also help rheumatoid arthritis. The studies aren't as strong, but on the other hand, GLA is very safe and is less likely to upset your digestion than fish oil. If you want to try it, the usual dose is between 1.4 and 2.8 g daily. As with fish oil, it can take up to 12 weeks for the effects to be felt.

Healing Herbs for Aching Joints

There's hardly an herb that hasn't been recommended for arthritis at some point. Frankly, people with arthritis can get a little desperate. Why else would some of them believe that sitting in a former uranium mine soaking up the radiation would help their symptoms? (We're not making this up.) Most of the miracle herbs that are said to cure arthritis don't do much of anything to help. There are a few, however, that do offer some relief.

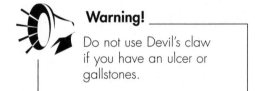

Warning! _____

Do not use Devil's claw if you have an ulcer or gallstones.

Devil's claw (*Harpagophytum procumbens*) is a plant found in South Africa. The name comes from the clawlike hooks that cover the plant's fruit. It's the large, thick roots of this plant that are used medicinally, however. Several studies have shown that devil's claw helps relieve the pain of arthritis safely, with no side effects. Unlike glucosamine, however, there's no evidence that devil's claw helps heal the damaged cartilage in the arthritic joint.

If you want to try devil's claw, look for a product that has been standardized to contain 3 percent iridoid glycosides. The usual dose is 750 mg three times a day.

At least some scientific evidence backs up the claims for these herbs:

◆ **Boswellia.** A gummy resin that comes from a tree found in India, boswellia may help relieve inflammation and may also protect your cartilage. The studies have been with patients suffering from rheumatoid arthritis, a severe form of arthritis. If you want to try it, look for an extract standardized to 37.5 percent boswellic acids. Take 400 mg three times daily.

◆ **Bromelain.** An enzyme found in pineapples, bromelain is approved by the German Commission E as a treatment for swelling and athletic injuries. Bromelain's anti-inflammatory properties may also be helpful for rheumatoid arthritis. The daily dose is anywhere from 1,200 to 1,800 mg a day. Although bromelain seems to be pretty safe at that dosage level, some researchers worry that it could cause bleeding problems if you take it with blood-thinning drugs such as warfarin (Coumadin), aspirin, or even ginkgo or high doses of Vitamin E.

◆ **Turmeric/curcumin.** Turmeric is a bright-yellow spice widely used in Indian cooking. Curcumin, the main component of turmeric, turns out to be a fairly powerful anti-inflammatory agent. It's widely used in India as a treatment for rheumatoid arthritis, although there aren't many studies to prove its effectiveness. The usual dose is 400 mg of curcumin three times daily. Don't use it if you have gallbladder trouble.

There's practically no evidence that the Peruvian herb cat's claw (*Uncaria tomentosa*) does anything for arthritis—and there's no evidence at all that it cures cancer or prevents pregnancy. Some of Dr. Pressman's arthritis patients have benefited from sea cucumber, but this doesn't seem to work for everybody.

How Do You Spell Relief?

Try DMSO, MSM, or CMO. We'll spell it out for you:

◆ **DMSO.** Dimethyl sulfoxide, or DMSO, is a very controversial supplement. It's been extensively studied for a wide variety of health problems, but the FDA has approved it for only one, the treatment of a painful bladder condition called interstitial cystitis. Professional sports trainers often use DMSO cream to treat sprains and aching joints.

- **MSM.** A close cousin of DMSO, methyl sulfonyl methane, or MSM, is a sulfur-containing compound (check back to Chapter 21 for more about why you need sulfur). MSM is found naturally in many foods, including milk, meat, seafood, and fruits and vegetables. On the basis of very little evidence, it's said to help relieve not just arthritis pain but also muscle aches, allergies, and inflammation in general. Does it? Well, it does seem to help some of Dr. Pressman's arthritis patients, but others don't seem to benefit. You need to take a fair amount—up to 3 g a day. (Doses much larger are safe.) MSM is said to help glucosamine work better, but again, there's no real evidence for this. If you want to try a combination formula, choose one from a reliable manufacturer.

- **CMO.** Cetyl myristoleate (CMO) is a mixture of a fatty acid and cetyl alcohol. A major European study in 1994 showed that it helped relieve pain and swelling in rheumatoid arthritis patients. The usual dose is two to four 100 mg capsules daily.

We need to spell something else out for you: these are unconventional treatments that should be used with caution. Talk to your doctor before you try them.

Managing Migraines

If you've ever had one, you know how painful and debilitating a migraine headache is. Some 26 million Americans, many of them young adult women, suffer from migraines at least occasionally. Prevention is a big part of managing migraines. As we discussed back in Chapter 6, taking supplements of this B vitamin is often very helpful for preventing migraines.

The herb feverfew is another helpful migraine preventive. A number of strong studies show that migraine sufferers who take feverfew leaves regularly have fewer headaches, and that the ones they do have are less severe. In some cases, patients who take feverfew stop having migraines altogether.

If you want to try feverfew for your migraines, talk to your doctor first. The usual daily dosage is 80 to 100 mg of powdered whole feverfew leaf in capsule form. You have to take it every single day for it to work. Don't take feverfew extract—parthenolide, the active ingredient in the extract, turns out not to be the beneficial ingredient of feverfew.

 Warning!

Do not use feverfew if you are pregnant or have liver or kidney disease. Do not give feverfew to young children.

An extract from the root of the butterbur plant may help reduce how often people get migraines, although it doesn't seem to help the headache itself that much. The studies on butterbur are limited, but this is a promising area that's now getting a fair amount of attention.

The Least You Need to Know

◆ Glucosamine and chondroitin can not only relieve arthritis pain, but also can help heal injured cartilage.

◆ The supplement SAMe is useful for relieving arthritis pain.

◆ Herbs such as devil's claw, boswellia, bromelain, and turmeric are also helpful for arthritis pain.

◆ The supplements DMSO, MSM, and CMO can be helpful for a variety of aches and pains.

◆ The herb feverfew is an effective treatment for migraine headaches.

Chapter 30

Smart Supplements

In This Chapter

- ◆ Staying smart as you age
- ◆ Learning about vitamins for the brain
- ◆ Having supplements for short-term memory
- ◆ Helping Alzheimer's the natural way
- ◆ Finding supplements for smarter kids

Have you reached the age where you can't always remember where you left the car keys? Have you started having a little trouble recalling the names of people? Do you sometimes find yourself staring into a closet and wondering what it was you were looking for? Is your forgetfulness starting to worry you a little bit?

Relax. Researchers still don't know why it happens, but mild short-term memory loss starts to hit just about all of us by the time we're 45 or so. But does that mean you have to spend the rest of your life searching for your reading glasses? No—find those glasses and read on.

I'll Never Forget Old What's His Name

Your short-term memory is exactly that: your ability to remember recent events, including things such as what you ate for breakfast, the phone number of someone you call fairly often, the title of a book you read last week, the date of your upcoming dentist visit, and so on. It's perfectly normal for your short-term memory to falter. One theory is that as we get older, we literally have less storage space left in our brains for details such as the names that go with new faces. (It's sort of like the baldness theory: only smart men go bald because grass doesn't grow on a busy street.)

Whatever the reason for mild short-term memory loss, there are some simple steps you can take to help you cope and keep the problem from getting worse. The simplest step of all? Write things down. Keep to-do lists, shopping lists, an appointment book, and so on. Two other steps are crucially important: good nutrition and exercise. As we'll discuss in the following sections, good nutrition from regular meals and enough vitamins are essential for maintaining mental alertness. And a number of recent studies have shown that regular exercise—both physical and mental—makes a big difference. Older adults who take regular walks have a sharply reduced risk of heart disease, stroke, and mental impairment. Older adults who stay mentally active by reading, taking classes, participating in social events, and so on also are healthier and smarter. And older adults who combine the two are the healthiest and smartest of all. Our advice? Eat well, take your vitamins, walk at least a mile a day, and keep your mind busy. (Maybe that walk should be to the library.)

Vitamins on the Brain

All through Part 1, we talked about the importance of vitamins for your brain. All the B vitamins, for instance, are crucial for keeping your brain functioning properly. And as you'll recall from our discussions in Chapters 4 through 12, you don't absorb the B vitamins all that well as you get older. A shortage of Bs can make you depressed and forgetful—symptoms that could be taken for senility. If you're not already taking a complete B-vitamins supplement, check back to these chapters and think again.

The antioxidant Vitamins C and E are also crucial for protecting your brain as you age. Your delicate brain cells need all the help they can get to fight off the effects of free radicals. High levels of these vitamins can help.

C for Comprehension

In 1998, researchers in Australia published the results of a four-year study of a group of retired people. The participants fell into three groups: those who didn't get much Vitamin C from their diets, those who got a lot of Vitamin C from their diets, and those who took Vitamin C supplements. At the start of the study, the participants were tested for their levels of cognitive function; they were tested again at the end. We bet you can guess who had the best results. You're right. After four years, the group that took Vitamin C supplements had 60 percent less mental impairment compared to the low Vitamin C group.

Excellent for the Aging Memory

Vitamin E has been shown to be particularly important for warding off memory loss. In an important 1999 study of nearly 5,000 people aged 60 and older, researchers found a strong connection between poor memory and low blood levels of Vitamin E. The lower the Vitamin E level, the more severe the memory loss problems were. In fact, in the group with the lowest Vitamin E levels, 11 percent had such poor memory that they had trouble preparing their meals and handling their money. Among the groups with the highest Vitamin E levels, only 4 percent had memory problems that severe. As we discussed back in Chapter 15, other studies have backed this up. Taking Vitamin E can help keep your brain function high.

Food for Thought

We can't stress enough the importance of good, nutritious meals on a regular basis for older adults. In the Vitamin E study we mentioned, 20 percent of the people who skipped meals or didn't eat enough food had serious memory problems. Among the people who ate regularly and took in enough calories, only 7 percent had memory problems.

Ginkgo: Skipping Those Senior Moments

One of the best-selling herbs on the market today is an extract made from the leaves of the ginkgo biloba tree. What makes this stuff so popular? Flavonoids. The flavonoids in ginkgo are safe, very powerful antioxidants that can boost your memory and mental alertness.

def•i•ni•tion

> **Cerebral insufficiency** is a general term for problems caused by poor blood circulation to your brain. It's most common in older people, where it often causes symptoms of senility such as memory loss, poor concentration, confusion, anxiety, and depression.

Ginkgo can also be very helpful for *cerebral insufficiency*, or poor bloodflow to your brain, and for poor circulation in your feet, legs, and hands. Ginkgo can also help some cases of male impotence by improving circulation to the penis.

Ginkgo's powerful antioxidant action is particularly good for squelching free-radical attacks on your cell membranes. In fact, some researchers think ginkgo can actually reverse free-radical damage to brain-cell membranes. And as we'll explain later in this chapter, ginkgo is being carefully studied as a treatment for Alzheimer's disease.

There have been literally thousands of studies showing the effectiveness and safety of ginkgo. In Europe, doctors are allowed to prescribe ginkgo—and they do. It's one of the most widely prescribed medicines in Germany, for example. In the United States, ginkgo is sold over-the-counter in pharmacies and health-food stores. Look for a standardized tablet or capsule that contains 24 percent flavone glycosides and 6 percent terpene lactones (the scientific terms for the active flavonoids in ginkgo). In a 40 mg gingko tablet, this might be listed as 9.6 mg of flavone glycosides and 2.4 mg of terpene lactones; the product might also be labeled GBE, for ginkgo biloba extract. Don't buy products that contain anything less—and make sure you buy them only from reputable manufacturers. Lab tests have shown that some producers cheat and use less ginkgo than they claim on the label.

The usual dose for cerebral insufficiency is 40 mg three times a day. This would also be a good dose for other circulatory problems. Doses of up to 240 mg a day are routinely prescribed in Europe for severe cases. A dose this high is generally safe. If you take any sort of blood-thinning drug such as aspirin or warfarin (Coumadin), however, talk to your doctor first.

A lot of people take anywhere from 40 to 120 mg of ginkgo daily as a preventive measure to keep their mental function high. Does this work? It sure does for us. If you try it, you'll probably find that it gives your short-term memory and overall alertness a definite boost.

Ginkgo can be helpful for situations in which you want to be mentally alert—before a big exam or interview, for example. A recent study in England found that taking a dose of 360 mg in the morning caused an all-day improvement in reaction times and short-term memory.

Ginkgo is very, very safe and is unlikely to cause any side effects. It works by improving the bloodflow through the tiny blood vessels of your brain, so you get more oxygen and other nutrients. As it improves circulation to your brain, though, you might get some dizziness or even a mild headache. To be on the safe side, start with smaller doses and gradually build up the amount over several weeks. It can take six weeks or even longer before you start to notice any improvement from taking ginkgo. Stick with it.

Food for Thought

Tinnitus, or ringing in the ears often accompanied by dizziness, is a fairly common problem among older adults. Several studies have shown that taking ginkgo regularly can reduce or even eliminate the symptoms.

PS: SOS for Aging Brains

Phosphatidylserine (PS) is a fatty substance found in all your cell membranes. It's involved in keeping the cell membranes, especially the ones in your brain, stable.

Because the membrane not only protects the cell but also controls what goes into it (such as nutrients) and what comes out of it (such as waste products), you can see why PS is so important.

PS is widely used in Europe, especially in Scandinavia and Italy, as a brain booster to improve short-term memory and overall alertness and a supplement to slow the mental decline of Alzheimer's disease. There's some pretty solid evidence to back this up, so you might want to give it a try.

def•i•ni•tion

Phosphatidylserine, or **PS** (pronounced *fos-fa-TIDE-ul-ser-een*), is a type of fat called a phospholipid. Your body manufactures PS from the B vitamins, particularly folic acid, cobalamin, and choline, so it's not an essential nutrient.

You can't raise your PS level through your diet—no food contains it in high enough amounts. You'll need to take supplements. The usual dose is 100 mg two or three times a day. PS supplements used to be made from cow brains. Because of the threat of disease, however, these supplements are no longer sold. Today PS supplements are generally made from soybean oil. PS is very safe even in large doses, although it may cause some mild stomach upset in a few people.

Right now there's a lot of interest in PS as a treatment for Alzheimer's disease. We'll talk about that in just a minute.

Carnitine for Cognition

The amino acid carnitine, in the form of acetyl-L-carnitine (ALC), is needed to produce the neurotransmitter acetylcholine, which in turn plays an important role in memory and overall cognitive ability. (See Chapter 22 for more about amino acids.) A number of studies have shown that ALC levels in your brain decline as you age. Will taking ALC supplements raise those levels up again and improve your memory? Quite possibly, especially if you also take PS supplements—the two seem to boost each other's effect.

ALC comes as a powder that you can stir into water or juice. The usual dose is 750 mg two or three times a day. We suggest taking a combination formula that contains both ALC and PS.

Natural Help for Alzheimer's Disease

Sadly, there's no cure for *Alzheimer's disease*. The most we can hope to do is slow it down and help the patient stay independent as long as possible. In 1997, medical researchers showed that there's an easy, inexpensive, and effective way to do exactly that: Vitamin E. In fact, high doses of Vitamin E work as well as the prescription drug selegiline (also called deprenyl or Eldepryl). The study, which appeared in the prestigious *New England Journal of Medicine*, showed that Vitamin E slowed the pace of the disease so much that the patients involved were able to delay entering a nursing home by about seven months.

def•i•ni•tion

Alzheimer's disease (AD) is a degenerative disease of the brain that causes the slow, progressive loss of memory and mental function. AD strikes mostly adults older than age 65; nearly half of all people in the United States older than age 85 suffer from it to some degree. About half of all the people in nursing homes are there because of AD.

In 1997, a serious study of ginkgo biloba as a treatment for Alzheimer's disease appeared in the *Journal of the American Medical Association*. The study showed that ginkgo biloba in the form of EGb (an extract made in Germany) slowed the progression of the disease in about a third of the patients. The dosage in the study was 40 mg three times a day over a year-long period—an amount that had no side effects and worked almost as well as the prescription drug tacrine (THA or Cognex). The researchers think that the antioxidant powers of gingko are probably responsible for the improvement.

Now You're Cooking

We don't recommend tea made from crushed ginkgo leaves—it's extremely bitter and you won't get very much of the active ingredients. To get the most from ginkgo, buy it in capsules or tablets standardized to 24 percent flavone glycosides and 6 percent terpene lactones. Skip products such as beverages and chewing gum that contain ginkgo—there's not enough of the active ingredients in them to have any effect.

Phosphatidylserine has been extensively studied as a treatment both for AD and for dementia in the elderly from other causes. The results suggest strongly that PS is quite helpful in slowing mental deterioration. The usual dose is 100 mg three times a day. The effects take several weeks to kick in. After a few months, the dose can be lowered to 100 mg daily for some patients. PS is generally safe even in large doses, but don't use it if you are also taking a prescription blood-thinning drug such as heparin or warfarin (Coumadin).

Food for Thought

Phosphatidylserine is a hot supplement today among bodybuilders and other athletes who work out intensely with weights. PS is said to help boost the benefits from a weight-training session and to help reduce muscle soreness afterward. There's not a whole lot of evidence for this, but if you want to try it, take 800 mg of PS daily.

Huperzine A and vinpocetine are two substances, for lack of a better word, that are touted as treatments for AD and memory decline. Huperzine A is a supplement made from club moss. It may come from a natural source, but Huperzine A is highly refined in the laboratory, to the point that it's basically a drug that works in very much the same way as the prescription drugs tacrine (Cognex) and donepezil (Aricept). Similar to these drugs, Huperzine A helps improve memory in patients with AD. But just because Huperzine A is sold as a dietary supplement and is basically safe doesn't make it something we recommend you use on your own. It's a drug and should be used only with a doctor's advice.

Vinpocetine is another "natural" drug—it's made from the leaves of the common periwinkle plant. In Europe, vinpocetine is a prescription drug that's quite effective for Alzheimer's. In the United States, vinpocetine is sold as a dietary supplement. As with Huperzine A, vinpocetine is highly processed and can't really be called anything but a drug. It's safe and effective, but again, use it only after consulting a doctor.

Supplements for Smarter Kids

Wouldn't it be great if you could give your kids a pill that made them get better grades? Well, it's not quite that simple, but there are two extremely important supplements that can help babies grow up to be smarter kids.

Human breast milk naturally contains two fatty acids, docosahexaenoic acid (DHA) and arachidonic acid (AA). When babies were fed formula supplemented with these fatty acids, they did better on standard tests of mental development than did the control group of babies that got just regular formula. The spread was pretty impressive—26 percent of the babies fed the fortified formula scored IQs higher than 115, compared to just 5 percent of those on the plain formula. The results of the study are very encouraging, but they're hardly a revelation—throughout Europe and Asia, DHA and AA have been routinely added to infant formulas for years. Could that be one reason these kids consistently do better than American kids on standardized math tests? But maybe not for much longer—in 2002 the FDA approved baby formulas that contain both AA and DHA.

DHA isn't just for kids, however. It's essential for brain development and mental functioning at all ages. In fact, a 1999 study in Japan showed that DHA supplements improve dementia symptoms in the elderly. Later studies in 2004 in the United States showed that DHA has a protective effect against Alzheimer's disease. The retina in your eye is high in DHA, so taking supplements may also be helpful for your eyesight.

Because DHA is actually an omega-3 fatty acid, you get some whenever you eat fish or take omega-3 supplements (check back to Chapter 23 for more information). Other dietary sources of DHA include eggs, red meat, and organ meats. If you're a vegan or vegetarian or limit your intake of these foods, you might be low on DHA; nursing mothers might be low as well. Even if you do eat foods high in DHA, taking supplements might be something to consider. DHA supplements are quite safe, even in large doses. For kids ages 6 through 12, the usual dose would be 100 mg daily, taken with food. Adults can take up to 300 mg daily. When buying DHA supplements, look for the Neuromins trademark on the label.

Food for Thought _____

Your brain is actually 60 percent fat—and DHA is the most abundant fat in your brain. (Remember this fact the next time someone calls you a fathead!) It's also the most abundant fat in breast milk, because babies need it to nourish their growing brains. DHA seems to be important mostly for connecting brain cells to each other and making sure the signals get through correctly. Because you have 10 *billion* nerve cells in your brain (roughly the same number of cells as there are stars in our galaxy, the Milky Way), you can see how important DHA is.

The Least You Need to Know

◆ Antioxidant vitamins such as Vitamin C and Vitamin E help protect your brain from free-radical damage as you age.

◆ Gingko biloba supplements are useful for improving your short-term memory.

◆ Phosphatidylserine is a valuable supplement that helps preserve brain function.

◆ Vitamin E, ginkgo, and phosphatidylserine are all valuable natural treatments for Alzheimer's disease.

◆ The supplement DHA is valuable for improving the brain power of infants and children—and it helps adults, too.

Quick Reference Chart of Ailments and Suggested Supplements

Problem	Supplement	Chapter
Acne	Zinc	19
Aging	Vitamin C	13
	Vitamin D	14
Allergies	Quercetin	25
	Vitamin C	13
Alzheimer's disease	Choline	12
	Ginkgo biloba	30
	Phosphtidyl serine	30
	Vitamin E	15
Anemia	Cobalamin	10
	Iron	21

continues

continued

Problem	Supplement	Chapter
Arthritis	ASU	29
	Chondroitin	29
	Devil's claw	29
	Fish oil	23 and 29
	Glucosamine	29
	MSM	29
	SAMe	29
Asthma	Magnesium	18
	Pyridoxine	8
	Quercetin	25
	Vitamin C	13
Breast cancer	Beta carotene	3
	Vitamin D	14
Cancer	Folic acid	9
	Selenium	21
	Vitamin A	3
	Vitamin C	13
	Vitamin D	14
	Vitamin E	15
Carpal tunnel syndrome	Pyridoxine	8
Cataracts	Lycopene	25
	Riboflavin	6
	Vitamin A	3
	Vitamin C	13
	Vitamin E	15
Cervical dysplasia	Folic acid	9
Chronic fatigue syndrome	Carnitine	22
	DHEA	27
Colds	Vitamin C	13
	Zinc	19

Problem	Supplement	Chapter
Colon cancer	Calcium	17
	Fish oil	23
	Folic acid	9
	Vitamin D	14
Constipation	Fiber	28
Depression	Cobalamin	10
	Folic acid	9
	Pyridoxine	8
	SAMe	22
Diabetes	Chromium	21
	Fiber	28
	Fish oil	23
	Magnesium	18
	Niacin	7
	Thiamin	5
	Vitamin C	13
	Vitamin E	15
	Zinc	19
Diabetic neuropathy	Lipoic acid	24
	Pyridoxine	8
Eyesight problems	Bilberry	25
	Lutein	25
	Vitamin A	3
Gallstones	Vitamin C	13
Gingivitis	Vitamin C	13
Heart disease	Beta carotene	3
	Calcium	17
	Carnitine	22
	CoQ_{10}	26
	Fish oil	23
	Folic acid	9

continues

continued

Problem	Supplement	Chapter
	Garlic	25
	Magnesium	18
	Pyridoxine	8
	Selenium	21
	Soy isoflavones	27
	Vitamin C	13
	Vitamin E	15
Hemorrhoids	Fiber	28
Herpes	Lysine	22
High blood pressure	Calcium	17
	CoQ_{10}	26
	Fish oil	23
	Magnesium	18
	Potassium	20
	Vitamin C	13
High cholesterol	Fiber	28
	Niacin	7
	Pantothenic acid	11
	Vitamin C	13
Immune system support	Arginine	22
	NAC	24
	Pyridoxine	8
	Vitamin A	3
	Vitamin C	13
	Vitamin E	15
Infertility	Vitamin C	13
	Vitamin E	15
	Zinc	19
Inflammatory bowel disease	Fish oil	23
	Vitamin D	14
Insomnia	Melatonin	27
	Tryptophan	22

Problem	Supplement	Chapter
Intermittent claudication	Niacin	7
	Vitamin E	15
Interstitial cystitis	DMSO	29
Jet lag	Melatonin	27
Kidney stones	Calcium	17
	Magnesium	18
	Pyridoxine	8
	Vitamin C	13
Macular degeneration	Bilberry	25
	Lutein	25
	Lycopene	25
	Vitamin A	3
	Zinc	19
Memory loss	Ginkgo biloba	30
	Phosphatidyl serine	30
	Vitamin C	30
	Vitamin E	15
	Zinc	19
Menopause	Soy isoflavones	27
Menstrual problems	Manganese	21
Migraines	Butterbur	29
	Feverfew	29
	Magnesium	18
	Riboflavin	6
Nail problems	Biotin	12
	Zinc	19
Night blindness	Bilberry	25
	Vitamin A	3
Osteoporosis	Boron	21
	Calcium	17

continues

continued

Problem	Supplement	Chapter
Osteoporosis	Magnesium	18
	Vitamin C	13
	Vitamin D	14
	Vitamin K	16
Parkinson's disease	CoQ$_{10}$	26
	DHEA	27
	Soy isoflavones	27
	Vitamin C	13
	Vitamin E	15
Pregnancy	Folic acid	9
Premenstrual syndrome (PMS)	Calcium	17
	Magnesium	18
	Niacin	7
	Pyridoxine	8
Prostate problems	Lycopene	25
	Vitamin D	14
	Zinc	19
Skin cancer	Pyridoxine	8
	Vitamin A	3
Skin problems	Biotin	12
	PABA	12
	Zinc	19
Stroke	Potassium	20
	Quercetin	25
	Tea	25
	Vitamin E	15
Thyroid problems	Iodine	21
Tinnitus	Ginkgo biloba	30
	Niacin	7
Wound healing	Vitamin C	13
	Zinc	19

Web Resources

Useful Websites

Today there are literally thousands of websites that provide information about medical conditions, nutrition, supplements, and much more. Many of these sites, however, offer a lot of distorted or outright wrong information or are thinly disguised ways to sell you unnecessary supplements. When you check out a health-related website, look for the Health on the Net Foundation (HON) logo. Sites that carry the logo subscribe to the strict HON Code of Conduct for medical and health websites. (Go to www.hon.ch for more information.)

Here's our list of 25 top health sites on the Web. It's as current and accurate as we could make it; but remember, the Web changes faster than we can keep up.

Website	Web Address
American Botanical Council	www.herbalgram.org
Ask the Dietitian	www.dietitian.com
drkoop.com	www.drkoop.com
Dr. Weil	www.drweil.com

continues

continued

Website	Web Address
Food and Nutrition Information Center	www.nal.usda.gov/fnic
Harvard School of Public Health Nutrition Source	www.hsph.harvard.edu/nutritionsource
Health and Age	www.healthandage.com
HealthAtoZ	www.healthatoz.com
Healthfinder	www.healthfinder.gov
HealthierUS.gov	www.healthierus.gov
Healthline with Dr. Alan Pressman	www.drpressman.com
HealthScout	www.healthscout.com
Institute of Medicine	www.iom.edu
InteliHealth	www.intelihealth.com
Linus Pauling Institute	www.lpi.oregonstate.edu/infocenter
MayoClinic	www.mayoclinic.com
MDChoice.com	www.mdchoice.com
MedlinePlus	www.nlm.nih.gov/medlineplus/
MyPyramid.gov	www.mypyramid.gov
National Center for Complementary and Alternative Medicine	nccam.nih.gov
National Institutes of Health	www.nih.gov
New York Online Access to Health (NOAH)	www.noah-health.org
Office of Dietary Supplements, National Institutes of Health	www.dietary-supplements.info.nih.gov
SupplementQuality.com	www.supplementquality.com
WebMD	www.webmd.com

Glossary

acetylcholine   A neurotransmitter made using choline.

adenosine   A flavonoid found in onions. It may be helpful for lowering cholesterol.

Adequate Intake (AI)   The minimal amount, determined by the Institute of Medicine, of a vitamin, mineral, or other nutrient needed by most individuals. AIs apply to nutrients for which data is insufficient to make a more specific recommendation.

adrenal glands   There are two adrenal glands, one on top of each kidney. The adrenal glands produce a number of steroid hormones, including DHEA.

ajoene   A flavonoid found in garlic that may help thin blood and prevent blood clots.

alpha carotene   A carotene found in red- and orange-colored foods. It is a powerful antioxidant.

alpha linolenic acid (LNA)   Omega-3 fatty acids found in plant foods, especially nuts, soybeans, canola oil, and flaxseed oil.

alpha tocopherol   The most active form of Vitamin E.

Alzheimer's disease (AD)   Degenerative disease of the brain that causes the slow, progressive loss of memory and mental function. AD strikes mostly adults older than age 65; nearly half of all people in the United States older than age 85 suffer from it to some degree.

amino acids   The building blocks of protein. Twenty-two amino acids are necessary for life. *See also* essential amino acid; nonessential amino acid.

anemia   A general term meaning that red blood cells either don't have enough hemoglobin or that there's a below-normal number of them.

anthocyanins   Flavonoids found in blue foods such as blueberries and grapes. They help protect eyes against free radicals.

antioxidants   Enzymes that protect the body by capturing free radicals and escorting them out of the body before they do any more damage.

arachidonic acid (AA)   A type of omega-6 fatty acid.

arginine   A nonessential amino acid helpful for boosting the immune system.

arthritis   General term for pain and swelling in a joint. The word comes from the Greek *arthro*, meaning "joint," and *-itis*, meaning "inflammation" (pain and swelling). *See also* osteoarthritis.

ascorbic acid   Another name for Vitamin C.

atheroma   Fatty deposit in an artery; the first stage of plaque.

atherosclerosis   Fatty deposits, called plaque, built up inside arteries, often an artery that nourishes the heart or leads to the brain.

aura   Warning sign of a migraine headache, usually occurring an hour or two before the headache strikes. The aura is usually visual—many people see flashing lights or zigzag patterns. Also called a prodrome.

B vitamins   A group of related water-soluble vitamins. *See also* biotin; choline; cobalamin; folic acid; niacin; PABA; pantothenic acid; pyridoxine; thiamin.

benign prostatic hypertrophy (BPH)   A condition caused by an enlarged prostate gland, which presses on the urethra and causes a need to urinate frequently.

beriberi   A deficiency disease caused by a lack of thiamin.

beta carotene   A carotene found in abundance in many red- and orange-colored plant foods. The body easily converts beta carotene into Vitamin A.

beta-cryptoxanthin   A carotene found in some plant foods such as oranges and peaches. It's also used to color butter.

biotin   A B vitamin made in the body by friendly bacteria in the small intestine.

boron   An essential trace mineral needed for bone growth.

bran   The thin inner husk of grains such as wheat, rice, and oats. A good source of soluble and insoluble fiber as well as minerals and vitamins.

butterbur   An herb that may help prevent migraine headaches.

caffeine   Alkaloid chemical found in many plants; mild stimulant that improves alertness and concentration.

calciferol   Another name for Vitamin D.

calcifidiol   Another name for Vitamin D_2, the form of Vitamin D received from foods or supplements.

calcitrol   Yet another name for Vitamin D_2, the form of Vitamin D received from foods or supplements.

calcium   The most abundant mineral in the body, needed to build bones and teeth, make some hormones and enzymes, make muscles contract, and other functions.

capsanthin   A xanthophyll found in red peppers.

cardiac arrhythmia   Irregular heartbeat.

carnitine   An amino acid useful for people with heart disease.

carotenes   Carotenoids found in many red- and orange-colored foods. The body can convert carotenes into Vitamin A. *See also* alpha carotene; beta carotene.

carotenoids   Orange- or red-colored substances found in many fruits and vegetables such as carrots. *See also* carotenes; xanthophylls.

cartilage   The super-smooth, tough tissue attached to the ends of your bones. It forms joints and cushions the bones.

catechins   Antioxidant flavonoids found in tea.

cerebral insufficiency   Poor blood circulation to the brain, causing senility, memory loss, and depression.

chelation   Treating minerals to change their electrical charge, usually by binding them chemically to an amino acid or other harmless substance. This helps the body absorb the minerals better.

chloride   An electrolyte mineral needed to control blood pressure and for other body functions.

cholecalciferol   The form of Vitamin D made in the body from sunshine. Also called Vitamin D.

cholesterol   A waxy fat the body uses to make cell membranes, the sheaths that cover the nerves, and hormones, among other things.

choline   A substance closely related to the B vitamins.

chromium   A trace mineral needed to help the body use glucose in cells.

circadian rhythm   A body's 24-hour internal clock.

clotting factors   Substances in blood that help it clot and stop bleeding.

cobalamin   A B vitamin, also known as Vitamin B_{12}.

cobalt   An essential trace mineral used to make cobalamin.

coenzyme   A substance, usually a vitamin or mineral, needed to complete an enzyme.

coenzyme Q_{10}   A coenzyme the mitochondria need to produce energy. Supplements can be helpful for people with heart failure.

collagen   A protein used to make the connective tissue that holds cells together and makes up the bones, tendons, muscles, teeth, skin, blood vessels, and every other part of the body.

constipation   Having fewer bowel movements than normal or having stools that are hard, dry, and difficult to pass. Also called irregularity.

copper   An essential trace mineral needed to make enzymes that are important for blood vessels and nerves.

Crohn's disease   A serious inflammatory disease of the large intestine.

cyanocobalamin   The form of Vitamin B_{12} used in vitamin pills.

cysteine   A sulfur-containing nonessential amino acid.

deficiency disease   Illness caused by a deficiency of a vitamin. Classic deficiency diseases include scurvy and beriberi.

DHA (docosahexaenoic acid)   A fatty acid found naturally in breast milk and important for brain development in infants.

DHEA (dehydroepiandrosterone)   A steroid hormone made in the adrenal glands. The body converts DHEA into other hormones.

diabetes   Inability to use glucose for fuel in cells, sometimes because the body no longer makes the hormone insulin, but more often because the cells have become resistant to insulin. *See also* Type 2 diabetes.

diabetic neuropathy   A complication of diabetes that causes numbness, tingling, and pain in the nerves of the feet and legs; it sometimes spreads to the nerves of the arms and trunk.

diarrhea   Frequent passing of loose, watery stools.

diastolic pressure   The blood pressure when a heart is at rest between beats—the lower number in the blood pressure reading.

dietary fiber   The indigestible parts—mostly cell walls—of plant foods. *See also* insoluble fiber; soluble fiber.

diosgenin   A phytoestrogen found in Mexican wild yam root. It resembles the female hormone progesterone and was used to make the first birth-control pills.

diuretic   A drug or herb that makes kidneys produce more urine. Diuretics remove water—and also some minerals and vitamins—from the body.

docosahexenoic acid (DHA)   Omega-3 fatty acids found in cold-water fish and available in supplement form.

Dietary Reference Intake (DRI)   The benchmark nutrient-based reference values set by the Institute of Medicine for use in planning and assessing diet and for other purposes. The DRI for a nutrient includes the Recommended Dietary Allowance (RDA) or Adequate Intake (AI) amount.

echinacea   Herb also sometimes called purple coneflower (*Echinacea angustifolia* and *E. purpurea*), used as an immune-system stimulant. Pronounced *eh-kin-AY-sha*.

eicosapentenoic acid (EPA)   Omega-3 fatty acids found in cold-water fish.

electrolytes   Minerals that dissolve in water and carry electrical charges. In the body, potassium, sodium, and chloride are the electrolyte minerals.

elemental calcium   The actual amount of usable calcium in a supplement. It's usually given on the label as a percentage of the total calcium in the supplement.

endocrine gland   A gland, such as the thyroid or testes, that makes hormones.

enzyme   A chemical compound the body makes from various combinations of proteins, vitamins, and minerals. Enzymes speed up chemical reactions in the body.

epithelial tissue   The tissue that covers the internal and external surfaces of the body. Skin, the linings of the eyes and nose, the entire digestive tract, lungs, urinary tract, and reproductive tract are all epithelial tissue.

ergocalciferol   The form of Vitamin D received from foods or supplements. Also called Vitamin D$_2$.

essential amino acid   One of the nine amino acids needed from food.

essential fatty acid   A fat needed from food. *See also* linoleic acid; linolenic acid.

estrogen   The main female hormone, made by the ovaries and uterus.

fat-soluble vitamin   A vitamin that dissolves in fat and can be stored in the body's fatty tissues. Vitamin A, Vitamin D, Vitamin E, and Vitamin K are fat-soluble.

fiber   *See* dietary fiber.

flavin adenine dinucleotide (FAD)   A riboflavin-containing enzyme needed by the mitochondria to release energy.

flavin mononucleotide (FMN)   A riboflavin-containing enzyme needed by the mitochondria to release energy.

flavonoids   Substances found in fruits and vegetables. Flavonoids give these foods their color and taste. Flavonoids are also powerful antioxidants. *See also* anthocyanins; carotenoids; catechins; quercetin.

fluoride   A trace mineral that helps prevent tooth decay.

folacin   An old-fashioned name for folic acid.

folate   The natural form of folic acid found in foods.

folic acid   The synthetic form of one of the B vitamins.

fortified milk   Milk that has Vitamin D and (sometimes) Vitamin A added to it.

FOS   *See* fructooligosaccharides.

free-form amino acids   Amino-acid supplements in their pure form, sold as a powder.

free radicals   Unstable, destructive oxygen atoms created by the body's natural processes and also by the effects of toxins such as cigarette smoke.

fructooligosaccharides (FOS)   Natural sugars found in honey, garlic, and artichoke flour that help nourish desirable bacteria in the large intestine.

functional medicine   Another term for orthomolecular medicine. Functional medicine works to restore the body to its proper functioning with vitamins, minerals, and other supplements.

gamma linoleic acid (GLA)   Omega-6 fatty acid found in evening primrose and borage seed oil.

glucosamine   An amino-acid sugar found in the shells of shrimp and lobsters. Glucosamine supplements can be helpful for arthritis.

glutamine   A nonessential amino acid useful for intestinal problems.

glutathione   The body's most abundant natural antioxidant enzyme.

goiter   A swollen thyroid gland forming a lump in the neck. It's caused by a shortage of iodine.

guar gum   A type of soluble fiber found in beans and also in grains, seeds, and nuts.

heart failure   A condition occurring when the heart is damaged or weak and can't pump blood efficiently.

heme iron   The iron found in hemoglobin.

hemoglobin   The oxygen-carrying protein that gives red blood cells their color. Every molecule of hemoglobin has four atoms of iron in it.

hemorrhoids   Itchy, enlarged, or swollen veins in the rectum. Also called piles.

herpes   A group of viruses. *Herpes simplex* type 1 causes cold sores. *Herpes simplex* type 2 causes genital herpes. *Herpes zoster* causes chicken pox and shingles.

hesperidin   A flavonoid found in citrus fruits. It's helpful for improving circulation in small blood vessels.

high-density lipoprotein (HDL)   One form of cholesterol. It's often called "good" cholesterol because it can help remove LDL cholesterol from blood.

high blood pressure   Blood pressure—the pressure of blood against the arteries as the heart beats and contracts—that is too high. Also called hypertension. If blood pressure is 140/90 or more, you have hypertension. *See also* diastolic pressure; systolic pressure.

homocysteine   An amino acid formed when other amino acids in blood are broken down by normal body processes. Too much homocysteine in blood can cause heart disease. Folic acid breaks down the homocysteine and prevents a toxic buildup.

hormone   A chemical messenger the body makes to tell the organs what to do. Hormones regulate many activities, including growth, blood pressure, heart rate, glucose levels, and sexual characteristics.

human papillomavirus (HPV)   A sexually transmitted virus that causes venereal warts, which can cause cervical dysplasia and cancer of the cervix.

hyperhomocysteinemia   The medical term for too much homocysteine in the blood.

hypertension   *See* high blood pressure.

hypothyroidism   An underactive thyroid gland.

inositol   A substance closely related to the B vitamins that is needed to make neurotransmitters and cell membranes.

inositol hexaniacinate (IHN)   A form of niacin that also contains inositol.

insoluble fiber   Dietary fiber that is mostly cellulose from the cell walls of plants. Insoluble fiber absorbs water.

insulin   A hormone made by the pancreas and needed to carry glucose into cells for fuel.

intrinsic factor   A special substance secreted by the stomach to allow the absorption of cobalamin from food.

iodine   An essential trace mineral needed to make thyroid hormones.

iron   An essential trace mineral needed to make hemoglobin.

isoflavones   Hormonelike substances found in soybeans.

jet lag   Fatigue and insomnia caused by traveling rapidly through several time zones.

linoleic acid   An essential fatty acid found in many plants and in fish, especially cold-water fish such as mackerel and cod. *See also* omega-3 fatty acids.

linolenic acid   An essential fatty acid found in many seeds, including corn. *See also* omega-6 fatty acids.

lipoic acid   A vitaminlike substance needed to make energy in the mitochondria. It's also a powerful antioxidant.

low-density lipoprotein (LDL)   One form of cholesterol. It's often called "bad" cholesterol because excess amounts in blood can lead to health problems, including heart disease.

lutein   Xanthophyll that helps protect eyes against free radicals. Lutein is found in dark-green, leafy vegetables.

lycopene   A carotene found in tomatoes. It's a very powerful antioxidant and may help prevent prostate cancer.

lysine   An essential amino acid that may be helpful for treating herpes.

magnesium   A mineral needed for many body functions, including relaxing muscles and regulating heartbeat.

manganese   A trace mineral needed for many body functions, including blood clotting and digesting proteins.

marginal deficiency   The early stages of a vitamin or mineral deficiency.

megablastic or **macrocytic anemia**   Anemia from cobalamin deficiency.

melanoma   The most dangerous type of skin cancer. It can quickly spread to other parts of the body.

melatonin   A hormone made by the pineal gland. Melatonin regulates the sleep-wake cycle.

menadione   The synthetic form of Vitamin K. Also called Vitamin K_3.

menaquinone   The form of Vitamin K made in the intestines by friendly bacteria. Also called Vitamin K_2.

metabolism   The chemical reactions inside cells that create energy.

methionine   An essential sulfur-containing amino acid.

migraine   A very severe headache usually felt on just one side of the head. Other symptoms include nausea, vomiting, sensitivity to light, and cold hands and feet.

mitochondria   Tiny, rod-shaped structures found in all cells. They function as miniature power plants where glucose is converted to energy, with the help of oxygen and a group of enzymes.

molybdenum   An essential trace mineral important for making some enzymes and for normal growth and development.

mucilage   Soluble fiber found in beans, seeds, grains, and nuts.

NAC (N-acetyl cysteine)   A form of the amino acid cysteine.

naringin   A flavonoid found in citrus fruits.

neurotransmitter   A chemical the body makes to transmit messages along the nerves and among the brain cells. The body makes a number of different neurotransmitters, including serotonin.

niacin   A B vitamin also known as Vitamin B$_3$.

niacinamide   Another name for niacin.

nicotinamide   Another name for niacin.

nicotinic acid   Another name for niacin.

nonessential amino acid   One of the 11 amino acids received from food or made in the body from the 9 essential amino acids.

nonheme iron   The iron found naturally in plant foods such as spinach and whole grains.

nonsteroidal anti-inflammatory drugs (NSAIDs)   A large group of medications that relieve pain, help reduce swelling and redness (inflammation), and lower fevers. Aspirin, ibuprofen (Advil), acetaminophen (Tylenol), and naproxen (Aleve) are widely used nonprescription NSAIDs.

oligomeric proanthocyanidins (OPCs)   Flavonoids found in many plants and red wine. OPC supplements are usually made from grape seeds or pine bark. *See also* pycnogenol.

omega-3 fatty acids   Another name for linolenic fatty acids, found in plants and cold-water fish. *See also* alpha linolenic acid; docosahexanoic acid; eicosapentenoic acid.

omega-6 fatty acids   Another name for linoleic fatty acids. *See also* arachidonic acid; gamma linoleic acid.

orthomolecular medicine   Treating the underlying causes of illness with vitamins, minerals, and other supplements. The phrase was coined by Nobel Prize–winning scientist Linus Pauling. *See also* functional medicine.

osteoarthritis   The most common form of arthritis. If you have osteoarthritis, the cartilage that lines and cushions your joints gradually deteriorates, causing pain, swelling, and stiffness.

osteomalacia   Soft, weak bones in adults caused by a shortage of Vitamin D.

osteoporosis   Bones that break easily because they are thin, porous, and brittle. Osteoporosis has several related causes, but too little calcium in the diet plays a big part in causing it.

PABA   An abbreviation for para-aminobenzoic acid. PABA makes up part of the folic acid molecule.

pantothenic acid   One of the B vitamins. Pantothenic acid is found in every food.

pectin   Soluble fiber found in the skins and rinds of plant foods.

pellagra   A deficiency disease caused by a serious lack of niacin.

peptide   A small protein made from a very short chain of amino acids—usually only two or three.

pernicious anemia   Anemia caused when the stomach stops making intrinsic factor and the body stops being able to absorb cobalamin from food.

phenylalanine   An essential amino acid.

phosphatidylcholine (PC)   A fatty substance made from choline that is needed to make the walls of cells.

phosphatidylserine (PS)   A fatty substance the body uses to make cell walls, particularly in the brain.

phosphorus   The second-most abundant mineral in the body, used to make teeth and bones and for many metabolic processes.

phylloquinone   The form of Vitamin K found in plant foods. Also called Vitamin K_1.

phytoestrogens   Hormonelike compounds found in plant foods, especially soybeans.

pineal gland   A small gland found inside the brain. It produces melatonin and regulates the internal clock.

plaque   Fatty deposits of cholesterol and other substances that build up inside arteries and block them.

potassium   An electrolyte mineral needed to control blood pressure and regulate heartbeat.

preformed Vitamin A   The Vitamin A found in animal foods such as egg yolks. The body can use preformed Vitamin A as soon as it's eaten.

prodrome   *See* aura.

progesterone   A female steroid hormone.

prostate gland   A small male organ wrapped around the urethra. The prostate makes some of the fluids found in semen.

protein An organic substance made from hydrogen, oxygen, carbon, and nitrogen. Proteins are needed to live; most of the body is made of it. Proteins are made from strings of amino acids.

prothrombin The most important clotting factor. Vitamin K is needed to make it.

psyllium powder Soluble fiber made from the husks of plantago seeds and sold as a fiber supplement.

pteroylglutamic acid or **pteroylmonoglutamate** Scientific names for folic acid.

pycnogenol A type of OPC made from pine bark.

pyridoxal Another name for pyridoxine.

pyridoxamine Another name for pyridoxine.

pyridoxine A B vitamin also known as Vitamin B_6.

quercetin An antioxidant flavonoid found in onions.

quinones Brightly colored organic substances found in all living plants and animals.

Recommended Dietary Allowance (RDA) The intake of a nutrient that meets the needs of almost all healthy individuals in a specific age and gender group, as set by the Institute of Medicine.

resveratrol A flavonoid found in red wine. It may help lower cholesterol and prevent blood clots.

retina The thin, light-sensitive layer of cells at the back of the eyes.

retinoid, retinol, retinaldehyde, or **retinoic acidretinoic acid** Different names for the same thing: preformed Vitamin A.

rickets Crippling bone deformities in children caused by a shortage of Vitamin D.

rutin A flavonoid found in citrus fruits, buckwheat, berries, and red wine. It's helpful for improving circulation in small blood vessels.

s-adenosylmethionine (SAMe) A form of the amino acid methionine. SAMe supplements are used to treat depression and arthritis pain.

scurvy A deficiency disease caused by a prolonged lack of Vitamin C in the diet.

selenium An essential trace mineral needed to make glutathione and to help Vitamin E work more effectively.

serotonin A neurotransmitter that plays a role in mood and emotions.

sodium   An electrolyte mineral needed to control blood pressure and the amount of water in the body.

soluble fiber   Dietary fiber that dissolves in water to form a soft gel. *See also* guar gum; mucilage; pectin.

steroid hormones   Hormones the body makes in the adrenal glands from cholesterol.

stool   Human solid waste; feces.

sulfur   A mineral found in every tissue of the body. It's needed to make proteins and many vitamins, hormones, and enzymes.

systolic pressure   The blood pressure when a heart beats to pump out blood—the higher number in a blood pressure reading.

taurine   An amino acid that contains sulfur.

thiamin   A B vitamin, also called Vitamin B_1.

thiamin pyrophosphate (TPP)   An enzyme the body needs to convert carbohydrates into energy. Thiamin is needed to make it.

thioctic acid   Another name for lipoic acid.

thymus gland   A small organ found in the neck just above the breastbone. It makes some of the hormones that tell the immune system what to do.

thyroid gland   A small, butterfly-shaped gland found in the neck just below the Adam's apple. It produces hormones that regulate metabolism.

thyroxin   A hormone made in the thyroid gland.

tocopherol   Another name for Vitamin E. *See also* alpha tocopherol.

tocotrienols   Forms of Vitamin E found in some plant foods such as rice and barley.

tryptophan   An essential amino acid used in the body to make niacin, among other things.

Type 2 diabetes   The most common type of diabetes. It happens when cells become resistant to insulin, a hormone made in the pancreas.

tyrosine   A nonessential amino acid.

ubiquinone   *See* coenzyme Q_{10}.

urethra   The tube that carries urine from the kidneys to the bladder.

vegan   Someone who eats no animal foods.

vegetarian   Someone who doesn't eat meat. Some vegetarians limit or don't eat other animal foods either.

vitamin   An organic chemical compound essential for normal health. Vitamins must be received from outside the body—from the foods eaten and from any supplements taken.

Vitamin A   A fat-soluble vitamin needed for healthy epithelial tissues, eyes, growth, bone formation, and immunity.

Vitamin C   A water-soluble vitamin needed to make connective tissue and for many other functions. Vitamin C is also a powerful and abundant antioxidant.

Vitamin D   A fat-soluble vitamin the body makes from sunshine on the skin and also gets from some foods. It's needed to build healthy bones and to regulate the amounts of calcium in blood.

Vitamin E   A fat-soluble vitamin that is a powerful antioxidant.

Vitamin K   A fat-soluble vitamin needed to help blood clot.

water-soluble   Vitamins that dissolve in water and can't be stored in the body. The B vitamins and Vitamin C are water-soluble.

Wernicke-Korsakoff syndrome   Nerve damage caused by low thiamin levels from years of alcoholism.

wild yam   A tuberous plant found in the tropics. The roots contain a natural form of the female hormone progesterone. Wild yam cream or tincture can be helpful for relieving menopause symptoms.

xanthophylls   Carotenoids found in dark-green, leafy vegetables. *See also* lutein; zeaxanthin.

zeaxanthin   A carotenoid found in dark-green, leafy vegetables. It helps protect the eyes against free radicals.

zinc   A mineral needed to make many enzymes and hormones.

Index

Symbols

5-HTP (5-hydroxy-tryptophan), 292

A

A vitamin, 33-47, 50
AA (arachidonic acid), 298, 384
ABC study (Alpha-tocopherol Beta-carotene Cancer Prevention Study Group) study, 48, 181
Accutane (isotretinoin), 46
ACE inhibitors, influence on potassium level, 246
acerola, 145
acetyl-L-carnitine (ALC), 287, 382
acetylcholine, 135
acidophilus, 367
ACP (acyl carrier protein), 126
adenosine triphosphate (ATP), 288
Adequate Intake. *See* AI
adrenal glands, steroid hormones, 349
adult-onset diabetes, 27
Advicor, 62
aging, 62-63
Agriculture surveys (U.S. Department of), 201
AI (Adequate Intake)
    B vitamins, 57-58
    biotin, 132-133
    choline, 6, 135-136
    chromium, 264-265
    D vitamin, 165-166
    fluoride, 268-269
    K vitamin, 188-189

manganese, 269
molybdenum, 271
pantothenic acid, 126-127
trace minerals, 255
ajoene, 328
ALC (acetyl-L-carnitine), 287, 382
alcohol
    abuse
        B vitamin levels, 58
        niacin deficiency, 84
    calcium-robbing properties, 203
allergies, benefits of C vitamin, 154-155
alliin, 328-329
alpha-lipoic acid, 314
alpha-tocopherol, 175
alpha carotenes, 36, 320
alpha linolenic acid (LNA), 299
ALS (amytrophic lateral sclerosis), prevention, 184
alternative treatments, functional medicine, 21
aluminum, 273
aluminum antacids, calcium-robbing properties, 203
Alzheimer's disease, 382-383
    B vitamins and, 62
    prevention
        choline, 137
        niacin, 91
        vitamin E, 183
    homocysteine and, 62
American Diabetes Association, 28
amino acids, 277
    arginine, 285-286
    carnitine, 286-287
    cautions, 284-285
    creatinine, 288
    cysteine, 288-289

decarboxylation, 94
glutamine, 289
homocysteine, 111
lysine, 289-290
methionine, 61, 111, 290
necessity, 278-279
phenylalanine, 292-293
protein production, 279-280
racemization, 94
RI (recommended intake), 280-283
sources, 283-284
taurine, 290
tryptophan, 83, 86-87, 291
tyrosine, 292-293
amytrophic lateral sclerosis (ALS), 184
androstrenedione, 349-350
anemia, 120
animal foods, carotenes, 36
anthocyanins, 329-330
anti-infective agent (vitamin A), 34
"anti-stress" vitamin (pantothenic acid), 128
antibiotics, calcium-robbing properties, 204
Antioxidant Polyp Prevention Study. *See* APPS
antioxidants, 13-15, 319-320
    catechins, 324-327
    C vitamin, 151
    free radicals, 14
    power of carotenes, 36
    super antioxidants, 309
        glutathione, 310-314
        lipoic acid, 314-315
aphthous stomatitis (canker sores), 71
APPA (Antioxidant Polyp Prevention Study), 48